Practical Immunology

Frank C. Hay
PhD
Professor of Immunology
St. George's Hospital Medical School
Cranmer Terrace
London

Olwyn M.R. Westwood
PhD
Senior Lecturer in Immunology
University of Surrey Roehampton
and St. George's Hospital Medical School
London

with the assistance of
Paul N. Nelson
Wolverhampton University, Wolverhampton

FOURTH EDITION

Blackwell
Science

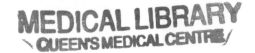
© 1976, 1980, 1989, 2002 by Blackwell Science Ltd
a Blackwell Publishing Company
Editorial Offices:
Osney Mead, Oxford OX2 0EL, UK
 Tel: +44 (0)1865 206206
Blackwell Science, Inc., 350 Main Street, Malden, MA 02148-5018, USA
 Tel: +1 781 388 8250
Blackwell Science Asia Pty, 54 University Street, Carlton, Victoria 3053, Australia
 Tel: +61 (0)3 9347 0300
Blackwell Wissenschafts Verlag, Kurfürstendamm 57, 10707 Berlin, Germany
 Tel: +49 (0)30 32 79 060

First published 1976
Second edition 1980
Third edition 1989
Reprinted 1991
Fourth edition 2002

Library of Congress Cataloging-in-Publication Data
Hay, Frank C.
    Practical immunology / Frank C. Hay, Olwyn M.R. Westwood;
  with the assistance of Paul N. Nelson. — 4th ed.
        p.;   cm.
    Rev. ed. of: Practical immunology / Leslie Hudson, Frank C. Hay. 3rd ed. 1989.
    Includes bibliographical references and index.
    ISBN 0-86542-961-8 (pbk.)
    1. Immunology—Laboratory manuals. I. Westwood, Olwyn M.R.
II. Nelson, Paul N.   III. Hudson, Leslie. Practical immunology.   IV. Title.
[DNLM: 1. Immunologic Techniques—Laboratory Manuals.   2. Allergy and
Immunology—Laboratory Manuals. QW 525 H412p   2001]
QR183 .H39 2001
616.07′9—dc21
                                                        2001035417

ISBN 0-86542-961-8

A catalogue record for this title is available from the British Library

Set in 8¹/₂/13¹/₄ Stone Serif by Graphicaft Limited, Hong Kong
Printed and bound in Great Britain by MPG Books Ltd, Bodmin, Cornwall

For further information on Blackwell Science, visit our website:
www.blackwell-science.com

CONTENTS

FOREWORD TO THE FIRST EDITION

Immunology might well claim to be the most popular and the most glamorous of biological sciences today. I suspect that there has been a sharper increase in the number of research workers in immunology over the last two decades than in any other scientific discipline.

Applied immunology, plus the intangibles we lump together as the rising standard of living, has virtually rid the world of smallpox, yellow fever, diphtheria and poliomyelitis and has helped in many other fields. Its prestige lingers on as the major tool of preventive medicine but, as one whose first immunological paper was published more than 50 years ago, I have seen a complete switch in the contemporary importance of immunology—but not a diminution.

Immunology today is a science in its own right. The enthusiasm of younger workers, like the authors of this book, is primarily directed toward understanding; medical applications of the new knowledge will be wholeheartedly welcomed but they are not central. For me, and to some extent all of us in immunology, the excitement is in the lead that our subject is giving toward a real understanding of the form and strategy of living process. Thanks to the *recognisability* of the significant molecules, antibody, antigen and the like, we have been able to apply the new techniques of molecular biology to the elucidation of one of the essential bodily functions. We are leading the field, for nowhere else have genetics, biochemistry and every other basic science that can help, been so effectively applied to living function. It is the first step toward a sophisticated understanding of what we are and how we became so.

This book is basically an introduction to the techniques and ideas on which immunology is based; to one who grew up with the older, predominantly medical approach, the new version can be sensed everywhere in the authors' approach.

I wish them every success.

F.M. BURNET
Basel, Switzerland
1976

ACKNOWLEDGEMENTS

Immunology has certainly changed since the first edition of *Practical Immunology*. Then laboratory workers had to produce virtually all their own antisera and much of the apparatus as well. Now the majority of reagents are bought ready made with appropriate fluorescent or enzyme labels attached. It was our policy from the start that the book should be complete, so that a technique could be performed without reference to numerous other texts. This has become increasingly difficult as each laboratory has its own preferred make of machine with associated reagents.

We have decided to continue with our original aim of assuming only basic equipment—such as might be available for a class practical. There are instructions for making reagents from first principles, to take account that not everyone using this book will have access to either the equipment or the funds to purchase everything to order.

Each previous edition has grown in size but we have been ruthless in cutting the length for this edition while including much new material. It is our firm intention that this should be an easily carried, working guide for undergraduates and research students. There are other reference tomes for the library shelf. With this edition Leslie Hudson has left for pastures new, and Frank Hay is delighted to welcome instead Olwyn Westwood, who has been extremely busy amassing new material. Paul Nelson has been most helpful in going through the completed text with us over several sessions and has supplied us with further useful material.

Immunology has become a very wide field and we have been grateful to other colleagues, particularly members of the immunology web news group, who helped us in the choice of methods to be included. Also, we are grateful to those who took the trouble to look through the draft manuscript, including Neville Punchard and Brian Ellis, who were most helpful in error trapping. Terry Poulton, Andy Soltys and Emma Frears were generous suppliers of help and advice. Special thanks are due to all our friends at Blackwell Science, especially Andrew Robinson, Fiona Goodgame and Karen Moore.

There are more references to the literature in this edition to guide the reader further, together with some key web sites. We have also set up a web site at http://www.sghms.ac.uk/depts/ immunology/frankhay to maintain updates to methods. Please check the site to look for any modifications and do send us your tips and suggestions so that we can make them available for the benefit of other immunologists.

It is our hope that experienced immunologists, students and their lecturers alike will find this text useful, and we look forward to helpful discussions via the World Wide Web.

1 Isolation and structure of immunoglobulins

The following characteristics of the immunoglobulin classes can be used for their isolation and fractionation:

- solubility in aqueous solution;
- molecular size;
- electrostatic density;
- isoelectric point; and
- affinity for other molecules, e.g. lectins.

1.1 Fractionation by solubility

The relative solubility of proteins in pure water, ethanol or various salt solutions may be used as a basic fractionation technique. Serum may be separated into its euglobulin (insoluble) and pseudoglobulin (soluble) fractions by dialysis against distilled water. Although this is often used as the first step in the purification of immunoglobulin M (IgM), the euglobulin fraction is always contaminated with some immunoglobulin G (IgG).

1.1.1 Euglobulin precipitation to prepare IgM

MATERIALS

Sample: *either* monoclonal antibody culture supernatant of known immunoglobulin (IgM) *or*
  30 ml serum derived from a subject who has fasted overnight (around 50 ml of whole blood)
Dialysis membrane tubing
Distilled water
Sephacryl S-200 HR in a column (100 × 2.5 cm) (see Appendix B.1.2)
0.1 M borate buffer, pH 7.4
UV spectrophotometer

Preparation of serum sample from whole blood

METHOD

1 Collect blood by venesection and allow to clot in a glass container without anticoagulant.
2 Once the clot has formed, separate the serum from the clotted cells by centrifugation at 1000 g for 15 min.
3 Transfer the serum (straw-coloured supernatant) to a suitable container, then proceed to isolation of the immunoglobulins.

Preparation of monoclonal antibody culture supernatant

METHOD

1 Centrifuge the sample at 10 000 g for 30 min at 4°C.
2 Save the supernatant and discard the cell debris, then proceed to next section.

Isolation of the immunoglobulins

METHOD

1 Secure one end of the dialysis tubing and decant in the spun supernatant or serum.
2 Dialyse against water to a volume that is 100 times the sample volume.
3 Collect the dialysed supernatant into a suitable test tube and centrifuge at 15 000 g for 60 min at 4°C.
4 Discard the supernatant.
5 Dissolve the pellet in 5 ml of borate buffer.
6 Prepare a column (100 × 2.5 cm) with Sephacryl S-200 HR and equilibrate with borate buffer.
7 Load the dialysed supernatant, and allow flow into the column.
8 Elute immunoglobulin with borate buffer, collecting 1 ml fractions, detecting the peaks by UV spectroscopy at 280 nm (IgM is eluted as the first peak).
9 Adjust the IgM to between 1 and 5 mg/ml and store at either 4°C or –70°C. See Appendix B.5.1 (methods for estimation of protein concentration).

TECHNICAL NOTES

- Increasing salt concentration of the medium leads to interference with the interaction of water molecules and the charged polar groups on protein molecules, i.e. rendering them less hydrophilic. This allows a greater hydrophobic interaction between protein molecules and they eventually become insoluble.
- The culture supernatant should contain around 1–50 mg/ml, therefore 500–1000 ml is required for a decent yield of IgM.
- The salt concentration at which each protein precipitates is different, but between closely related molecules such as immunoglobulins, the difference is not sufficiently great to give a precipitate with high-grade purity. However, it is often useful: (a) as a first step in isolation procedures as many serum proteins, e.g. albumin, will remain in solution when immunoglobulins are precipitated; and (b) for concentration of immunoglobulins from dilute solution.

1.1.2 Ammonium sulphate precipitation

Ammonium sulphate precipitation is a widely used for the preparation of a crude immunoglobulin fraction from whole serum. The use of ammonium rather than sodium sulphate as the precipitating salt offers the advantage of a high solubility that is only minimally dependent on temperature:

$(NH_4)_2SO_4$ ~ 3% variation between 0°C and 25°C;
Na_2SO_4 5 × more soluble at 25°C than at 0°C.

Relatively 'pure' IgG may be rapidly prepared by precipitation at a 33.3% saturation of ammonium sulphate. A higher yield of IgG at lower purity (i.e. containing other classes of immunoglobulin) is obtained at 50% saturation. However, smaller fragments of the molecule require higher salt concentrations for precipitation.

Preparation of serum immunoglobulin

MATERIALS AND EQUIPMENT
Ammonium sulphate
Dilute ammonia solution
Serum
UV spectrophotometer
0.14 M sodium chloride solution (saline)
Phosphate-buffered saline (PBS)

METHOD

1 Dissolve 1000 g ammonium sulphate in 1000 ml distilled water at 50°C, allow to stand overnight at room temperature and adjust to pH 7.2 with dilute ammonia solution.

2 Dilute 1 part serum with 2 parts saline and add an equal volume of saturated ammonium sulphate solution (prepared in step 1) to a final concentration of 45% saturated v/v.

3 Stir at room temperature for 30 min.

4 Centrifuge off precipitate (1000 g for 15 min at 4°C).

5 Wash precipitate with 45% saturated ammonium sulphate and recentrifuge.

6 Redissolve the precipitate in the same volume of PBS as the original serum.

7 Centrifuge to remove any insoluble material.

8 Reprecipitate the immunoglobulin using a final concentration of 40% saturated ammonium sulphate.

9 Centrifuge off the precipitate and wash with 40% saturated ammonium sulphate.

10 After centrifuging the washed precipitate, redissolve in a minimum volume of PBS.

11 Dialyse the immunoglobulins against five changes of PBS at 4°C (typically five changes of 1 litre). Centrifuge to remove any precipitate.

12 Prepare a 1 : 20 dilution of the immunoglobulins in PBS and determine the absorbance at 280 nm using a UV spectrophotometer. (Note the use of UV spectrophotometer requires pure immunoglobulin, as the technique is based on absorbance of UV light by aromatic amino acid residues in the protein.)

Calculation of protein content

At 280 nm, an absorbance of 1.0 (1-cm cuvette) is equivalent to an immunoglobulin concentration of 0.74 mg/ml.

Example:

if absorbance of sample diluted 1 : 20 = 0.95

immunoglobulin concentration = 0.95 × 0.74 × 20

$$= 14.1 \text{ mg/ml.}$$

TECHNICAL NOTES

- Use blood from a person who has fasted overnight as this has a low lipid content.
- Calculation of volume of saturated solution required to achieve a required concentration of ammonium sulphate:

$$V_r = \frac{100(S_f - S_i)}{1 - S_f}$$

  where V_r is volume of saturated solution (ml) to be added per 100 ml volume of protein solution, S_f is final saturation (fraction, not percentage) and S_i is initial saturation (fraction, not percentage).

  To minimize excessive volumes of solution when working in bulk, add solid ammonium sulphate according to the nomogram on the front inside cover.

- Determination of protein concentration by UV spectrophotometry is accurate down to about 0.05 mg/ml (see Technical note below).
- Use of protein solutions containing residual ammonium sulphate can interfere with some of the chemical reactions described in this book. It is good practice to test for residual ammonium sulphate by adding 1 drop of dialysate to 0.5 ml acidified barium chloride solution (use 1 M HCl to acidify a 10 mg/ml solution of barium chloride in water). If a precipitate forms, continue the dialysis of the protein solution.
- The extinction coefficient varies depending on the species. The figures quoted in Appendix B are for human immunoglobulins and provide a reasonable guide for immunoglobulins from other species. However, it is important to know that the UV absorption is dependent on the proportion of aromatic amino acids such as tryptophan. Polyclonal immunoglobulins will have an average content of these amino acids, but monoclonal antibodies are likely to give aberrant results owing to their unique composition.

Purification of mouse monoclonal antibodies

MATERIALS AND EQUIPMENT
Monoclonal antibody supernatant
Saturated ammonium sulphate solution, pH 7.2 (45–50% final saturation)
UV spectrophotometer

1   Collect the monoclonal antibody supernatant and remove any contaminating cells by centrifuging at 10 000 g for 30 min at either 4°C or room temperature.

2   Precipitate the immunoglobulin with ammonium sulphate as described above in Section 1.1.2, using 40–50% saturated solution depending on purity required.
    After dialysis determine the protein content of the solution using the following conversion factor: at 280 nm, absorbance of 1.0 (in a 1-cm cuvette) = 0.69 mg/ml immunoglobulin.

Rapid concentration of immunoglobulins

After column chromatography, samples are often recovered in dilute solution in large volumes of buffer. It is important to concentrate these rapidly as denaturation occurs in dilute solution. Ammonium sulphate precipitation is useful, using the solid salt to limit the total working volume of solution (nomogram, front inside cover).

The method described below is suitable for:

*   light chains (see Section 1.6);
*   Fab regions (see Section 1.7);
*   preparing Bence-Jones proteins from the urine of patients with multiple myeloma.

MATERIALS

Material for concentration, for example:
    Fab or light chains from column chromatography;
    urine from patient with multiple myeloma;
    urine from a mouse with a transplanted mineral oil-induced plasmacytoma or hybridoma
Solid ammonium sulphate
Phosphate-buffered saline (PBS)

Steps 1–2 are for urine samples only; otherwise start at step 3.

1   Dialyse the urine against cold, running tap water for 24 h to remove inorganic salts and urea.

2   Centrifuge at 1000 g for 15 min to remove any insoluble material.

3   Adjust to pH 5.5 (salt precipitation is most effective at the isoelectric point of the protein required).

4   Add solid ammonium sulphate to 75% saturation. At 25°C, 575 g solid ammonium sulphate is required for 1000 ml of solution (see also nomogram, front inside cover). Add the salt slowly with stirring, otherwise it will form lumps bound up with protein that are very difficult to dissolve.

5   When all the salt has been added, stir for 1 h at room temperature to equilibrate.

6   Centrifuge at 1000 g for 15 min and discard the supernatant. (Take care to wash any salt off the rotor head or corrosion will occur.)

7   Redissolve the precipitate in PBS.

- Ammonium sulphate precipitation is often used to prepare crude γ-globulin fractions from whole serum. For many applications this may provide protein of sufficient purity, but even if highly purified material is required, salt precipitation may provide a useful first step in the isolation procedure.
- The redissolved precipitates still containing residual ammonium sulphate can be stored at 4°C or dialysed against the appropriate buffer system before use.

Combined ammonium sulphate and polyethylene glycol precipitation of IgM

Euglobulin precipitation can produce pure IgM but tends to give low yields, but it can be of use when a source rich in IgM is available, e.g. Waldenström's macroglobulinaemia serum.

When using polyethylene glycol precipitation of serum proteins it is necessary to remove lipid, e.g. by adsorption to silicon dioxide.

Tatum (1993) developed a method involving:

- low strength ammonium sulphate precipitation to remove lipids and fibrinogen (e.g. useful for plasma samples);
- high strength ammonium sulphate to isolate immunoglobulins;
- subsequent separation of IgM with polyethylene glycol.

MATERIALS AND EQUIPMENT

Plasma or serum

Saturated ammonium sulphate (SAS)

Polyethylene glycol 6000 (PEG-6000), 24% w/v in distilled water

Phosphate-buffered saline (PBS)

Distilled water

Centrifuge

Conductivity meter

pH meter

Dialysis tubing

1 M phosphoric acid

METHOD

1 Add 42 ml of SAS to 100 ml plasma with gentle stirring over 5 min.
2 Continue stirring at room temperature for 30 min.
3 Centrifuge for 20 min at 4000 g.
4 Discard pellet.
5 Add a further 50 ml SAS to the supernatant with stirring over 5 min.
6 Continue stirring at room temperature for 30 min.
7 Centrifuge for 30 min at 4000 g.
8 Remove as much supernatant as possible.
9 Resuspend the precipitate in 100 ml 50% SAS and stir gently for 5 min at room temperature.
10 Centrifuge for 20 min at 4000 g.
11 Remove as much supernatant as possible and redissolve the precipitate by the slow addition of a minimal volume of distilled water.
12 Adjust the conductivity to 80 mÙ⁻¹/cm³.

Continued

13 Adjust the pH to 6.5–7.0 with 1 M phosphoric acid.

14 Add 1 volume 24% PEG-6000 for every 3 volumes of protein solution over 5 min with gentle stirring.

15 Continue stirring for 30 min.

16 Centrifuge at 4000 *g*.

17 Remove as much supernatant as possible and redissolve pellet in 5–10 ml PBS (or other desired buffer).

18 Dialyse to remove residual PEG and ammonium sulphate.

TECHNICAL NOTES

- The yield can be expected to be about 60–80% with a purity of over 90%, the major contaminants being IgG and IgA. These may be removed by gel filtration (Fig. 1.1; see Appendix B.1.2).
- Increasing the final PEG concentration from 6 to 7.5% will increase the yield of IgM at the expense of greater IgG contamination.
- Individual monoclonal antibodies, e.g. from patients with Waldenström's macroglobulinaemia, may need optimization of the method to get maximum yield. Lowering the temperature of PEG precipitation to 4°C can be helpful.

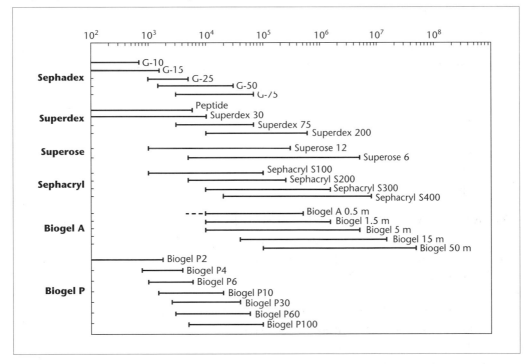

Fig. 1.1 Effective fractionation ranges for gel filtration media.
Sephadex G-10, G-50 and G-75: available in a range of bead sizes. The finest beads give better resolution but at the expense of slower flow rates.
Superdex Peptide and 30–200: prepacked columns.
Superose 6 and 12:
Sephacryl S100–S400:
Biogel A 0.5m–50m: for high resolution, narrow range fractionation.
Biogel P2–100: for small proteins and peptides.

1.2 Ultracentrifugation

Analytical and preparative ultracentrifugation have been widely applied in immunochemistry, for both molecular weight determinations and isolation procedures.

Preparative ultracentrifugation in sucrose density gradients is useful for the isolation of chicken IgM. Chicken IgM cannot be easily isolated by gel filtration as the IgG readily forms soluble aggregates, so appears within the excluded fraction of Sephacryl S-200 as a major contaminant of the IgM. However, the difference in size between the IgG dimers and the IgM is still sufficiently great to allow good resolution in the ultracentrifuge.

A detailed treatment of the basic techniques available, for example rate separation and isopycnic separation, both with and without a density gradient, is beyond the range of this book (see Lechner 1994).

1.3 Ion-exchange chromatography

Ion-exchange chromatography is an extremely useful method for the separation of proteins and the isolation of immunoglobulins. Proteins are bound electrostatically onto an ion-exchange matrix bearing an opposite charge. The degree to which a protein binds depends upon its charge density. Proteins are then eluted differentially by:

(a) increasing the ionic strength of the medium. As the concentration of buffer ions is increased they compete with the proteins for the charged groups upon the ion exchanger;

(b) alteration of the pH. As the pH of the buffer approaches the isoelectric point of each protein, the net charge becomes zero and so the protein no longer binds to the ion exchanger.

Both cation (e.g. carboxymethyl (CM)–cellulose) and anion exchangers (e.g. diethylaminoethyl (DEAE)–cellulose) are available. DEAE is used more widely for the fractionation of serum proteins. Cellulose remains the favoured support for the diethylaminoethyl group. Various forms are available to suit particular applications, and high-pressure liquid chromatography columns are available for analytical work.

1.3.1 Batch preparation of rabbit IgG with DEAE–cellulose

DEAE–cellulose and other ion exchangers can be used in columns or in batches. The batch technique is useful when large volumes of serum must be processed under standardized conditions. DEAE–cellulose is equilibrated under conditions of pH and ionic strength which allow all the serum proteins to bind except IgG. The serum must be pre-equilibrated to the same pH and ionic strength as the DEAE–cellulose, then simply stirred with the cellulose prior to recovering the supernatant containing IgG.

However, it should be noted that although this method is suitable for rabbit IgG, DEAE is not nearly as efficient for human IgG and so a gradient separation will be described for the latter.

Preparation of DE52 cellulose (DEAE)

MATERIALS
Diethylaminoethyl (DEAE)–cellulose DE52 (Whatman)
0.01 M phosphate buffer, pH 8.0
1.0 M HCl

METHOD

1 Place 100 g DE52 in a 1-l flask and add 550 ml 0.01 M phosphate buffer, pH 8.0.
2 Titrate the mixture back to pH 8.0 by adding 1.0 M HCl.
3 Leave the slurry to settle for 30 min, then remove the supernatant with any fines it may contain. Resuspend the cellulose in enough phosphate buffer to fill the flask.
4 Repeat this cycle of settling, decantation and resuspension twice.
5 Pour the slurry into a Buchner funnel containing two layers of Whatman no. 1 filter paper. Suck the cellulose 'dry' for 30 s to leave a damp cake of cellulose.

Preparation of IgG

The degree of purity of IgG is governed by the ratio of ion exchanger to serum; Fig. 1.2 illustrates the problems involved. For high purity, more cellulose is added but this leads to losses of IgG through binding to the ion exchanger. The precise proportions used depend upon the required purity of the IgG. Reasonable purity (about 96%) and good yield (about 70%) are obtained using 5 g (wet weight) cellulose for every ml of serum.

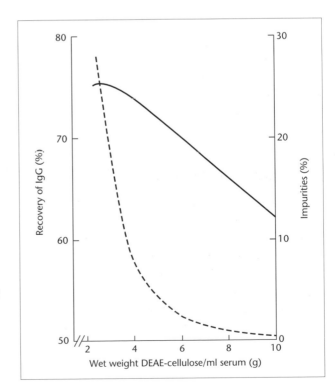

Fig. 1.2 Relationship of purity (dashed line) and yield (solid line) of IgG to the amount of ion exchanger used per ml of serum. This illustrates a universal rule of all protein purifications that the higher one tries to make the yield the lower will be the purity.

1 Weigh the cellulose into a beaker; for every 10 ml serum use 50 g wet weight of cellulose. Mix 10 ml serum with 30 ml distilled water, to lower its ionic strength, and add to the cellulose at 4°C.
2 To equilibrate stir thoroughly every 10 min for 1 h at 4°C.
3 Pour the slurry onto a Buchner funnel and suck through the supernatant; this contains the required IgG. Rinse the cellulose with 3 volumes of 20 ml 0.01 M phosphate buffer, pH 8.0.
4 Collect and combine all the filtrates.

Examination of IgG preparation

1 If a determination of yield is required, then the IgG content in the original serum and the filtrate may be measured immunologically; e.g. using either rate nephelometry (see Section 3.6) or radial immunodiffusion (see Section 3.4).
2 The purity of the preparation may be determined by comparing the IgG content (measured above) of the filtrate with its total protein content (determined by UV spectrometry).
3 Use SDS-PAGE or immunoelectrophoresis against anti-whole rabbit serum to identify the main contaminants of the IgG (see also Appendix B.2.1 and Sections 3.2–3.9).

1.3.2 Preparation of IgG with an ionic strength gradient

For maximum yield and purity a column technique using gradient elution is preferred for the preparation of IgG of any species. For human and mouse IgG gradient elution is essential. Initially, buffering conditions are adjusted such that virtually all the serum proteins bind to the ion exchanger. Proteins are then eluted sequentially by gradually increasing the ionic strength of the buffer running through the column.

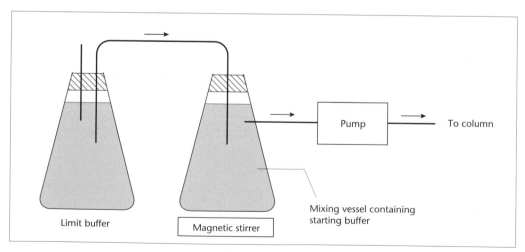

Fig. 1.3 Simple apparatus for the production of an exponential gradient. When the buffer concentration in the limit vessel is greater than the initial concentration in the mixing vessel a convex gradient is produced. Sophisticated pumps are now supplied for fast performance liquid chromatography (FPLC) and high performance liquid chromatography (HPLC) systems, with microprocessor controllers, which allow the programming of an almost limitless range of gradients. Arrows indicate the direction of flow.

Serum sample

Diethylaminoethyl (DEAE)–cellulose DE52 (Whatman)

Column and fraction collection apparatus (a short wide column is preferable; e.g. 25×3.3 cm; see Appendix B, Fig. B.1)

Gradient device (commercially available, or constructed as in Fig. 1.3)

Conductivity meter

Phosphate buffers, pH 8.0, 0.005 M and 0.3 M

METHOD

A Equilibration of ion exchanger

1 Place the ion exchanger in a beaker—use 2–5 g (wet weight) DE52 for every 1 ml of serum.

2 Add the basic component to the phosphate buffer (0.5 M disodium hydrogen phosphate) until the pH reaches 8.0.

3 Add 0.005 M phosphate buffer, pH 8.0. There should be 6 ml buffer for every 1 g of wet ion exchanger.

4 Disperse the cellulose and pour into a measuring cylinder and allow to settle (settling time [min] = $2 \times$ height of the slurry [cm]). Remove the supernatant that contains cellulose 'fines'; these may block the column.

5 Add a volume of 0.005 M buffer equal to half the volume of settled cellulose and resuspend.

6 Pour the slurry into the column with the flow-control valve open.

7 Pack the column by pumping 0.005 M, pH 8.0, phosphate buffer through at 45 ml/h for each cm^2 internal cross-section.

8 Monitor the buffer effluent with a conductivity meter. When the ionic strength of the effluent is the same as that of the original buffer, the ion exchanger is equilibrated. If a meter is not available, pass 2–3 l of buffer through the column.

B Running the column

1 Dialyse the sample against the starting buffer (0.005 M, pH 8.0 phosphate buffer).

2 Centrifuge the sample. (Some protein will precipitate at this low ionic strength.)

3 Apply the serum to the column and pump through the starting buffer (about 60–100 ml/h). Monitor the effluent for protein. Most of the proteins should bind to the ion exchanger.

4 Elute the proteins with a gradient of increasing ionic strength (see below). Collect fractions of approximately 5 ml.

TECHNICAL NOTE

If a high concentration of protein is detected in the column effluent prior to the application of the ionic strength gradient, either (a) the ion exchanger or serum was not fully equilibrated or (b) the absorbing capacity of the cellulose has been exceeded.

Ionic strength gradient

Gradients of varying shapes are used for different purposes. A great variety of commercial gradient-forming equipment is available, ranging from simple devices which are essentially two chambers joined together (similar to Fig. 1.3), to sophisticated electronic systems in which the rate of advance of the gradient is controlled by a monitor for protein in the column effluent. In this system a discontinuous gradient can be formed automatically and greatly increases the resolution of ion-exchange chromatography.

A continuous exponential gradient may be produced as shown in Fig. 1.3. The limit buffer enters the mixing vessel at the same rate as the buffer is pumped onto the column. The gradient is established according to the following equation:

$$C_m = C_1 - (C_1 - C_0)e^{-v/v_m}$$

where C_m is concentration in mixing vessel, C_1 is concentration in limit vessel, C_0 is initial concentration in mixing vessel, v is volume removed from mixing vessel and v_m is volume of the mixing vessel.

For ease of calculation this equation may be rewritten as:

$$2.303 \cdot \log\frac{C_1 - C_m}{C_1 - C_0} = \frac{-v}{v_m}$$

When $C_1 > C_0$ the gradient is convex; when $C_1 < C_0$ the gradient is concave. (The latter is used for density gradient formation not ion-exchange chromatography: the highest ionic strength buffer will emerge first and elute everything off the column.)

Linear gradients may be established using an open mixing vessel (Fig. 1.4a) or by means of a multichannel pump as shown in Fig. 1.4(b). In this case the equation for the gradient is:

$$C_m = C_0 + (C_1 - C_0)\frac{v}{2v_0}$$

where v_0 is initial volume of buffer in the mixing vessel and other symbols are as in the equation for exponential gradient above.

Distribution of serum proteins

Assuming that the ion exchanger has not been overloaded with protein the first peak should contain only IgG. This is the only pure protein that can be isolated under these conditions of pH and buffer molarity; the remaining peaks contain several proteins. Beta-lipoproteins, haptoglobin and α_2-macroglobulin will contaminate the IgA and IgM fractions.

Regeneration of the ion exchanger

1 Remove the ion exchanger from the column by washing out with distilled water.
2 Add 0.1 M HCl (0.5–1 × bed volume of cellulose).
3 Place on Buchner funnel and rinse through with distilled water.
4 Add 0.1 M NaOH (volume equivalent to the HCl used) and then rinse through with distilled water.
5 Wash through with full strength buffer and then re-equilibrate with low ionic strength buffer.

TECHNICAL NOTE

To store cellulose ion exchangers add chlorhexidine to a concentration of 0.002% for anion exchangers and sodium azide to 0.02% for cation exchangers.

Note: Azide is a dangerous chemical—do not discard down the sink.

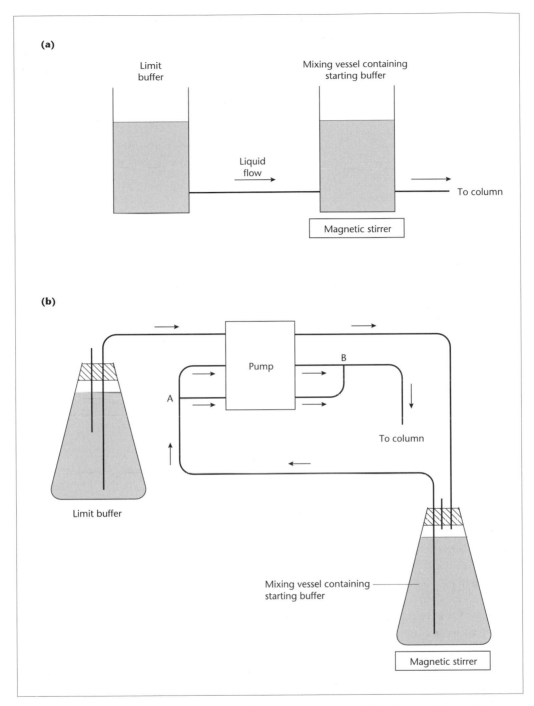

Fig. 1.4 (a) **Formation of a linear gradient using an open mixing vessel.** The effective volume of the mixing chamber reduces as the gradient is formed. (**b**) The production of a linear gradient by means of a multichannel pump. Tubing from B to the column must be of sufficient internal diameter to take twice the flow rate in the rest of the system. Arrows indicate direction of flow. A and B are 'h'-type functions.

1.3.3 Mass production and mini-column ion-exchange chromatography

Conditions for running ion-exchange columns are less critical than for gel filtration; it is therefore possible to set up large numbers of mini-columns in cheap apparatus such as disposable syringe barrels. The conditions are sufficiently reproducible that fixed volumes of cellulose, serum and buffer give reproducible preparations of IgG and are technically so simple that up to 20 syringe columns in a rack with gravity flow may be run simultaneously. The following procedure will rapidly give very pure IgG.

MATERIALS AND EQUIPMENT
Serum (human)
Saturated ammonium sulphate
Phosphate buffers 0.02 M and 0.2 M, pH 7.2
1 M potassium chloride in 0.02 M phosphate buffer, pH 7.2
Disposable syringe with a central nozzle (e.g. 10-ml hypodermic syringe)
Diethylaminoethyl (DEAE)–cellulose DE52
Glass or nylon wool, or sintered plastic disc

Caution: Wear gloves when handling glass wool.

METHOD

1 Add 1 ml saturated ammonium sulphate dropwise to 2 ml human serum to give a 33% saturation. Stir for 30 min. Precipitating the serum with ammonium sulphate eliminates much of the material which would otherwise bind to the ion exchanger and reduce its capacity.
2 Spin the precipitate at 1000 g for 15 min and resuspend the pellet in 40% saturated ammonium sulphate.
3 Stir for 10 min and then spin at 1000 g for 15 min.
4 Resuspend the pellet in 0.02 M phosphate buffer, pH 7.2.
5 Dialyse the sample against 0.02 M buffer overnight.
6 Block the outlet of a disposable syringe with a little glass or nylon wool or a sintered plastic disc.
7 Place 3 g (wet weight) of DEAE–cellulose in the syringe and wash through with 5 ml 0.02 M phosphate buffer containing 1 M KCl.
8 Wash the column with 20 ml 0.02 M phosphate buffer (without KCl).
9 Add the dialysed protein sample to the cellulose.
10 Elute the IgG with 15 ml 0.02 M phosphate buffer and collect 3 ml fractions.
11 Determine the absorbance at 280 nm of the fractions and pool those containing protein. These contain the IgG.
12 Calculate the yield of IgG using the extinction coefficient given in Appendix B.
13 Elute the bound protein from the column with 0.02 M phosphate buffer containing 1 M KCl.
14 Regenerate the DE52 column as in step 8 above.

TECHNICAL NOTE
Greater throughput efficiency may be achieved by combining the protein dialysis and ion-exchange media in the same column. Layer Sephadex G-25 on top of the DE52 cellulose

and equilibrate both as above. Filtration of the protein sample through the Sephadex G-25 will allow sample equilibration by buffer exchange prior to interaction with the DE52 cellulose. Using this procedure, many samples of highly purified IgG may be prepared during one working day.

1.3.4 QAE–Sephadex isolation of IgG

Quaternary aminoethyl (QAE)–Sephadex is a strongly basic anion exchanger that is particularly suitable for the column separation of proteins using pH gradient elution as the swelling of QAE–Sephadex is not affected by changes in pH. The advantage is that IgG may be prepared using a volatile buffer and freeze dried without prior salt removal. It is advisable to remove β-lipoproteins from the serum before chromatography, otherwise they may break through and contaminate the IgG.

MATERIALS AND EQUIPMENT

Human serum

Aerosil

Diamino ethane–acetic acid buffer, ionic strength 0.1, pH 7.0

Acetic acid–sodium acetate buffer, ionic strength 0.1, pH 4.0

Quaternary aminoethyl (QAE)–Sephadex A-50

Column and fraction collection apparatus

1.0 M sodium hydroxide

Polyethylene glycol 8000 (PEG-8000)

Dialysis membrane tubing

Centrifuge capable of 12 000 g

UV spectrophotometer

METHOD

1 Swell QAE–Sephadex A-50 in the diamino ethane–acetic acid buffer. A bed volume of 20 ml of swollen gel is required per 10 ml serum.

2 Pack the gel into a suitable chromatography column and equilibrate with the diamino ethane–acetic acid buffer.

3 Remove β-lipoprotein from the serum by adding 0.2 g Aerosil to 10 ml serum and stir at room temperature for 4 h.

4 Centrifuge the serum at 12 000 g for 30 min and remove the lipid layer.

5 Equilibrate the serum with the diamino ethane–acetic acid buffer by dialysis or column buffer exchange.

6 Dilute the equilibrated serum with an equal volume of diamino ethane–acetic acid buffer. (If column buffer exchange was used the sample will have already been diluted by passing through the column.)

7 Apply the sample to the column at a flow rate of 8 ml/cm^2/h and continue the elution with the diamino ethane–acetic acid buffer. IgG will come straight through the column while other proteins will be retained. Assess completion of the elution by monitoring the optical density (OD) of elute using a UV spectrophotometer.

8 Elute the other proteins with the acetate buffer, pH 4.0.

Continued on p. 16

9 Regenerate the column by running through two bed volumes of diamino ethane–acetic acid buffer.

10 Concentrate the IgG in the first peak to 1/10 volume as quickly as possible; e.g. using dialysis tubing and PEG-8000.

11 The concentrated sample may now be freeze dried without removing salt as the buffer is volatile.

TECHNICAL NOTES

- It is important to concentrate the sample prior to lyophilization otherwise an insoluble precipitate may form.
- The yield of IgG should be about 70% of the serum IgG.
- Conditions should be optimized when preparing immunoglobulins from other species.

1.4 Affinity techniques for immunoglobulins and other molecules

The series of techniques described in this chapter combine the two most sought-after attributes in any purification procedure: (i) large gains in purity in single-step procedures; and (ii) technical simplicity.

In affinity chromatography the technique (summarized in Fig. 1.5) is (a) achieved by the selection of an affinity ligand that shows strong, selective and reversible binding to the molecule being purified (in operational terms, the ligand's substrate) and (b) facilitated by the use of an insoluble (and, preferably, chemically inert) affinity matrix thus permitting rapid partitioning of the ligand and its substrate.

Axen, Porath and Ernbach introduced a general technique for affinity chromatography whereby molecules containing primary amino groups could be coupled to insoluble polysaccharide matrices activated by cyanogen bromide. This route of derivatization is still the most widely employed today, even though the matrix so formed has the disadvantage of charged isourea groups, leading to a bioselective matrix with ion-exchange properties, and unstable covalent bonds between the matrix and ligand, which are susceptible to nucleophilic attack.

Support matrices such as beaded agarose gels may be used. Commercially prepared agarose beads consist of linear chains of agarobiose units in which the ionic charge of the repeating

---

Fig. 1.5 (*opposite*) **Affinity chromatographic separation of substrate molecules. (a)** Preparation of the affinity matrix. Although we have chosen to illustrate cyanogen bromide activation of Sepharose, there is an enormous range of different solid supports and derivatization reactions available (see Further reading at end of chapter). The solid support should be chemically and biologically inert (before and after derivatization); it should have a large surface area and a physical form (e.g. beaded) that will permit a high flow rate; and its physical and chemical stability should not be affected by the conditions used for desorption (treatment with free ligand, chaotropic agents, agents which disrupt hydrogen bonding detergents, etc., or changes in pH and ionic strength). The derivatization reaction should result in an uncharged covalent bond between the ligand and solid support which is stable during both desorption and long-term storage. It should not inactivate the ligand! Sometimes the ligand is sterically hindered by the support, resulting in a low adsorptive capacity

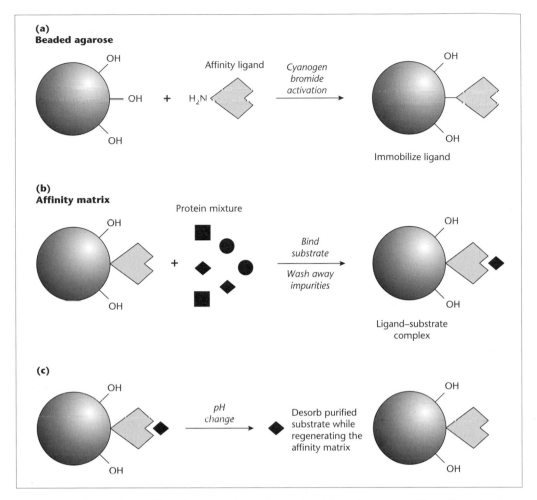

(a)
Beaded agarose

OH

OH + H₂N ⟨ Affinity ligand → *Cyanogen bromide activation* →

OH

OH

OH

OH

Immobilize ligand

(b)
Affinity matrix

Protein mixture

OH

+

→ *Bind substrate* → *Wash away impurities*

OH

OH

OH

Ligand–substrate complex

(c)

OH

→ *pH change* →

Desorb purified substrate while regenerating the affinity matrix

OH

OH

OH

(the theoretical upper limit of the affinity matrix may be calculated from the amount of ligand bound and the stoichiometry of the ligand–substrate interaction). This can be frequently overcome by the use of a 'spacer arm' between the support and ligand (see Further reading at end of chapter).

(**b**) Capture of the substrate molecules. Practical considerations are very important at this stage: e.g. the mixture containing the substrate should be in complete solution (this can be a particular problem with detergent-solubilized cells); the insolubilized ligand and substrate should have sufficient time to interact (do not run the columns too fast and recycle the column effluent several times); and the final washing of the column should be exhaustive to ensure that no unbound or weakly bound material is trapped in the interstices of the column.

(c) Desorption of the purified substrate. It is only rarely possible to desorb the substrate purely by competition with free ligand. Consider, for example, a relatively simple system such as the purification of anti-dinitrophenyl (anti-DNP) antibodies on a DNP–bovine serum albumin affinity column. Even when using very small molecules for free ligand competition, such as DNP–lysine, it is impossible to achieve a sufficiently high local concentration of free ligand, in the environment of the affinity matrix and anti-DNP binding site of the antibody, to be able to compete with the high-avidity multipoint interaction. Instead it is necessary to reduce or neutralize the forces of interaction originally responsible for capturing the bound substrate. A reduction of the interactive forces will sometimes permit the final release of the bound substrate molecules by free ligand competition; this brings an additional specific desorption step to the whole technique and so gives greater purity of product. The simultaneous desorption of substrate and regeneration of the matrix is a particularly appealing feature of affinity chromatography; the column need only be returned to the adsorptive conditions to start the whole process again.

1,3-linked β-D-galactopyranose and 2,4-linked 3,6-anhydro-α-galacto-pyranose moieties is removed by reduction with sodium borohydride under alkaline conditions.

As there are no natural covalent bonds between the linear polysaccharides, these are introduced by treatment with epi-chlorohydrin, improving the mechanical and chemical properties of the gel, thus permitting higher flow rates without compression of the gel bed and leading to improved stability at higher temperatures and in the presence of denaturing or chaotropic agents, etc. (Sepharose CL-4B is a commercially available gel with these physical and chemical properties.)

Matrix derivatization–cyanogen bromide activation

Cyanogen bromide reacts with the vicinal diols of agarose (also dextran and cellulose) to produce an activated matrix which will react with ligands (or spacer arms) containing unprotonated primary amines as summarized in Fig. 1.6. The isourea group is positively charged at physiological pH and can act as an ion-exchange matrix with negatively charged proteins.

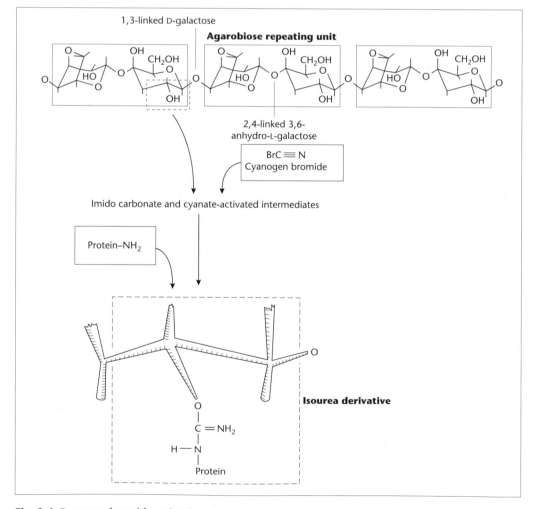

Fig. 1.6 Cyanogen bromide activation of agarose.

1.4.1 Preparation of immunoglobulin isotypes by affinity chromatography

Affinity chromatography may be used to purify immunoglobulin isotypes as an alternative to the physical chemical methods. The most obvious way to use affinity adsorption: prepare an insoluble antibody specific for the required isotype. However, this requires that the purified isotype first be available to prepare the antibody for immunosorption. Fortunately, immunoglobulins have affinity for a range of other molecules. For example:

IgG binds strongly to protein A, a cell-wall protein derived from *Staphylococcus aureus*;

IgM binds to mannan-binding protein;

IgA_1 binds to the lectin jacalin, and mouse IgD binds to *Griffonia simplicifolia* I lectin.

The above examples of affinity methods for isolating immunoglobulins largely (except for protein A and G) depend on the recognition of sugars. While particular sugars are associated with various immunoglobulin isotypes the relationship is not absolute and may be altered in disease. Using these methods always has some danger of contamination and yields will not be 100%.

1.4.2 Preparation of IgG on protein A–agarose

The IgG binding properties of protein A make affinity chromatography with protein A–agarose immunoadsorbents a very simple method for preparing IgG. IgG subclasses show differential binding: e.g. human IgG subclasses 1, 2 and 4 bind to protein A but IgG_3 does not.

MATERIALS
Human serum
Protein A–agarose, e.g. protein A–Sepharose CL-4B
Phosphate-buffered saline (PBS)
0.1 M glycine–HCl, pH 2.8
1 M sodium hydroxide or solid tris (hydroxymethyl)-aminomethane (Tris)

METHOD

1. Swell 1.5 g protein A–Sepharose CL-4B in 10 ml PBS for 1 h at room temperature and then pack it into a small chromatography column, e.g. a 10-ml disposable hypodermic syringe. Store and use this column at 4°C.
2. Dilute 10 ml human serum with an equal volume of PBS.
3. Filter the serum through the column at a flow rate of 30 ml/h.
4. Wash through unbound proteins with PBS until no more protein leaves the column (monitor the protein with a UV flow cell).
5. Elute the bound IgG with glycine–HCl buffer, pH 2.8.
6. Titrate the pH of the purified IgG solution to near neutrality with NaOH or solid Tris, and dialyse against PBS.
7. Regenerate the column by washing with 2 column bed volumes of PBS. Store the column at 4°C.

- The protein A content of the swollen gel is 2 mg/ml and the binding capacity for human IgG is approximately 25 mg/ml of packed gel.
- Small quantities of some types of IgM will bind to protein A. You should be aware of this possibility and monitor the IgG preparations if absolute purity is required. Remove the IgM by gel filtration.
- Protein G is also useful for preparing IgG. It has a slightly different range of subclass specificities and is particularly good for preparing rat IgG. Generally it has a high capacity for binding IgG and similar conditions may be used as for protein A isolation of IgG.

As well as IgG, protein A binds to the V_H3 region of other immunoglobulin subclasses.

Protein G shows greater specificity for IgG. Protein L, derived from *Peptostreptococcus magnus*, binds to immunoglobulins through interaction with κ light chains, particularly human κI, κIII and κIV and mouse κI. It therefore binds all immunoglobulin classes, but omits all antibodies with λ light chains. Protein L can be bound to agarose gels using cyanogen bromide and used as for protein A. (See De Chateau *et al.* (1993) which discusses the interaction between protein L and immunoglobulins of various mammalian species.)

1.4.3 Isolation of IgG subclasses using protein A–agarose

Although in both human and mouse the IgG subclasses differ markedly from each other in their biological properties, they are structurally very similar. This similarity has made it almost impossible to isolate single subclasses using physical chemical techniques. Fractionation of the IgG subclasses is possible using protein A affinity chromatography and pH gradient elution.

Isolation of mouse subclasses

IgG is common to mammalian species, but further evolution has occurred since subclasses of IgG are present in many animals but there is no clear relationship between subclasses in different species. IgG_1, IgG_2, IgG_3 and IgG_4 are found in humans; IgG_1, IgG_{2a}, IgG_{2b} and IgG_3 in mice; and IgG_1, IgG_{2a}, IgG_{2b} and IgG_{2c} in rats.

Mouse serum may be fractionated on protein A–agarose by:

1 allowing all the IgG to bind to the adsorbent; and then
2 eluting the separate subclasses with a stepped gradient of increasing acidity.

MATERIALS AND EQUIPMENT
Mouse serum
Protein A–Sepharose CL-4B
Phosphate-buffered saline (PBS)
0.1 M phosphate buffer, pH 8.0
0.1 M citrate buffers, pH 6.0, 5.5, 4.5, 3.5
1.0 M tris (hydroxymethyl)-aminomethane(Tris)–HCl buffers, pH 8.5, 9.0
Chromatography column or 10-ml disposable syringe
Antisera to the mouse IgG subclasses

1 Swell 1.5 g protein A–Sepharose in 10 ml PBS for 1 h at room temperature and then pack it into a small chromatography column. Store and use this column at 4°C.

2 Equilibrate the column with 0.1 M phosphate buffer, pH 8.0.

3 Add 2 ml 0.1 M phosphate buffer, pH 8.0 to 4 ml mouse serum and adjust to pH 8.1 with 1 M Tris–HCl buffer, pH 9.0.

4 Apply the diluted serum to the column and wash through with 30 ml 0.1 M phosphate buffer, pH 8.0 (flow rate 0.4–0.5 ml/min throughout).

5 Elute the IgG_1 with 30 ml 0.1 M citrate buffer, pH 6.0.

6 Wash the column with 25 ml 0.1 M citrate buffer, pH 5.5.

7 To minimize the denaturation of the IgG_{2a} and IgG_{2b} antibodies, collect the eluates from steps 7 and 8 into tubes containing 1.0 M Tris–HCl buffer, pH 8.5.

8 Elute the IgG_{2a} with 30 ml 0.1 M citrate buffer, pH 4.5.

9 Elute the IgG_{2b} with 25 ml 0.1 M citrate buffer, pH 3.5.

10 Re-equilibrate the column to pH 8.0.

11 Determine the composition of each fraction with specific antisera, preferably using immunoassay.

Figure 1.7 shows the purity of fractions obtained from a protein A fractionation of mouse serum. An enzyme-linked immunosorbent assay has been used to examine the protein fractions dot blotted onto nitrocellulose.

TECHNICAL NOTE

IgG_3 usually elutes with the IgG_{2a} fraction. Immunoaffinity chromatography on subclass-specific antibody affinity columns is required to remove this contamination.

Isolation of human IgG subclasses

Protein A may be used to obtain fractions of human IgG which, although not completely pure, are certainly much enriched for individual subclasses. IgG_3 does not bind to protein A, so if total IgG is filtered through a column of protein A–Sepharose, IgG_1, IgG_2 and IgG_4 will bind to the adsorbent but IgG_3 will come straight through. IgG_1 and IgG_2 may be differentially eluted from the adsorbent with a pH gradient of increasing acidity. Although IgG_4 is a slight contaminant in the IgG_2 fractions, this problem may be reduced by starting with IgG prepared using DEAE–cellulose ion-exchange chromatography (see Section 1.3); this is relatively deficient in IgG_4.

MATERIALS AND EQUIPMENT

Protein A–Sepharose CL-4B

Human IgG, DEAE–cellulose purified or human serum

0.15 M citrate–phosphate buffers, pH 7.0, 5.0, 4.5

0.1 M citric acid, pH 2.2

Antisera to human IgG subclasses

Chromatography column or 10-ml disposable syringe

UV flow cell

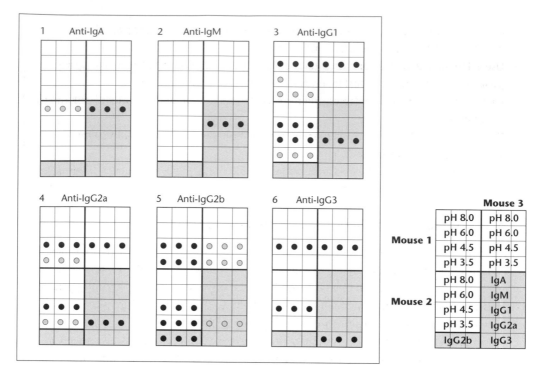

Fig. 1.7 Protein A fractionation of mouse IgG subclasses. Sera from MRL/lpr mice (an inbred mouse strain characterized by lymphoproliferation and high immunoglobulin levels) have been fractionated on protein A–agarose. The material coming straight through the column at pH 8.0 and fractions eluted at pH 6.0, 4.5 and 3.5 have been collected and dot blotted, in triplicate, on to six nitrocellulose membranes. Each membrane has been incubated with a biotinylated specific anticlass or subclass antibody. The blots (1–6) were then incubated with streptavidin labelled with peroxidase. Grid key to each blot shown on right of main figure. Commercially obtained, purified myeloma IgA, IgG_1, IgG_{2a}, IgG_{2b}, IgG_3 and HPLC-purified IgM were included on the blots as standards. The blots show that it is possible to considerably enrich fractions for single subclasses from whole mouse serum. Some slight cross-reactivity is seen with the antibodies reacting with the myeloma proteins. Here there is the problem of determining whether the myeloma proteins or the antisera (all obtained commercially) are impure, or even possibly both. This experiment cautions the reader against always taking manufacturers' publicity at face value.

METHOD

1 Swell 1 g protein A–Sepharose with 10 ml citrate–phosphate buffer, pH 7.0.

2 Pack the swollen gel into a small chromatography column and equilibrate with citrate–phosphate buffer, pH 7.0.

3 Load either 5 mg human IgG or 0.5 ml human serum (premixed with 0.5 ml buffer, pH 7.0) onto the column.

4 Wash the column through with pH 7.0 buffer. If purified IgG was used on the column, pure IgG_3 will come out with the washing buffer. Otherwise, it will come out mixed with all the other non-IgG serum proteins.

5 Elute the IgG_2 and IgG_1 with a pH gradient of citrate–phosphate buffer. This is constructed by using a gradient maker of three equivolume chambers connected in series. The first chamber should contain 6 ml 0.1 M citric acid, pH 2.2, the middle chamber 6 ml of

Continued

citrate–phosphate buffer, pH 4.5, and the final chamber, which is connected to the column, 6 ml of citrate–phosphate buffer, pH 5.0.

6   Use a flow rate of 12 ml/h and monitor the eluate with a UV flow cell. Two overlapping peaks will be obtained, the first being enriched for IgG_2, the second for IgG_1.

7   Each peak should be concentrated and recycled on the re-equilibrated protein A column to increase resolution.

8   To re-equilibrate the column, wash sequentially with 6 ml 0.1 M citric acid and 30 ml citrate–phosphate buffer, pH 7.0.

9   Check the purity of the IgG subclasses with specific antisera, preferably using immunoassay.

1.4.4 Preparation of human IgA_1 on jacalin–agarose

IgA is a comparatively difficult immunoglobulin to isolate by physicochemical methods. The lectin jacalin, obtained from the seeds of the jackfruit, *Artocarpus integrifolia*, binds human IgA_1, but not IgA_2. Binding is through O-glycosidically linked oligosaccharides containing galactosyl (β-1,3) N-acetylgalactosamine, in the presence or absence of sialic acid. This lectin is available conjugated to agarose for use in affinity chromatography methods.

An immunoglobulin fraction prepared with ammonium sulphate must be applied to the column, as non-immunoglobulin serum proteins also bind to the lectin. Bound IgA_1 is then eluted with melibiose or galactose.

MATERIALS

Jacalin–agarose

Jacalin storage buffer: (4-(2-hydroxyethyl)piperazine-1-ethane sulphonic acid) HEPES 10 mM, pH 7.5, containing 150 mM sodium chloride, 100 mM calcium chloride, 20 mM galactose and 0.08% w/v sodium azide

175 mM tris(hydroxymethyl)-aminomethane (Tris)–HCl buffer, pH 7.5

Immunoglobulin preparation, e.g. 45% saturated ammonium sulphate precipitate of human serum

Melibiose 0.1 M or galactose 0.8 M in 0.175 M Tris–HCl buffer

Chromatography column or 10-ml disposable syringe

Note: Azide is a dangerous chemical—do not discard down the sink.

METHOD

1   Pour 2 ml of jacalin–agarose gel into a small chromatography column (or 5-ml disposable syringe barrel with the outlet covered by glass or nylon wool).

2   Wash the gel thoroughly with 50 ml of Tris buffer to remove the sugars used to stabilize the lectin during storage.

3   Slowly add 5 ml of human immunoglobulin (10 mg/ml) in Tris–HCl buffer.

4   Wash the column through with 20 ml Tris–HCl buffer (or until the absorbance returns to base line, if you are using a flow-through UV monitor).

5   Elute the IgA with 5 ml 0.1 M melibiose or 0.8 M galactose (if using a UV monitor, elute until the protein peak has been collected).

6   Collect fractions of 1 ml and determine their protein content by spectrophotometry at 280 nm.

Continued on p. 24

7 Pool the fractions containing protein and examine for IgA$_1$ content and purity by SDS-PAGE (see Appendix B.2.1) and Western blotting (see Section 4.11) with isotype-specific antisera, or alternatively by immunoelectrophoresis with antisera to IgA and whole human serum.

8 Regenerate the column by washing through with 20 ml storage buffer and store the jacalin–agarose gel at 4°C.

TECHNICAL NOTES

- The binding capacity of the jacalin–agarose gel will vary between batches but is typically 4.0 mg monomeric IgA$_1$ per ml of gel.
- IgA$_2$ is lost with other immunoglobulins which do not bind to jacalin. Loomes *et al.* (1991) provide a method for the purification and characterization of IgA$_1$ and IgA$_2$ from serum that requires a series of column preparations including gel filtration, DEAE and affinity chromatography on jacalin sepharose.

1.4.5 Preparation of IgM on mannan-binding protein (MBP)

Immobilized mannan-binding protein is commercially available from Pierce (Rockford, Illinois, USA) but can be prepared in-house by immobilizing mannan for isolation of MBP, then coupling the MBP to cyanogen bromide-activated Sepharose 4B (adapted from Nevens *et al.* 1992).

Preparation of immobilized mannan for isolating MBP

Activation of Sepharose 4B with cyanogen bromide

MATERIALS

Sepharose 4B
Cyanogen bromide (*this chemical is very toxic and must be handled in a fume cupboard*)
Crushed ice
5 M sodium hydroxide
0.1 M sodium bicarbonate solution
Yeast mannan
1.0 M ethanolamine, pH 9.0
1.25 M NaCl containing 20 mM CaCl$_2$ and 10 mM imidazole, pH 7.8

METHOD

1 Wash 100 ml Sepharose 4B in 1.6 l of distilled water, then remove the water by suction until it is dried.

2 Transfer the Sepharose 4B into a beaker and suspend in 100 ml of distilled water.

3 Put beaker containing the Sepharose 4B and water onto a magnetic stirrer and insert a pH meter probe.

Next step (4) using cyanogen bromide must be performed in a fume cupboard (owing to possible release of cyanide gas). It is essential that the slurry is maintained at about 20°C and an alkaline pH.

Continued

4 Slowly add 20 g of solid cyanogen bromide over a 20-min time period, maintaining the temperature at around 20°C by adding crushed ice to the stirring slurry.

5 Keep the pH of the slurry between 10.5 and 11.0 by adding a concentrated solution of sodium hydroxide (dropwise).

6 Wash the cyanogen bromide-activated Sepharose using a glass Buchner funnel with around 2 l of ice-cold 0.1 M sodium bicarbonate, then dry by suction.

7 Dissolve 1.78 g of yeast mannan in 100 ml 0.1 M sodium bicarbonate solution, add to the activated Sepharose beads and stir overnight at room temperature.

8 Wash the activated Sepharose beads with 1 litre of distilled water, then suspend in 160 ml 1.0 M ethanolamine, pH 9.0, at room temperature for 60 min.

9 Wash with 1 litre of distilled water and pack into a glass column—the Sepharose is now ready for isolating the MBP.

10 Equilibrate the column with 10 column volumes of 1.25 M NaCl containing 20 mM $CaCl_2$ and 10 mM imidazole, pH 7.8.

Coupling of cyanogen bromide-activated Sepharose 4B and MBP

MATERIALS

Sepharose 4B

Solid cyanogen bromide (*this chemical is very toxic and must be handled in a fume cupboard*)

0.1 M sodium bicarbonate buffer, pH 8.5

1.0 M NaCl

10 mM tris(hydroxymethyl)-aminomethane (Tris) containing 1.25 M NaCl and 2 mM ethylene diamine tetra-acetic acid (EDTA), pH 7.4

Mannan-binding protein (MBP) solution

Coomassie protein assay reagent

1 Activate the Sepharose 4B with cyanogen bromide by the same procedure as in steps 1–5 (above).

2 Wash the activated Sepharose with 200 ml of ice-cold distilled water followed by 100 ml 0.1 M sodium bicarbonate buffer, pH 8.5, then dry by suction.

3 Mix the MBP solution and activated Sepharose and stir overnight at 4°C.

4 Filter the gel suspension and wash with 200 ml 1.0 M NaCl, followed by 200 ml water.

5 Block the excess reactive groups on the MBP coupled to cyanogen bromide-activated Sepharose 4B column with 10 ml 1.0 M ethanolamine, pH 9.0, and stir at room temperature for 60 min.

6 Wash with 200 ml of distilled water followed by 200 ml 10 mM Tris containing 1.25 M NaCl and 2 mM EDTA, pH 7.4.

Note: Test the coupling of MBP with the activated Sepharose by mixing 200 µl of immobilized MBP suspension and 2 ml of Coomassie protein assay reagent into a test tube. If the gel remains blue and the supernatant is colourless it indicates there is no unbound MBP present.

Isolation of IgM using MBP coupled to cyanogen bromide-activated Sepharose 4B

MATERIALS

Sample: serum or monoclonal antibody culture supernatant

MBP coupled to cyanogen bromide-activated Sepharose 4B

Hypodermic syringe and glass wool (Caution: Wear gloves when handling glass wool)

10 mM tris(hydroxymethyl)-aminomethane (Tris) containing 1.25 M NaCl with 0.02% w/v sodium azide, pH 7.4

10 mM Tris containing 1.25 M NaCl, 20 mM $CaCl_2$ with 0.02% w/v sodium azide, pH 7.4

10 mM Tris containing 1.25 M NaCl, 2 mM EDTA with 0.02% w/v sodium azide, pH 7.4

Note: Azide is a dangerous chemical—do not discard down the sink.

METHOD

Steps 1–8 are performed at 4°C; therefore all buffers must be ice cold.

1 Dialyse the monoclonal antibody supernatant or sample containing IgM overnight against two changes of 1000 ml 10 mM Tris containing 1.25 M NaCl with 0.02% w/v sodium azide, pH 7.4. (This step is to remove any phosphate ions that could form a precipitate with the calcium ions in subsequent steps.)

2 Dilute the sample with an equal volume of 10 mM Tris containing 1.25 M NaCl, 20 mM $CaCl_2$ with 0.02% w/v sodium azide, pH 7.4.

3 Load the MBP coupled to cyanogen bromide-activated Sepharose 4B into a 100-ml hypodermic syringe plugged with glass wool.

4 Wash the column with 5 column volumes of 10 mM Tris containing 1.25 M NaCl, 20 mM $CaCl_2$ with 0.02% w/v sodium azide, pH 7.4.

5 Apply the diluted sample, allow to flow completely into the column, collect the eluate and re-apply to the column.

6 Repeat step 5 around five times for the best yield of IgM antibodies.

7 Allow the sample to incubate on the column for about 30 min by clamping the eluate tubing, and keep the top of the gel from drying by adding 200 μl of 10 mM Tris containing 1.25 M NaCl, 20 mM $CaCl_2$ with 0.02% w/v sodium azide, pH 7.4.

8 After the incubation, wash the column with 10 column volumes of 10 mM Tris containing 1.25 M NaCl, 20 mM $CaCl_2$ with 0.02% w/v sodium azide, pH 7.4, monitoring the fractions spectrophotometrically at 280 nm.

Steps **9** onwards are performed at room temperature; therefore buffers **must not** be ice cold.

9 Take the column into room temperature and allow to stand for 60 min (do not allow the column to dry out).

10 Wash with 3 column volumes of 10 mM Tris containing 1.25 M NaCl, 20 mM $CaCl_2$ with 0.02% w/v sodium azide, pH 7.4.

11 Elute the IgM with 10 mM Tris containing 1.25 M NaCl, 2 mM EDTA with 0.02% w/v sodium azide, pH 7.4, monitoring the fractions spectrophotometrically at 280 nm. An absorbance of 1.18 at 280 nm is equivalent to an IgM concentration of 1 mg/ml.

12 Store the IgM-containing fractions at –20°C.

13 Wash the column with 3 column volumes of distilled water followed by 3 column volumes of 10 mM Tris containing 1.25 M NaCl, 20 mM $CaCl_2$ with 0.02% w/v sodium azide, pH 7.4, and store at 4°C.

1.4.6 Purification of IgD on *Griffonia simplicifolia* I lectin

MATERIALS

Monoclonal antibody culture supernatant derived from an IgD-secreting hybridoma

5-ml hypodermic syringe

Glass wool (Caution: Wear gloves when handling glass wool)

GS-I lectin–Sepharose (purchase coupled or linked as above)

Phosphate-buffered saline (PBS) containing 1 mM $CaCl_2$

PBS containing 1 mM $CaCl_2$ and 0.1 M D-galactose

UV spectrophotometer

Dialysis membrane tubing

METHOD

1 Centrifuge monoclonal antibody culture supernatant at 10 000 g for 30 min at 4°C or room temperature.

2 Save the supernatant and discard the cell debris.

3 Dilute the supernatant with 10 volumes of PBS containing 1 mM $CaCl_2$ and centrifuge at 15 000 g for 30 min at 4°C and save the supernatant for step 7.

4 Prepare a mini-column such as a 5-ml hypodermic syringe plugged with glass wool (use gloves when handling glass wool).

5 Pour in 3 ml of GS-I lectin–Sepharose and maintain at a temperature of 4°C.

6 Wash GS-I lectin–Sepharose with the following ice-cold buffers:

12 column volumes PBS containing 1 mM $CaCl_2$;

12 column volumes PBS containing 1 mM $CaCl_2$ and 0.1 M D-galactose;

12 column volumes PBS containing 1 mM $CaCl_2$.

7 Load the supernatant and allow to flow into the GS-I lectin–Sepharose.

8 Wash the column with sufficient ice-cold PBS containing 1 mM $CaCl_2$, monitoring the fractions spectrophotometrically at 280 nm, until a baseline is reached.

9 Elute the IgD antibodies with ice-cold PBS containing 1 mM $CaCl_2$ and 0.1 M D-galactose. Around 3–5 column volumes should be enough to elute the IgD, but it is advised that the eluate is monitored spectrophotometrically at 280 nm.

10 The column may be regenerated with 2 column volumes PBS containing 1 mM $CaCl_2$ and 0.1 M D-galactose, then 10 column volumes PBS containing 1 mM $CaCl_2$. To preserve the column add 0.02% w/v sodium azide to the final wash and store at 4°C.

11 Dialyse the IgD sample against 500 ml ice-cold PBS, pH 7.3, at 4°C with five changes of buffer.

12 Estimate the IgD concentration of the dialysed sample by measuring at 280 nm with a UV spectrophotometer.

1.5 Purification of antibodies

An antibody reacts specifically with its own antigenic determinant to form an antigen–antibody complex. An animal immunized with an antigen will respond to produce antibodies all reacting with the antigen to some degree. Serum from this animal will have the usual range of immunoglobulins but those reacting with this antigen will be at a relatively higher concentration, compared to normal serum.

An animal receiving a transplantable plasmacytoma or hybridoma will produce large amounts of the monoclonal immunoglobulin or antibody, but there will still be a significant background of normal serum proteins and immunoglobulins, even in ascitic fluid.

To study a particular antibody in detail it is of great advantage to be able to separate it from the surrounding non-specific antibody molecules using the antigen. Then to obtain reactive purified antibody we must separate the complex and remove the antigen.

The forces binding antibody to antigen are those involved in any protein–protein interaction:

(a) coulombic;

(b) dipole;

(c) hydrogen bonding;

(d) van der Waals';

(e) hydrophobic bonding.

All these forces depend upon the charge of the molecules taking part in the reaction. The net charge of the molecules in turn depends on the pH of the medium. If the pH of the medium is lowered sufficiently the protein molecules change conformation, gain H^+ ions and so repel each other. We are now faced with the problem of physically removing the antigen or the antibody, because when the pH is returned to neutrality the complexes will re-form.

If the antigen is insoluble it can be easily separated from soluble antibody. There are many methods available for rendering either the antigen or antibody insoluble, some of which are described in the following sections.

1.5.1 Preparation of a protein immunoadsorbent

In this experiment antibodies to mouse immunoglobulin are purified but the identical method can be used for other proteins.

MATERIALS AND EQUIPMENT

Sepharose 4B

Cyanogen bromide (*this chemical is very toxic and must be handled in a fume cupboard*)

2.0 M sodium hydroxide

Phosphate-buffered saline (PBS)

Borate–saline buffer, pH 8.3, ionic strength 0.1

Mouse immunoglobulin

Sintered glass funnel

UV spectrophotometer

METHOD

1 Pipette 14 ml of Sepharose (about 200 mg) into a 50-ml glass beaker and add 10 ml of distilled water.

   All procedures must now be carried out in a fume cupboard.

2 Weigh a stoppered tube, add some solid cyanogen bromide, replace the stopper and reweigh the tube.

Continued

---

3 Dissolve the cyanogen bromide in distilled water to a final concentration of 50 mg/ml.
4 Place the Sepharose beads on a magnetic stirrer and titrate the pH to 11.0–11.5 with 2.0 M sodium hydroxide.
5 Add 10 ml of the cyanogen bromide solution.
6 Maintain the pH at 11.0–11.5 by dropwise addition of sodium hydroxide for 5–10 min until the pH becomes stable.
7 Wash the activated beads on a sintered glass funnel with 100 ml of water, and then 100 ml of borate–saline buffer.
8 Wash the beads into a glass beaker, allow them to settle and remove the supernatant.
9 Add 100 mg of mouse immunoglobulin at 5–10 mg/ml (initial concentration).
10 Leave the beads stirring with the protein overnight at 4°C (most of the uptake occurs within the first 4 h and so this stage can be abbreviated).
11 Wash the beads on a sintered glass funnel with 10 ml PBS and collect the washings. (Use negative pressure and collect washings in a tube standing in a side-arm flask.)
12 Wash the beads thoroughly with PBS to remove the rest of the unbound immunoglobulin.
13 A UV spectrophotometer reading of the washings will give the amount of unbound protein and so the approximate quantity of protein bound to the column can be calculated. The immunoadsorbent is now ready for use. Store in PBS containing azide (0.1 M).
Note: Azide is a dangerous chemical—do not discard down the sink.

TECHNICAL NOTES
- In step 6, wash the gel with borate–saline buffer as soon as the pH becomes stable. The rate of inactivation by hydrolysis is highly pH dependent and increases sharply above pH 9.5.
- For maximum uptake, the coupling pH should be above the pK_a of the protein, but below pH 10.0.
- Avoid buffers containing amines; they will compete with the amino function on the protein for the activated groups on the gel. Borate and bicarbonate buffers are the most useful; however, Tris buffers may be used as the amino group on the Tris moiety is sterically hindered.
- After coupling, it is possible to add 1.0 M glycine, pH 8.0, for 6 h at 4°C if you wish to be completely sure that all the activated hydroxyls have been derivatized.

1.5.2 Use of immunoadsorbent for antibody purification

MATERIALS AND EQUIPMENT
Rabbit anti-mouse immunoglobulin
Immunoadsorbent mouse immunoglobulin on Sepharose 4B (20 ml)
0.1 M glycine–HCl buffer, pH 2.5
Trichloroacetic acid (TCA), 10% aqueous solution
Tris-(hydroxymethyl) aminomethane (Tris)
Phosphate-buffered saline (PBS)
Chromatography column or 20-ml disposable syringe
Glass wool

Preparation of the column and antigen–antibody complex

METHOD

1 Pour the immunoadsorbent into the column and equilibrate with 20 ml PBS. Close the column.
2 Run 20 ml of antiserum through the column—do not use positive pressure; allow to run under gravity.
3 Wash the unbound protein from the column until the absorbance measured in a flow through a UV cell is < 0.1, otherwise wash with 200 ml PBS. Close the column.

We now have the antigen–antibody complex.

Dissociation of complex

METHOD

1 Pipette out 20 × 0.5 ml aliquots of TCA into small glass tubes. (Use this to sample the effluent for protein elution if a flow-through UV cell is not available.)
2 Add glycine–HCl buffer to the top of the column and collect the effluent when protein is first detected.
3 Stop collecting the effluent when protein is no longer detectable.
 The first stage of the elution is now complete and part of the antibody has been recovered. The acid elution buffer will, however, eventually denature the antibody so we must raise the pH.
4 Titrate the protein to pH 8.5 with solid Tris. Mix thoroughly and monitor with a pH meter or indicator papers.
 The elution conditions are altered to recover a second batch of antibody.
5 Add glycine–HCl plus 10% dioxane to the column. Monitor the effluent and collect the second batch of antibody.
6 Adjust the pH to 8.5 with solid Tris.
7 Read the absorbance of each protein solution at 280 nm and calculate the recovered protein. (Remember to use the buffer plus dioxane as reference for the spectrophotometer.)
8 Concentrate the samples in dialysis tubing with either sucrose or polyethylene glycol 40 000 or by negative-pressure dialysis (see also Appendix B.1.4).
9 When the sample volume has been reduced to 3.0–5.0 ml, dialyse against 5 × 1 litre PBS.
10 Spin off the precipitate and determine the protein content of each sample.

This method of antibody purification is highly reproducible and so it is not necessary to calculate the antibody content of the sample routinely. However, a specimen calculation is given below.

TECHNICAL NOTES

- Under the conditions described, the Sepharose should bind 90–100 mg of mouse immunoglobulin. Approximately the same uptake can be expected with other common protein antigens, with the notable exception of bovine serum albumin where only 20–30 mg are bound.

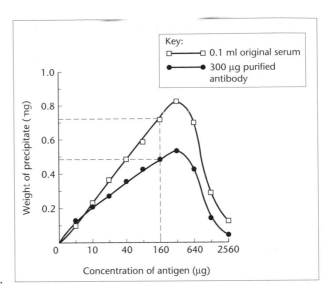

Fig. 1.8 Precipitin curves of anti-immunoglobulin serum and antibody.

- Although the proportion of antibody in the final sample is fairly constant, the actual yield of antibody relative to the serum concentration varies with serum pool and species. The greatest loss of antibody occurs due to denaturation and precipitation after elution, concentration and dialysis.
- In the experiment, the immunoadsorbent has been used below its maximal capacity; in general it should be able to deplete 1 ml of antiserum for each mg of antigen on the column.
- Pre-activated Sepharose is available commercially; this avoids the use of cyanogen bromide. For large-scale preparations, however, it is relatively expensive.

1.5.3 Calculation of recovery from immunoadsorbent

Total weight of immunoglobulin on column = 92.0 mg on 200 mg of Sepharose 4B.
Volume of antiserum for antibody purification = 10 ml.
Antibody content of serum calculated from Fig. 1.8, at equivalence condition.
Antibody content of serum = 5.2 mg/ml.
% yield of antibody protein from serum: immediately 81.5%; after concentration and dialysis 47.8%.

Eluates from immunoadsorbent
Total protein concentration in eluate:

Eluant	Immediately		After concentration and dialysis	
Glycine–HCl	36.4 mg	} 42.4 mg	23.0 mg	} 25.0 mg
Glycine–HCl + 10% dioxane	6.0 mg		2.0 mg	

Calculation of antibody content of eluate:

From Fig. 1.8: weight of antibody in around 300 µg of eluted protein = 490 – 160

$$= 330 \text{ µg.*}$$

* Within limits of experimental error

Hence, all the recovered protein has retained antibody activity. (In general, at least 90% of the recovered protein should be antibody.)

1.5.4 Elution conditions

Antibodies with high-affinity antigen-binding sites are the essential constituents of a 'strong' high-titred antiserum. When these antibodies are linked to Sepharose and used as solid-phase immunoadsorbents they give virtually irreversible binding to antigen. It is rarely possible to isolate antigen or antibody by true affinity methods, simply because a sufficiently high concentration of free competitor cannot be obtained to compete effectively with the solid-phase reagents.

Most techniques for the release of material from antibody affinity columns rely on deforming agents to alter the shape of the reacting molecules and so lower their net binding affinity. Acid or alkaline buffers are usually sufficient to release an acceptable proportion of bound material, most of which will regain full activity when a near-neutral pH is restored.

The addition of dioxane to an acid buffer increases yield from an affinity column (by reducing hydrophobic interactions) but with additional loss of recovered material due to irreversible denaturation. Other eluting buffers are more effective because they deform (and denature) to a greater extent but may produce an unacceptably high proportion of denatured material.

In order of increasing harshness they are:

(a) 3.5 M potassium thiocyanate in 0.1 M phosphate buffer, pH 6.6;

(b) 8.0 M urea; and

(c) 7.0 M guanidine hydrochloride.

When using anti-immunoglobulin affinity columns to isolate a particularly valuable antibody, e.g. a monoclonal antibody produced by a hybridoma cell line, it is good practice to saturate high-affinity anti-immunoglobulin sites by a cycle of pretreatment with normal mouse immunoglobulin and acid elution.

1.5.5 Practical applications of immunoadsorbents

Immunoadsorbents are widely used to render antisera specific by depletion of cross-reacting antibodies, and for quantitative adsorption. Although the method above used an antigen immunoadsorbent to isolate antibody, it is possible to prepare antigen or immunoglobulin by the same procedure using an antibody immunoadsorbent column or a cellular immunoadsorbent column.

1.6 Reduction of IgG to heavy and light chains

The heavy and light chains of IgG are covalently linked by disulphide bonds which may be broken by reduction. Intrachain disulphide links are less easy to break. Thus a balance has to be found whereby enough interchain bonds are broken to permit chain separation, but the number of intrachain bonds broken is limited so that biological activity is retained.

The reduced heavy and light chains are still held together by non-covalent forces but can be dissociated by fractionation in an acid medium.

MATERIALS AND EQUIPMENT

IgG

0.15 M tris(hydroxymethyl)-aminomethane (Tris)–HCl buffer, pH 8.2

2-mercaptoethanol (toxic chemical that must be handled with gloves and in a fume cupboard)

0.1 M iodoacetamide

1 M propionic or acetic acid

Trimethylamine

Nitrogen cylinder

Polyethylene glycol 8000 (PEG-8000)

Supadex-200 column, equilibrated with 1 M propionic or acetic acid at 4°C (100 ml column; 100 × 2.5 cm)

Dialysis tubing

METHOD

1 Dialyse the IgG against Tris–HCl buffer and adjust the protein concentration to 30 mg/ml.

2 De-gas the IgG solution with a vacuum pump and then bubble in nitrogen.

3 Add 2-mercaptoethanol to a final concentration of 0.75 M; *2-mercaptoethanol is toxic and so this procedure must be carried out in a fume cupboard.* (The solution is de-gassed and the reduction carried out in the presence of nitrogen as 2-mercaptoethanol is oxidized by atmospheric oxygen. Alternatively, reduction may be carried out with 0.02 M dithiothreitol which is less susceptible to oxidation. *Again, this agent is dangerous and will cause a severe headache if inhaled.*)

4 Incubate at room temperature for 1 h.

5 Cool the mixture in ice water and add iodoacetamide to a final concentration of 0.75 M. This prevents re-association of the reduced interchain S–S bonds by alkylating the liberated sulphydryl groups.

6 Maintain the pH at 8.0 by the dropwise addition of trimethylamine.

7 Concentrate the sample e.g. by placing in dialysis tubing and covering with PEG-8000.

8 Apply the sample to the Supadex-200 column equilibrated with 1 M propionic or acetic acid at 4°C and collect fractions of 5 ml.

9 Concentrate and return the fractions to neutrality.

TECHNICAL NOTE

A similar procedure may be followed for the reduction of the other immunoglobulin classes.

Analysis of the fractions

The success of the reduction can be assessed by SDS-PAGE (see Appendix B.2.1) in non-reducing conditions. Alternatively, the samples can be examined immunologically by Western blot analysis using specific antilight chain and anti-Fc antisera (see Section 4.11).

1.7 Cleavage of polyclonal IgG by proteolytic enzymes

In the pre-antibiotic era a major use of immunoglobulins was in immunotherapy. Immunoglobulins from animals immunized with antigens such as tetanus and diphtheria toxin were used to passively immunize patients suffering from diseases caused by these toxins. Unfortunately, these foreign immunoglobulins were themselves immunogenic and could often provoke a type III hypersensitivity serum sickness. To try to reduce the immunogenicity of these foreign immunoglobulins, they were treated with a range of proteolytic enzymes including pepsin and papain. These enzymes were known to cleave the antibodies into active and inactive fragments. In 1958 Porter exploited these observations in his Nobel prize-winning studies on antibody structure.

Many enzymes have now been introduced for the production of immunoglobulin fragments, but papain and pepsin are still the two most commonly used in the immunology laboratory. Most of the accumulated wisdom on enzymic fragmentation applies to human and rabbit immunoglobulin. Digestion conditions have been determined using biochemically heterogeneous polyclonal antibodies and so relate only to the average properties of the mixture.

With the advent of the hybridoma technique for producing monoclonal immunoglobulins it has become necessary to produce similar fragments from mouse immunoglobulins.

Two problems thus present themselves in that: (i) far less is known about the fragmentation of mouse immunoglobulins in general; and (ii) each monoclonal antibody is unique and requires its own digestion conditions.

1.7.1 Papain digestion

Papain is an enzyme that contains active site cysteine. It splits the IgG molecule to the N-terminal side of the disulphide bonds linking the two heavy chains, thus giving rise to two Fab fragments and one Fc fragment.

Soluble papain is perfectly adequate for most uses but does result in some contamination with residual papain.

Insoluble papain can be prepared by attaching the enzyme to a support such as agarose using cyanogen bromide. Alternatively it may be purchased attached to agarose or CM–cellulose (carboxymethyl cellulose) from Sigma. Insoluble enzymes may use the same conditions as soluble enzymes for protein degradation experiments and often result in more discrete fragments. The advantage of the insoluble enzyme preparations is that the reaction may be easily stopped by centrifugation at slow speed to pellet the enzyme.

Rabbit IgG

MATERIALS AND EQUIPMENT
IgG (rabbit)
Papain
Cysteine
Ethylene diamine tetra-acetic acid (EDTA), disodium salt
Carboxymethyl cellulose (CM–cellulose) (30 × 2.5.cm)
Sodium acetate buffers, 0.01 M and 0.9 M, pH 5.5

Phosphate-buffered saline (PBS)
Chromatography column or 40-ml disposable syringe
Fraction collector

METHOD

1 Adjust the concentration of the IgG to 20 mg/ml in PBS.

2 Add cysteine to a final concentration of 0.02 M.

3 Add EDTA to a final concentration of 0.002 M.

4 Add 1 mg papain for every 100 mg IgG used.

5 Incubate at 37°C for 4 h.

6 Dialyse the digest against 0.01 M sodium acetate buffer, pH 5.5.
   When the cysteine and EDTA are removed by dialysis, the enzyme is inactivated. More controlled termination of the reaction can be obtained by adding iodoacetamide to a final concentration of 0.1 mg/ml.

7 Apply the dialysate to a CM–cellulose column. This column should be prepared as for DEAE–cellulose (see Section 1.3) but should be pre-equilibrated with 0.01 M sodium acetate buffer, pH 5.5.

8 Allow 200 ml 0.01 M sodium acetate buffer, pH 5.5, to run through the column.

9 Apply a linear gradient of increasing ionic strength (starting buffer 0.01 M sodium acetate, pH 5.5; limit buffer 0.9 M sodium acetate, pH 5.5).

10 Collect and concentrate each peak. The first two peaks contain Fab, while the third smaller peak contains the Fc.

11 Dialyse against PBS. Crystals of the Fc fragment may form at this stage.

Note: It is possible to obtain pure fragments by a two-stage ion-exchange separation; the fractionation of the products of digestion is more complex. The first is on CM–cellulose followed by refractionation on DEAE–cellulose (see Section 1.3 and Fig. 1.9).

Human IgG

Human IgG subclasses differ in their sensitivity to papain, in the order: $IgG_3 > IgG_1 > IgG_4 > IgG_2$. Any one set of conditions will have a tendency to overdigest some subclasses while underdigesting

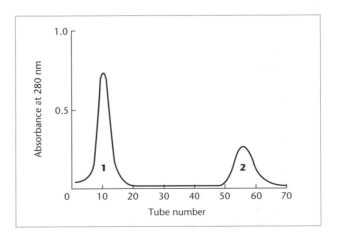

Fig. 1.9 Elution profile of papain digest of mouse IgG from DEAE–cellulose. After digestion with papain the sample was equilibrated in 0.005 M phosphate buffer, pH 8.0, and applied to a DEAE–cellulose column equilibrated in the same buffer. The column was eluted with a linear gradient, limit buffer 0.2 M phosphate, pH 8.0 (see also Fig. 1.10.)

others. Excessive digestion results in the further fragmentation of the Fc portion. The same digestion conditions may be used here as described for rabbit IgG. Although it is possible to obtain pure fragments by a two-stage ion-exchange separation, the fractionation of the products of digestion is more complex, i.e. the first on CM–cellulose followed by refractionation on DEAE–cellulose. It is easier to take advantage of the ability of staphylococcal protein A to bind to IgG Fc regions. Protein A has no affinity for the Fab region. As IgG_3 does not bind to protein A, the IgG preparation should be selected for protein A-binding species before digestion. Some of the IgG invariably remains undegraded after digestion so it is necessary to remove this on a gel filtration column before use of the protein A column.

MATERIALS AND EQUIPMENT
Supadex-75
Chromatography column and fraction collection apparatus
Polyethylene glycol 8000 (PEG-8000)
Protein A–Sepharose CL-4B
Phosphate-buffered saline (PBS)
1.0 M sodium hydroxide
0.1 M glycine–HCl buffer, pH 2.8
Dialysed digest (human IgG papain digest prepared as for rabbit IgG, steps 1–6, previous page)

METHOD

 1 Prepare a Supadex-75 column and equilibrate with PBS (see Appendix B.1).
 2 Pass the dialysed digest through the column and collect fractions.
 3 Any undigested IgG will come through in the breakthrough volume. The Fab and Fc will come later in one peak.
 4 Concentrate the Fab/Fc peak to the pregel filtration volume, e.g. by placing in a dialysis bag and covering with PEG-8000.
 5 Prepare a protein A–Sepharose CL-4B column (see Section 1.4.2).
 6 Apply the Fab/Fc peak to this column and wash through with PBS. The capacity of the column for binding Fc is 8 mg/ml of swollen gel.
 7 Collect the Fab which comes straight through the column.
 8 Elute the bound Fc with glycine–HCl buffer, pH 2.8.
 9 Titrate the pH of the purified Fc to near neutrality with NaOH and then dialyse against PBS.
 10 Regenerate the column by running through 2 column volumes of PBS. Store the column at 4°C.

Examination of fragments

The fragments can be analysed by either:
(a) SDS-PAGE (both under reducing and non-reducing conditions) (see Appendix B.2.1) to determine the molecular weights of the fragments. Then blot the fragments onto nitrocellulose and confirm their immunological identities with specific antisera (see Section 4.11); or alternatively:
(b) immunoelectrophoresis which is a simple technique for examining fragments (see Section 3.7.2; see Fig. 1.10 illustrating mouse fragments), although this will have less sensitivity for detecting contaminants.

Fig. 1.10 Immunoelectrophoresis of fractions from DEAE–cellulose chromatography of papain digest of mouse IgG (from Fig. 1.9). Sample a: peak 1, DEAE–cellulose, Fab fragments. Sample b: original IgG. Sample c: peak 2, DEAE–cellulose, Fc fragments. The proteins were visualized by precipitation with rabbit anti-mouse whole IgG. (Photograph of unstained preparation.)

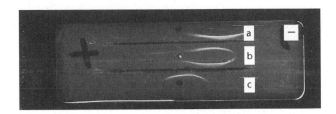

1.7.2 Pepsin digestion

Digestion of IgG yields a fragment with two-thirds the molecular weight of the original molecule but with intact, divalent antigen-binding activity. This is the $F(ab')_2$ fragment. The other one-third of the IgG molecule is digested into a smaller pFc′ fragment corresponding to the C_H3 domains held together non-covalently, while the C_H2 domains are digested away to small peptides.

MATERIALS AND EQUIPMENT

IgG (rabbit or human)

Pepsin

0.1 M sodium acetate

Phosphate-buffered saline (PBS)

Acetic acid, glacial

Sephacryl S-200 column equilibrated with PBS

METHOD

1 Adjust the IgG solution to 20 mg/ml and dialyse 10 ml against 0.1 M sodium acetate for 3 h.
2 Adjust the dialysate to pH 4.5 with acetic acid.
3 Add 2 mg pepsin for each 100 mg of IgG used.
4 Incubate at 37°C overnight.
5 Adjust the supernatant to pH 7.4. This inactivates the enzyme.
6 Centrifuge at 1000 g for 15 min and discard any precipitate that may form.

Analysis and isolation of fragments

Apply the digest to a gel filtration column, e.g. Sephacryl S-200, and equilibrate the column with PBS, monitor the eluate and collect fractions. Generally this will give fragments of sufficient purity but recycling on a column will get rid of any remaining contamination (see Fig. 1.11).

Peak 1 contains some undigested IgG; the amount will vary from preparation to preparation and may only show as a slight bulge on the leading edge of the second peak.

Peak 2 contains the $F(ab')_2$.

Peak 4 contains pFc′, the small C_H3 fragment, while the remaining material is composed of small peptides.

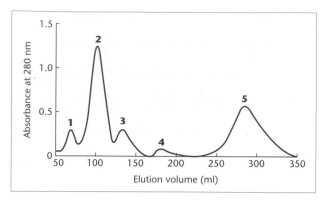

Fig. 1.11 Elution profile of a pepsin digest of IgG on gel filtration. A 2 ml sample of digest (20 mg/ml) was applied to gel filtration column (bed volume 90 × 2.5 cm) and equilibrated with phosphate-buffered saline.

1.8 Enzymic digestion of IgA and IgM

Enzymic fragmentation of IgA and IgM is possible but is not nearly so well established. Pepsin digestion is effective but needs to be monitored continually. Short digestion times can yield small amounts of F(ab')$_2$ from IgM but longer digestion proceeds to a Fab-like fragment.

IgA is a suitable substrate for pepsin digestion but, from work with myeloma proteins, there appears to be considerable variation in sensitivity between different IgA preparations.

1.9 Further reading

Affinity Chromatography—Principles and Methods. Available from Amersham Biotech Limited. Pharmacia; Amersham.

Aybay, C. & Imir, T. (2000) Development of a rapid, single-step procedure using protein G affinity chromatography to deplete fetal calf serum of its IgG and to isolate murine IgG$_1$ monoclonal ntibodies from supernatants of hybridoma cells. *J Immunol Meth* **233**, 77–81.

Bailon, P., Ehrlich, G.K., Fung, W.-J. & Wolfgang Berthold, B. (eds) (2000) *Affinity Chromatography: Methods and Protocols*. Humana Press, New Jersey.

Boden, V., Winzerling, J.J., Vijayalakshmi, M. & Porath, J. (1995) Rapid one-step purification of goat immunoglobulins by immobilized metal ion affinity chromatography. *J Immunol Meth* **181**(2), 225–32.

Bond, A., Jones, M.G. & Hay, F.C. (1993) Human IgG preparations isolated by ion-exchange chromatography differ in their glycosylation profiles. *J Immunol Meth* **166**, 27–33.

Bottomley, S.P., Sutton, B.J. & Gore, M.G. (1995) Elution of human IgG from affinity columns containing immobilized variants of protein A. *J Immunol Meth* **182**(2), 185–92.

Caponi, L. & Migliorini, P. (ed.) (1999) *Antibody Usage in the Lab* (Springer Lab Manual). Springer Verlag, New York.

Dainiak, M.B., Muronetz, V.I., Izumrudov, V.A., Galaev, I.Y. & Mattiasson, B. (2000) Production of Fab fragments of monoclonal antibodies using polyelectrolyte complexes. *Anal Biochem* **277**(1), 58–66.

De Chateau, M., Nilson, B.H., Emtell, M. *et al.* (1993) On the interaction between Protein L and immunoglobulins of various mammalian species. *Scand J Immunol* **37**, 399–305.

Deutscher, M.P., Simon, M.I. & Abelson, J.N. (eds) (1997) *Guide to Protein Purification: Methods in Enzymology,* Vol. 182. Academic Press, London.

Fassina, G. (2000) Protein A mimetic (PAM) affinity chromatography. Immunoglobulins purification. *Methods Mol Biol* **147**, 57–68.

Hames, B.D. & Glover, D.M. (1996) *Molecular Immunology: Frontiers in Molecular Biology*. Oxford University Press, Oxford.

Hames, B.D. (1998) *Gel Electrophoresis of Proteins: A Practical Approach*, 3rd edn. Oxford University Press, Oxford.

Herzenberg, L.A., Weir, D.M. & Blackwell, C. (1997) *Weir's Handbook of Experimental Immunology*, 5th edn. Blackwell Science Ltd, Oxford.

Howard, G.C., Bethell, D.R. & Vilsaint, F. (eds) (2000) *Basic Methods in Antibody Production and Characterization*. Cambridge University Press, Cambridge.

Jensen-Jarolim, E., Vogel, M., de Week, A.L. & Stadler, B.M. (1992) Anti-IgE autoantibodies mistaken for specific IgG. *J Allergy Clin Immunol* **89**(1), 31–43.

Kastner, M. (ed.) (1999) *Protein Liquid Chromatography* (Journal of Chromatography Library, 61) Elsevier Science Ltd, Kidlington.

Kleine-Tebbe, J., Hamilton, R.G., Roebber, M., Lichtenstein, L.M. & MacDonald, S.M. (1995) Purification of immunoglobulin E (IgE) antibodies from sera with high IgE titres. *J Immunol Meth* **179**(2), 153–64.

Lechner, M.D. (1994) *Ultracentrifugation*. Steinkopf Verlag, Darmstadt.

Lefkovits, I. (1997) *Immunological Methods Manual: A Comprehensive Source of Techniques*. Academic Press, London.

Llames, L., Goyache, J., Domenech, A., de Avila, A., Suarez, G. & Gomez-Lucia, E. (1999) Rapid detection of specific polyclonal and monoclonal antibodies against bovine leukaemia virus. *J Virol Meth* **82**(2), 129–36.

Loomes, L.M., Stewart, W.W., Mazengera, R.L., Senior, B.W. & Kerr, M.A. (1991) Purification of IgA$_1$ and IgA$_2$ isotypes from serum. *J Immunol Meth* **141**, 209–218.

Neoh, S.H., Gordon, C., Potter, A. & Zola, H. (1986) The purification of mouse monoclonal antibodies from ascitic fluid. *J Immunol Meth* **91**, 231–5.

Nevens, J.R., Mallia, A.K., Wendt, M.W. & Smith, P.K. (1992) Affinity chromatographic purification of immunoglobulin M antibodies utilizing immobilized mannan binding protein. *J Chrom* **597**, 247–256.

Parr, E.L., Bozzola, J.J. & Parr, M.B. (1995) Purification and measurement of secretory IgA in mouse milk. *J Immunol Meth* **180**(2), 147–57.

Rosenberg, I.M. (1996) *Protein Analysis and Purification: Benchtop Techniques*. Springer Verlag, New York.

Scholz, G.H., Vieweg, S., Leistner, S., Seissler, J., Scherbaum, W.A. & Huse, K. (1998) A simplified procedure for the isolation of immunoglobulins from human serum using a novel type of thiophilic gel at low salt concentration. *J Immunol Meth* **219**(1–2), 109–18.

Scopes, R.K. (1994) *Protein Purification: Principles and Practice*, 3rd edn. Springer-Verlag, Berlin.

Staak, C., Salchow, F., Clausen, P.H. & Luge, E. (1996) Polystyrene as an affinity chromatography matrix for the purification of antibodies. *J Immunol Meth* **194**(2), 141–6.

Stanworth, D.R. & Turner, M.W. (1997) Immunochemical analysis of human and rabbit immunoglobulins and their subunits. In: *Weir's Handbook of Experimental Immunology* (eds D.M. Weir, L.A. Herzenberg & C. Blackwell), 5th edn. Blackwell Science Ltd, Oxford.

Tatum, A.H. (1993) Large scale recovery of biologically active IgM (95% pure) from human plasma obtained by therapeutic plasmapheresis. *J Immunol Meth* **158**, 1–4.

Teng, S.F., Sproule, K., Husain, A. & Lowe, C.R. (2000) Affinity chromatography on immobilized 'biomimetic' ligands. Synthesis, immobilization and chromatographic assessment of an immunoglobulin G-binding ligand. *J Chromatogr B Biomed Sci Appl* **740**(1), 1–15.

Yan, Z. & Huang, J. (2000) Cleaning procedure for protein G affinity columns. *J Immunol Meth* **237**(1–2), 203–5.

2 Monoclonal antibodies: production, purification and enzymatic fragmentation

2.1 What is the difference between monoclonal and polyclonal antisera?

Monoclonal antibodies have the obvious advantages of single specificity, and have been produced out of a need for homogeneous antibodies as reproducible reagents, i.e. standardizable reagents.

Polyclonal antibodies are a minor component in a complex mixture of serum proteins and are a heterogeneous mixture of molecules with a wide range of binding affinities. Therefore such antisera lack the degree of definition required for many of the current molecular techniques, where an increase in assay sensitivity is often counteracted by a decrease in serological specificity.

Nonetheless, the fact that polyclonal antibodies can bind a particular antigen from so many different perspectives is of great technical advantage and they are therefore excellent for: (a) routine affinity purification of the native antigen; and (b) relating an expressed partial gene sequence to the mature gene product. However, they have the disadvantage that non-specific or cross-reactive binding reactions can be a serious problem when antisera are used to identify or quantify antigens, e.g. the study of differentiation or tumour antigens, or in the clinical laboratory for immunodiagnosis of disease. This is because of other components in an antiserum.

Standardization may be achieved through careful controls or cross-absorption so that an antiserum is 'monospecific'; such standardization is usually limited to one test system and, indeed, often only to one laboratory.

Monoclonal antisera are produced by:

1   the rescue and propagation of hybrid cell tumours representing clones of single plasma cells;

2 fusion of plasmacytoma cells with normal plasma cells to produce hybrid cells (later called hybridomas) that secrete both myeloma and antibody immunoglobulin and are grown as a transplantable tumour (Köhler & Milstein 1975); and

3 screening for antigen-specific culture supernatants and cloning of secreting cells to isolate potentially immortal cell lines synthesizing homogeneous antibody of exquisite specificity.

2.2 Outline of B-hybridoma production

Spleen cells, prepared from immunized mice or rats, are induced to fuse with murine plasmacytoma cells using polyethylene glycol.

Many cells show cytoplasmic fusion; a lower proportion complete the nuclear fusion required to produce tetraploid hybrids (or a greater ploidy, depending upon the number of fusing cells). This procedure results in a heterogeneous mixture of fused and unfused cells, although there is a preferential association of ontogenetically similar cells: plasmacytoma cells tend to 'rescue' large, recently activated B lymphocytes.

After dispensing into culture wells, the cell mixture is cultured in a selective medium that positively selects for fusion hybrids. Culture supernatants are tested for antibody activity after 1–3 weeks. Positive cultures are cloned by conventional cell cloning techniques.

2.2.1 Basis of fusion and selection

To understand the choice of cells and manipulation of the system, consider the contribution of each component of the hybrid cell:

1 The plasmablast parent is terminally differentiated and dies in culture but provides the genetic information for the required antibody.

2 The plasmacytoma parent confers potential immortality on the hybrid cell, but will itself grow in culture.

Once plasma cells from an appropriately immunized animal have been fused with tumour cells *in vitro* it is necessary to eliminate unfused tumour cells (or tumour–tumour hybrids), then select the hybrid cells secreting antibody of the required specificity.

2.2.2 Elimination of plasmacytoma cells

This is done by the use of a plasmacytoma cell line deficient in the enzyme responsible for incorporation of hypoxanthine into DNA.

Briefly, cells can synthesize DNA in two ways, either by *de novo* synthesis or via the so-called 'salvage' pathway using exogenous or endogenous sources of preformed bases, as summarized in Fig. 2.1(a). If plasmacytoma cells are grown in the presence of a purine analogue, for example 8-azaguanine or 6-thioguanine, the hypoxanthine guanine phosphoribosyltransferase (HGPRT) enzyme catalyses the incorporation of the purine analogue into DNA where it interferes with normal protein synthesis and so the cells die. Gene coding for the HGPRT enzyme is on the X chromosome, so only a single copy per cell is expressed. Cells will arise that are deficient in the HGPRT gene and therefore do not incorporate the purine analogue, i.e. HGPRT-deficient cells

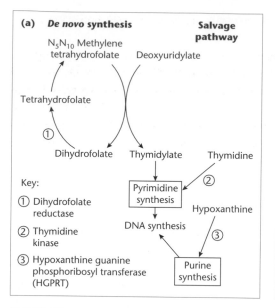

(a) *De novo* synthesis   **Salvage pathway**

N_5N_{10} Methylene tetrahydrofolate   Deoxyuridylate

Tetrahydrofolate

①   Dihydrofolate   Thymidylate   Thymidine

②

Key: Pyrimidine synthesis

① Dihydrofolate reductase   Hypoxanthine

② Thymidine kinase   DNA synthesis   ③

③ Hypoxanthine guanine phosphoribosyl transferase (HGPRT)   Purine synthesis

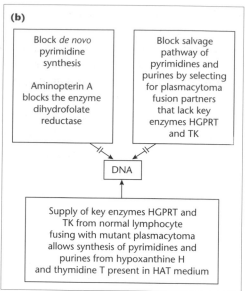

(b)

Block *de novo* pyrimidine synthesis

Aminopterin A blocks the enzyme dihydrofolate reductase

Block salvage pathway of pyrimidines and purines by selecting for plasmacytoma fusion partners that lack key enzymes HGPRT and TK

DNA

Supply of key enzymes HGPRT and TK from normal lymphocyte fusing with mutant plasmacytoma allows synthesis of pyrimidines and purines from hypoxanthine H and thymidine T present in HAT medium

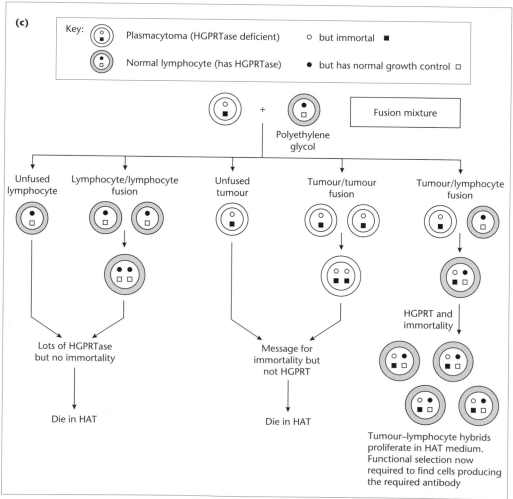

(c)

Key:

Plasmacytoma (HGPRTase deficient) ○   but immortal ■

Normal lymphocyte (has HGPRTase) ●   but has normal growth control □

\+   Polyethylene glycol   Fusion mixture

Unfused lymphocyte   Lymphocyte/lymphocyte fusion   Unfused tumour   Tumour/tumour fusion   Tumour/lymphocyte fusion

Lots of HGPRTase but no immortality

Message for immortality but not HGPRT

HGPRT and immortality

Die in HAT

Die in HAT

Tumour–lymphocyte hybrids proliferate in HAT medium. Functional selection now required to find cells producing the required antibody which are unable to utilize hypoxanthine and therefore can only synthesize ribonucleotides by *de novo* synthesis (Fig. 2.1b).

A selective medium containing aminopterin (or amethopterin, methotrexate), hypoxanthine and thymidine (HAT medium) is used. Aminopterin (analogue of folic acid) binds folic acid reductase and blocks the coenzymes required for *de novo* synthesis of DNA. To grow in this medium a cell must make DNA via the 'salvage' pathway. If HGPRT-deficient plasmacytoma cells are fused with normal lymphoid cells and then placed in HAT medium, only the hybrids between plasmacytoma and normal cells will grow (plasmacytoma cell provides immortality; plasma cell provides the HGPRT enzyme—Fig. 2.1c).

2.2.3 Origin of plasmacytoma lines for fusion

The majority of fusion experiments have been performed using sublines of P3/X63-Ag8 which is an 8-azaguanine-resistant subline of the plasmacytoma MOPC 21 (induced in a BALB/c mouse by the injection of mineral oil). Moreover, it tends to fuse spontaneously (with itself) and can grow at very low cell densities, thus facilitating the recovery of fusion hybrids. It also has the disadvantage that it synthesizes and secretes the MOPC 21 myeloma protein (a fully sequenced IgG_1, κ) and so hybrid cells will secrete myeloma and antibody molecules, as well as inactive hybrid molecules.

Spontaneous variants of P3/X63-Ag8 have been selected that neither synthesize nor secrete immunoglobulin molecules, but retain the ability to rescue normal antibody-producing cells. These are listed below; all are resistant to 8-azaguanine.

1   *NS1-Ag4-1* synthesizes, but does not secrete, κ light chain. Hybrids can still secrete a mixed molecule of antibody heavy chains with myeloma light chains.
2   *P3/X63-Ag8-6.5.3* does not synthesize or secrete immunoglobulin chains.
3   *SP2/0-Ag14* is a non-synthesizing and non-secreting variant of a hybrid cell formed by the fusion of a lymphoid cell (secreting antisheep erythrocyte antibody) with P3/X63-Ag8.

We would recommend that you use one of the non-synthesizing, non-secreting variants for any fusion work; these may be acquired from commercial suppliers or a friendly research laboratory doing routine fusions. It should be noted that cells from commercial suppliers are generally cloned and passaged through 6-thioguanine to maintain their HAT sensitivity.

Fig. 2.1 (*opposite*) **DNA synthesis and the selection of HAT-sensitive mutants. (a)** Most cells can make DNA either by *de novo* synthesis or via the so-called 'salvage' pathway, using an endogenous or exogenous source of preformed bases. **(b)** In order to select cells which are solely the result of fusion with a normal antibody-forming cell with a myeloma cell, *de novo* DNA synthesis is partially stopped with aminopterin A. This reagent blocks the enzyme dihydrofolate reductase, while the salvage pathway is blocked by preselecting for the myeloma cells that can survive in the presence of the lethal purine analogues, 8-aza- or 6-thioguanine. These cells lack the key salvage pathway enzymes HGPRT and TK. These enzymes are then supplied by the normal antibody-forming partner cell. **(c)** The tumour 'parent' used in the hybridoma technique (× 63) is HGPRT deficient and so is unable to grow in HAT medium; HAT contains either the folic acid analogue aminopterin or the amination inhibitor, azaserine, which block *de novo* synthesis; as these cells cannot use hypoxanthine they die. Hybrid cells grow out from HAT medium because DNA from the normal partner provides the information to synthesize HGPRT and the tumour cell DNA provides the 'message' for unrestricted proliferation.

2.3 Maintenance of plasmacytoma cells for fusion

Efficiency of fusion and recovery of hybrids is greatest when the plasmacytoma 'parent' cells are uniformly viable and growing exponentially. Incubation times and cell densities given below are a guide, but it is necessary to determine the growth characteristics of each plasmacytoma line.

2.3.1 Plasmacytoma cells for fusion

MATERIALS AND EQUIPMENT

Plasmacytoma line e.g. SP2 (if necessary, recover from frozen state)

Tissue culture medium RPMI 1640 (500 ml) supplemented with 5 ml 200 mM L-glutamine, 5000 units penicillin, 5 mg streptomycin, 10 ml 6.6 mM 8-azaguanine and 10–20% (v/v) fetal bovine serum (FBS)

Plastic culture flasks (75 cm^2), 10 ml culture volume

Incubator, humidified and gassed with 5% CO_2 in air

METHOD

1 Add 10^5 plasmacytoma cells to 10 ml of tissue culture medium and place in a humid incubator gassed with 5% CO_2 in air.
2 Each day, resuspend the cells and determine the number per ml using a haemocytometer.
3 Plot a growth curve of cell number versus time (see Fig. B2 in Appendix B).
4 As soon as the growth rate starts to decline, dilute the cells by transferring 0.2–1.0 ml aliquots of the resuspended culture to flasks containing 10 ml of fresh medium.
5 When the cells have again reached their exponential growth phase, select viable cultures for storage under liquid nitrogen.

TECHNICAL NOTES

- To remove the dimethyl sulphoxide (DMSO), thaw cell rapidly under running warm water, wash and resuspend in tissue culture medium.
- These cell lines will reach a maximum density of approximately 10^6 cells/ml. Exponential growth should be maintained by diluting the culture 1 : 10 with fresh medium every 3–5 days. Under these conditions the cells will have a doubling time of 16–20 h.
- The plasmacytoma cells grow either in suspension or lightly adherent. Release the adherent cells by gently tapping the culture flask or by gentle pipetting.
- Check by phase-contrast microscopy that the cells are 'healthy'. They should be phase-bright and of regular shape with clear outlines. Even in cloned lines size variation is common. Cell viability should be between 90 and 95%.
- As with all cell lines in long-term culture care must be taken to avoid cross-contamination between cultures.
- The rate of reversion to HAT resistance varies with cell lines and is a relatively rare event. Eliminate revertants by culturing the cells in medium containing 8-azaguanine or 6-thioguanine (2×10^{-5} M) every 3–6 months. Alternatively, import a 'seed' culture from a commercial

supplier, grow up into a large batch in the minimum number of subpasses and freeze for cryopreservation.

- As with all long-term maintenance of cell lines *in vitro* it is advisable to check periodically for *Mycoplasma* infection. Commercial kits are available for the demonstration of *Mycoplasma* DNA using a fluorescent dye. A rapid, but non specific, indication of potential *Mycoplasma* contamination may be obtained by culturing supernatant, obtained by centrifugation (150 g for 15 min) of a 5-ml sample of the suspected culture, with 3.7×10^3 Bq ^{3}H-thymidine overnight at 37°C. Incorporation of label into trichloroacetic acid (TCA)-precipitable material indicates contamination. More sensitive tests use DNA probes and can be performed within hours. Removing *Mycoplasma* infection is generally not worth the considerable effort involved, but antibiotics such as erythromycin and ciprofloxacin can help.

2.3.2 Preparation of cell for storage

MATERIALS AND EQUIPMENT
Viable cells in growth phase
Freezing medium (90% (v/v) fetal bovine serum (FBS) and 10% (v/v) dimethyl sulphoxide (DMSO))
Vials for freezing
Ice

METHOD

Steps **1–3** are performed at 4°C (step 1) or on ice (steps **2** and **3**).

1 Collect 10^7 cells and centrifuge at 1000 g for 15 min at 4°C to remove the excess supernatant containing the monoclonal antibody, but leave a residue of medium.
2 Resuspend the cells in the freeze-down medium by gently flicking of the centrifuge tube.
3 Load into the vial for freezing and ensure thorough mixing of the cells with the medium.
4 Slowly freeze the vial as follows:
   vial at –20°C for 2–4 h;
   vial at –70°C overnight;
   transfer into a Dewar flask containing liquid nitrogen.

TECHNICAL NOTES
- Hybridoma cells can be unstable; therefore, to ensure adequate storage, store in more than one aliquot and in different banks.
- Freeze the vials in a polystyrene box to allow the cells to freeze slowly.

2.4 Target cells for fusion

Most of the plasmacytoma cells used as fusion 'parents' have a BALB/c haplotype, but will fuse efficiently and productively with mouse or rat cells without regard to histocompatibility barriers. If you intend to propagate the hybridoma cells *in vivo*, it is technically simpler to use immunized BALB/c mice as spleen-cell donors. Although murine plasmacytoma lines can fuse to almost any species, e.g. human, frog or carrot, stable hybrid lines are only rarely obtained in other than rodent–rodent fusions (see Technical notes below).

Immunization protocols should be determined empirically, for they will vary depending on (a) the type of antigen used and (b) the 'folklore' of the laboratory where the experiments are being performed.

Plasmacytoma cells seem to fuse preferentially with recently activated B lymphoblasts, rather than plasma cells, so the immunization scheme giving the highest serum antibody titres might not necessarily give the highest rate of positive hybrids.

Note: Few problems have been encountered with immunization against cell or particulate antigens; almost any immunization scheme will give a 10–20% recovery of positive hybrids.

There follows an outline of a suggested protocol for soluble antigens, e.g. human IgG or γ-globulin:

- 100 µg i.p. human IgG in Freund's complete adjuvant (or substitute, such as Optivant) 7 days before fusion (see Section 11.1);
- i.v. boost with 100 µg soluble IgG 4 days before fusion. Most investigators tend to fuse 2–4 days after a final intravenous injection of antigen with the rationale that this should localize recently activated B lymphocytes in the spleen;
- The ultimate splenic localization protocol is the so-called 'intrasplenic immunization':
  (i) the spleen of an anaesthetized mouse is injected with soluble antigen via a fine 23 gauge needle;
  (ii) the wound is closed with two discontinuous sutures or Michel clips, and the spleen used for fusion 3–5 days later.

IMPORTANT: *This technique must be learnt from an experienced laboratory worker.*

This procedure is similar to the classical intra lymph-node injections performed to spare precious antigen and boost the immune response.

Some antigens of interest may be toxic to whole animals and *in vitro* immunization may be successfully used to get over this difficulty. With pressures to reduce the use of animals this can be a preferred option (Bonwick *et al.* 1996).

2.5 **Fusion protocol**

Preparations in advance

MATERIALS AND EQUIPMENT
Plasmacytoma cells in culture
Tissue culture medium
Serum
Tissue culture flasks
Polyethylene glycol 1500 (PEG-1500)
Phosphate-buffered saline (PBS)
Animals and cells

1. Immunize mice against required antigen (see Section 11.2).
2. Prepare plasmacytoma cell cultures for fusion by centrifugation (150 g for 10 min at room temperature) followed by reculture in an equal volume of tissue culture medium plus serum supplement. (Set up a sufficient culture volume to yield 10^7 cells for each spleen to be fused.) For efficient fusion, the plasmacytoma cells should be uniformly viable and in the exponential phase of growth. To ensure that this is so we routinely replace the culture medium, at the same cell density, the day before the cells are used for fusion.

PREPARATION OF POLYETHYLENE GLYCOL SOLUTION

1. Add 50 g PEG to warm PBS (in a 37°C water bath) and adjust to 100 ml.
2. Dispense 5 ml aliquots into 10 ml glass bottles and autoclave at 120°C for 15 min.
3. Store at 4°C for use.

Techniques

MATERIALS AND EQUIPMENT

Mice (immunized as above)

Plasmacytoma cells in culture (as above)

Tissue culture medium and serum

L-glutamine (200 mM initial concentration)

Polyethylene glycol 1500 (PEG-1500), 50% w/v in phosphate–saline buffer (as above)

Ethanol, 70% v/v in distilled water

Water bath at 37°C

Culture plate, 96 microwells (flat bottomed)

Conical polypropylene test tubes, 50 ml, sterile

Conical polypropylene test tubes, 15 ml, sterile

Petri dishes, 5 cm, sterile

Pasteur pipettes, sterile

Scissors, two pairs, sterile

Forceps, fine, sterile

Forceps, blunt, two pairs, sterile

Time clock

Prepare two types of tissue culture medium as follows:

(a) 100 ml medium: add 10 ml fetal calf serum (FCS) and 1.0 ml L-glutamine, i.e. serum-supplemented

(b) 200 ml medium: add 2.0 ml L-glutamine, i.e. serum-free

2.5.1 Preparation of spleen cells

Traditional method

1. Kill mouse by cervical dislocation and swab its left side with ethanol.
2. Open skin to expose peritoneum, discard scissors and forceps.
3. Use fresh forceps and scissors to open the peritoneum and remove the spleen, transfer to a Petri dish containing serum-free tissue culture medium.

4   Prepare a suspension of spleen cells free of clumps (see Section 6.3).

5   Wash spleen cells three times by centrifugation (250 g for 10 min at 4°C) and resuspend in 5 ml of serum-free tissue culture medium.

6   Determine the number of viable lymphoid cells/ml (see Section 11.8).

Alternative method for perfusing hyperimmunized spleen

Using an aseptic technique and sterilized equipment and solutions.

MATERIALS AND EQUIPMENT

Spleen

10-ml hypodermic syringes

Petri dishes

Needles 25 gauge, 21 gauge

Tissue culture medium RPMI 1640 (500 ml) supplemented with 5 ml 200 mM L-glutamine, 5000 units penicillin, 5 mg streptomycin

Tissue culture medium RPMI 1640 (500 ml) supplemented with 5 ml of 200 mM L-glutamine, 5000 units penicillin, 5 mg streptomycin and 20% (v/v) fetal calf serum (FCS)

50 ml Falcon or Universal tubes (sterile)

0.8% (w/v) polyethylene glycol 8000 (PEG-8000)

METHOD

1   Place a few drops of RPMI 1640 medium containing streptomycin only in a sterile Petri dish.

2   Fill three 10-ml syringes with medium and attach a 25-gauge needle and maintain at room temperature.

3   Fill a 20-ml syringe with 20 ml medium and attach a 21-gauge needle and maintain at room temperature.

4   Fill a 20-ml syringe with 21 ml medium and attach a 21-gauge needle and maintain at 37°C.

5   Place 24 ml RPMI 1640 containing streptomycin and 20% v/v FCS in a sterile 50-ml tube and maintain at 37°C.

6   Fill a 1-ml syringe with 0.8 ml PEG (40%) and attach a 25-gauge needle and maintain at 37°C.

7   Aseptically remove spleen: place the cervically dislocated mouse in a supine position, dab fur on right hand side with methanol and cut skin with sterile scissors and forceps (tear open to allow easy removal of spleen). With a second set of sterile instruments, cut open the peritoneal membrane, remove spleen and place in the sterile Petri dish. Remove any adhering fat.

8   Perforate the spleen with multiple holes using the 25-gauge needle attached to the 10-ml syringe(s) and perfuse gently with medium from the syringes (30 ml is usually sufficient). The cell suspension will collect in the Petri dish and can be collected using a sterile plastic pipette. Ultimately, the spleen will become translucent as perfusion continues.

9   Collect cells in a sterile Universal.

10 Perform a viability count on an aliquot of cells using 0.4% w/v trypan blue (see Sections 11.8–11.10).

2.5.2 Preparation of plasmacytoma cells

METHOD

1 Resuspend the cells and pool the suspensions into a 50-ml conical tube.
2 Wash the cells three times by centrifugation (250 g for 15 min at room temperature) in serum-free tissue culture medium.
3 Resuspend the final pellet in serum-free tissue culture medium, count the number of viable cells and adjust to 1×10^6 cells/ml.

2.5.3 Fusion protocol

METHOD

1 Mix 10^8 spleen cells with 10^7 plasmacytoma cells in a 50-ml conical tube and centrifuge at 500 g for 7 min at room temperature.
2 Decant the supernatant carefully, finally inverting the tube to drain completely.
3 Mix cell pellet by gently tapping the tube and allow to equilibrate to 37°C in a water bath. Similarly allow PEG solution and tissue culture medium with 10% serum to equilibrate to 37°C.
4 Add 0.8 ml of PEG to resuspended cells, mix gently and incubate at 37°C for 1 min.
5 Add 1.0 ml of serum-free medium over 1 min with gentle shaking.
6 Add 20 ml of serum-free medium over 5 min. Dilution must be done very slowly as the cells are very sensitive to mechanical damage when in the PEG solution.
7 Centrifuge at 200 g for 10 min at room temperature.
8 Remove supernatant and resuspend the cell pellet in 10 ml of tissue culture medium containing 10% serum.
9 Dispense 50 μl aliquots of cell suspension into each well of a 96-well culture plate.
10 Dilute the remaining cell suspension with 2 volumes of medium containing 10% serum and dispense 50 μl aliquots into each well of a second 96-well culture plate.
11 Dilute the remaining cell suspension with 2 volumes of medium containing 10% serum and dispense 50 μl aliquots into each well of a third 96-well culture plate.
12 Place all the plates in a humid 37°C incubator gassed with 5% CO_2 in air.
  The plates are now incubated for 24 h before the addition of the HAT selective medium.

TECHNICAL NOTES

• Although murine plasmacytoma cells have been fused with avian, amphibian and human lymphocytes in a similar manner, they rarely produce stable, antibody-secreting hybrids because of a rapid loss of chromosomes. Indeed, in mouse–human hybrids, the elimination of human, but not mouse, chromosomes occurs so frequently that this is one of the techniques used for mapping the human genome.
• The method of plating out the fusion mixture may be varied depending on the frequency of hybrid formation, the frequency of hybrids secreting the desired type of antibody and the method of detecting antibodies. If the frequency of hybrids is low, as with soluble proteins for example, then 2 ml cultures can be dispensed into 24-well culture plates. We have found that

dilution plating as described above limits the number of independent clones that grow out and so reduces the chance of a positive clone (secreting the desired antibody) being lost by 'overgrowth' of non-secreting hybrids.

2.5.4 Preparation of stock solution of HAT medium

This is the method for preparing HAT medium from individual reagents; alternatively, HAT medium is now available commercially, e.g. from Sigma, UK.

MATERIALS
Hypoxanthine (6-hydroxypurine) (molecular weight 136.1) 10×10^{-2} M
Thymidine (molecular weight 242.2) 1.6×10^{-3} M
Aminopterin (4-amino-folic acid; 4-aminopteroyl glutamic acid) (molecular weight 440.4)
    4.0×10^{-5} M
Sodium hydroxide (NaOH) 1 M
Hydrochloric acid (HCl) 1 M

Note: Aminopterin is highly toxic and a potent carcinogen, therefore wear gloves.

METHOD

A 100-fold concentrated stock solution of hypoxanthine and thymidine
1 Dissolve 136.1 mg hypoxanthine and 38.8 mg thymidine in 100 ml twice-distilled water at 50°C.
2 Sterilize by membrane filtration and store in 2–5 ml aliquots at –20°C.
   The hypoxanthine may precipitate out of solution during storage. Redissolve by heating in a boiling water bath.

B 100-fold concentrated solution of aminopterin
1 Add 1.76 mg aminopterin to 90 ml of twice-distilled water.
2 Add 1 M NaOH dropwise until the aminopterin dissolves and then titrate to pH 7.5 with 1 M HCl.
3 Adjust final volume to 100 ml with twice-distilled water.
4 Sterilize by membrane filtration, dispense into 2–5 ml aliquots and store at –20°C.

TECHNICAL NOTES
- Aminopterin must be protected from light.
- This stock can be frozen and thawed several times for use, provided sterility is maintained.
- The technique is so well established that reagents may be purchased ready-prepared, e.g. from Sigma.

2.5.5 Use of HAT medium

MATERIALS AND EQUIPMENT
Stock solution of hypoxanthine and thymidine (HT) as above.
Stock solution of aminopterin (A) as above

RPMI 1640 (500 ml) supplemented with 5 ml 200 mM L-glutamine, 5000 units penicillin, 5 mg
   streptomycin and 10–20% (v/v) fetal bovine serum (FBS)
Plates containing fused cells (see above)

METHOD

1   Add 2 ml of HT and 2 ml of A stock solutions to 100 ml of tissue culture medium containing
    10% serum.
2   Add 50 µl of HAT medium to each well containing fused cells.
3   Return plates to 37°C incubator.

TECHNICAL NOTES

- The HAT medium used above is double strength so that the final concentration in the cultures is
  as follows:
  hypoxanthine 1.0×10^{-4} M
  thymidine 1.6×10^{-5} M
  aminopterin 4.0×10^{-7} M
  This medium will appear to kill all the cells in the plate but do not despair: hybrids usually grow
  without any problem.
- You will need to feed each well with 25 µl of single strength medium only once per week. Prepare single strength medium by adding 1 ml of each of the HT and A stock solutions to 100 ml
  of tissue culture medium containing 10% serum.
- Vigorously growing hybrids are usually visible in the high cell density plates, i.e. those prepared
  from the undiluted suspension of fused cells, at 1–2 weeks after fusion (indicated by a change in
  the pH indicator dye). Examine all the plates under an inverted microscope and select the plate
  containing the cell dilution that shows growth every second to third well. Discard the plates that
  received the more concentrated cell suspensions; they will probably have several clones per
  well.
- After the 'selection phase' is complete, it is necessary to grow the hybrids onto normal tissue
  culture medium. However, do not transfer the hybrids directly from HAT to normal tissue
  culture medium as sufficient aminopterin may be carried over to prevent a resumption of
  de novo synthesis of DNA. Instead, grow the cells in HT and tissue culture medium for 3–5 days
  before transferring to tissue culture medium alone. Depending on the source of plasmacytoma
  cells and the frequency of fusion, hybrids may not show optimal growth when cultured alone.
  This problem may be overcome by plating onto feeder layers of macrophages. Macrophages
  are especially useful as they phagocytose the debris from the dying cells as well as providing the
  enhanced growth conditions for the hybridomas.

2.5.6 Preparation of macrophage feeder layers

MATERIALS AND EQUIPMENT
Mice
Tissue culture medium containing 10% serum
96-well microtitre culture plates (flat bottomed)
Incubator, humidified and gassed with 5% CO_2 in air

1   Prepare a suspension of peritoneal cells from untreated mice (see Section 6.1).

2   Wash the cells once in tissue culture medium by centrifugation (150 g for 10 min at room temperature).

3   If the cells are not histocompatible with the fusion hybrids, irradiate the peritoneal cells with 20 Gy.

4   Count and adjust the cells to 2×10^5/ml.

5   Dispense 100 µl aliquots into each well of a culture plate.

6   Incubate in a humid 37°C incubator gassed with 5% CO_2 in air.

   The feeder layers are optional and may be used for plating out of fusion mixtures after 24 h or up to 7 days (see below).

TECHNICAL NOTE

Each mouse should yield about 5×10^6 peritoneal cells of which about 50% will be lymphocytes.

2.5.7 Notes on screening of fusion wells for antibody activity

The initial screen for antibody activity should be carried out as soon as growth of hybrid cells is seen under the microscope or when the pH indicator dye has become yellow. Although cells are diluted to limit the number of independent hybrid cells per well, several hybrids may grow, perhaps at different rates, each producing their own clone of cells. This might affect the screening assay in two ways:

(i) A positive clone (secreting the desired antibody) may be detected soon after fusion, but then might be lost by overgrowth of a negative or other positive clones.

(ii) No activity may be detected during the first assay due to the cells of a positive clone being in a minority.

It is therefore essential to test negative supernatants from actively growing cultures on two or three occasions.

   Once antibody activity has been detected in any particular well, it is essential to clone and retest the cells as soon as possible. The type of assay used to detect antibody is determined by the nature of the antigen and the type of antibody desired.

   When designing the initial screening for selecting positive hybrids for cloning: (a) speed, convenience and reproducibility are essential; and (b) positive wells must be detected rapidly and then cloned out immediately to avoid overgrowth.

   It is essential that the screening assay is established and standardized before any hybridization is undertaken.

   Binding assays will, by definition, detect all antibody activity against a particular antigen and can be modified for the use of isotype-specific anti-immunoglobulin antibodies. Thus, if the antibody is being used to screen for a specific effector function, e.g. agglutination or complement fixation, then solid-phase radio- or enzyme-linked immunoassays are preferable (see also Chapter 5).

   The early determination of antibody isotype is important: (a) if you wish to select for or against specific isotypes; and (b) to ensure that an appropriate antibody purification protocol is used.

2.6 Cloning of hybrids

Antibody-secreting hybrid cells from positive culture wells must be cloned to ensure that the antibody is homogeneous and monospecific. Cloning is necessary to ensure that non-producers, arising either in the original fusion wells or as spontaneous variants, do not outgrow the antibody-secreting hybrids. If continuous growth of a hybrid line is required, it will be necessary to repeat the cloning and positive selection procedure at regular intervals.

Alternatively: prepare a large batch of cryopreserved cloned cells, and discard and replace growing lines at regular intervals. Cloning the initiation of a cell line from a single progenitor may be achieved either (a) in soft agar, (b) by limiting dilution, or (c) by using the continuous-flow cytometer (see also Section 8.5), but obviously the finer points of the technique are apparatus-dependent.

2.6.1 Cloning in soft agar

This is the original method used by Köhler and Milstein but usually limiting dilution is now the method of choice.

Preparation of soft agar stock solution

MATERIALS
Agarose (Sigma Type 1X-A)
Water, twice distilled

METHOD
1 Prepare a 2% w/v solution of agarose in twice-distilled water and dispense into glass bottles.
2 Autoclave at 120°C for 15 min and store at 4°C for use.

Cloning technique

MATERIALS AND EQUIPMENT
Hybrid cells
Agarose solution, 2% w/v, as above
Tissue culture medium, double strength, with 20% serum
24-well culture plates
Water bath at 44°C
Microwave oven

METHOD
1 Melt the agarose in the microwave oven and allow it to equilibrate in a 44°C water bath. Similarly, equilibrate the tissue culture medium to 44°C.
2 Mix equal volumes of agarose and tissue culture medium, and return the mixture to the water bath. The agarose will solidify if this is not done rapidly.

Continued on p. 54

3   Dispense 1 ml of the agarose tissue culture medium into each well of the tissue culture plate and allow it to solidify (subbed wells). Allow two cloning wells for each positive hybrid culture.

4   Count the hybrid cells and prepare suspensions at 2×10^3 cells/ml and 1×10^3 cells/ml.

5   For each cell suspension: mix 0.5 ml of cells with 1.0 ml of the agarose–tissue culture medium mixture.

6   Add 0.6 ml of the cell–agarose mixture to each of two subbed wells.

7   Repeat for all cells to be cloned.

8   Allow the agarose to solidify and incubate the plate in a humid incubator gassed with 5% CO_2 in air.
    Cell colonies will grow within 1–2 weeks and will be visible as white spots in the agarose; each discrete spot represents an individual clone.

9   Pick off 10 discrete colonies per well using sterile Pasteur pipettes and transfer to separate 200 µl microcultures.

TECHNICAL NOTES

• The underlay agarose is used to ensure that the cell colonies grow away from the well bottom. This aids manipulation of clones during isolation.

• Only discrete cell colonies must be isolated.

• The cloning efficiency of this technique is usually between 20 and 70% (percentage of original cells that grow as colonies). If growth is poor, a feeder layer of macrophages may be used, under the agarose.

• Not all of the colonies isolated will grow to produce lines of antibody-secreting cells. It is necessary therefore to screen and select for antibody activity. If the screening assay can be designed around the agar cloning plate, for example a modification of the Jerne plaque assay (see Section 9.1.1), it is possible to select antibody-secreting clones directly.

• The precision of cloning can be greatly enhanced by the direct selection of single hybrid cells from colonies growing in a primary fusion well detected as antibody positive. Cells can be picked by means of a micromanipulator and grown up either in agarose, as here, or in macrophage-supplemented microcultures.

2.6.2 Cloning by limiting dilution

The direct counterpart of the limiting dilution technique used to estimate the frequency of antigen-reactive lymphocytes. This is based on the same principle of random dispersion of rare elements, in this case hybrid cells, according to the Poisson distribution (see also Section 9.11).

Preparation in advance

Prepare macrophage feeder layers in 96-well, flat-bottomed microculture plates. Allow one plate for each positive hybrid well to be cloned.

MATERIALS AND EQUIPMENT

Hybrid cells for cloning

Microculture plates with macrophage feeder layers

Incubator, 37°C, humidified and gassed with 5% CO_2 in air

For each positive hybrid well:

1 Harvest and count the cells.
2 Prepare cell suspensions at 10 and 5 cells/ml.
3 Add 100 µl aliquots of the 10 cells/ml suspension to each of 48 wells. Repeat into remaining wells for the suspension at 5 cells/ml.
4 Incubate the plates in a humid 37°C incubator gassed with 5% CO_2 in air. Colonies should be visible after 1–2 weeks.
5 Test supernatants for antibody activity and select positive wells for culture.

TECHNICAL NOTES

- The initial distribution of cells per well follows Poisson statistics, thus although about 40% of the wells will receive only one cell (and therefore initiate a true clone), a significant proportion will receive two or more cells. Cloning must be repeated to ensure the homogeneity of any interesting hybrid line.
- It is advisable to reclone both the plasmacytoma and hybridoma lines at regular intervals. This will eliminate any variant cells, especially spontaneous non-secreting hybridoma variants, before they overgrow the culture.

2.7 Initiation and maintenance of B-hybridoma cell lines

2.7.1 Original method for the propagation of hybridomas

An outline of this procedure is included for historical reasons; however, it is no longer allowed in the UK owing to changes in the animal welfare regulations.

Freshly isolated hybrid cell cultures often grow slowly and are less tolerant of low cell densities than their plasmacytoma parent. The volume of the cell culture must be expanded slowly, at a rate that can only be determined empirically because hybrid lines show different growth rates. Colonies or cloning wells should be transferred to a maximum of 0.2–0.5 ml of medium (again with a feeder layer if necessary) and diluted with an equal volume of fresh medium as the pH indicator dye just begins to turn an orange-yellow. Hybridoma lines grown up to stationary phase in static flasks or spinner culture vessels can produce up to 1 µg/ml of antibody protein. Although the antibody is pure, the spent medium contains many other serum proteins. Large amounts of hybridoma-derived antibody may be prepared by injecting these tumorigenic lines into histo-compatible (or immunoincompetent) mice.

2.7.2 Alternative method for the propagation of hybridomas

Selected hybridomas in HT medium may be expanded from a 96-well microtitre plate to a 24-well plate and finally a 75-cm² flask. Hybridomas may also be propagated in tissue culture using hollow-fibre technology, e.g. MAbMAX, Bio Whittaker; Harvest Mouse, Serotec; Technomouse, Northumbria Biologicals. This approach avoids the necessity of ascites production.

2.7.3 Production of monoclonal antibodies from a hybridoma line within *in vitro* culture

MATERIALS
Mice (histocompatible with hybridoma or nude, athymic)
Hybridoma line from *in vitro* culture
Pristane (2,6,10,14-tetramethylpentadecane)

METHOD

1   Inject 0.5 ml Pristane into the peritoneal cavity of each mouse.
2   After 7 days, inject 10^7 hybridoma cells i.p. into each mouse.
    Most hybridoma lines will produce solid tumours or ascites within 2–3 weeks.
3   Use a syringe and 19-gauge needle to drain off the ascitic fluid. Clarify the ascitic fluid by centrifugation (500 g for 15 min at 4°C).
4   If desired, screen the ascitic fluid from individual mice by electrophoresis and store those samples showing a prominent peak of paraprotein in the γ-globulin region (see Section 3.7).
5   Repeat steps **3** and **4** for the lifetime of the mouse.

TECHNICAL NOTES

- Ascitic fluid often contains up to 1 mg/ml of specific antibody protein. There are, of course, other proteins, including immunoglobulins of unknown specificity.
- The serum of these tumour-bearing mice also contains large quantities of hybridoma-derived antibody.
- It is inadvisable to maintain a hybridoma by serial passage in mice because of the risk of accumulating non-secreting cells. Instead, inject large batches of mice with recently cloned cells from *in vitro* culture.
- Immunoincompetent nude or severe combined immunodeficient (SCID) mice will also be required if the hybrid line was derived from a mouse–rat fusion. Some investigators prefer to immunize rats, rather than mice, for fusion, as it is possible to obtain significant volumes of antisera in test bleeds prior to fusion.
- Passage through an animal can be helpful for a valuable monoclonal, to remove mycoplasma infection.

2.8 Human monoclonal antibodies

Monoclonal antibody production from human B lymphocytes is more difficult than from rodent cells. Antigens which may ethically be used to immunize people are largely limited to standard vaccines. In many cases cells spontaneously produce interesting immunoglobulins, such as autoantibodies which are likely to be of a low frequency within the B lymphocyte pool. It is not generally possible to remove the spleen to obtain a large number of lymphocytes! Therefore peripheral blood must be used instead, but this is not a very good source of antibody-secreting cells.

To increase the number of B lymphocytes for immobilization some researchers transform the cells with Epstein–Barr virus (EBV), but this can lead to selection of a subset of B lymphocytes. B lymphocytes are then immobilized by fusion with a myeloma clone as for mouse hybridomas, e.g. X63-Ag8.653, SP2/0-Ag14, or a pregenerated mouse/human hybridoma partner such as K6H6/B5 or SPAZ4 cells. The procedures for fusion, selection and cloning are then identical to the protocol for mouse–mouse hybridomas.

2.8.1 Generation of Epstein–Barr virus-immortalized human B-cell lines

MATERIALS AND EQUIPMENT
RPMI 1640
Fetal calf serum (FCS)
Cyclosporin A
Absolute ethanol (Analar)
B95-8 cells (Marmoset cell line)
Hank's balanced salt solution
Phosphate-buffered saline (PBS)
30 ml heparinized blood
Ficoll–Hypaque
75-cm^2 tissue culture flasks for 25 ml cultures

Preparation of the culture medium

METHOD

1 Prepare a culture solution of RPMI 1640 medium containing 20% v/v FCS.
2 In a separate flask, prepare a stock solution of cyclosporin A in ethanol to concentration of 1 mg/ml.
3 Supplement the culture medium with the solution prepared in step 2 to make a final concentration of 1 µg/ml of cyclosporin A, i.e. 1 : 1000 dilution.
4 Inoculate the prepared culture medium with 1×10^6 B95-8 cells/ml and incubate for 3 days at 37°C in a humidified 5% CO_2 incubator.

Preparation of human lymphocytes

METHOD

1 Make a 1 : 2 dilution of the heparinized blood with PBS.
2 Underlay 15 ml of the diluted blood with 15 ml of Ficoll–Hypaque and centrifuge at room temperature for 10 min at 1500 *g*.
3 Transfer the buffy coat (at the interface) into another tube, add 30 ml of PBS and centrifuge at room temperature for 15 min at 300 *g*.
4 Discard the supernatant and resuspend the pellet in 10 ml of Hank's balanced salt solution.
5 Centrifuge at room temperature for 10 min at 300 *g*.
6 Repeat steps 8 and 9.
7 Following the two washes in Hank's balanced salt solution, resuspend the pelleted cells in the 3 ml of modified RPMI 1640 culture medium (prepared in steps **1–3**).

Note: Cyclosporin A is added to inactivate the cytotoxic lymphocytes in the preparation isolated from heparinized blood which would otherwise kill the EBV-infected B lymphocytes.

Infection and culture of the B lymphocytes

METHOD

1 Count the mononuclear cells.
2 Place 1×10^7 cells in a tissue culture flask and add 3 volumes of modified RPMI 1640 culture medium containing the B95-8 cells following the 3 days of culture (steps **1–4**).
3 Incubate at 37°C in a humidified 5% CO_2 for 3 weeks.
4 Change the culture medium every 3 days by making a 1 : 3 dilution of the cells in supplemented RPMI 1640 culture medium.

Note: B95-8 cells are a biohazard (category II) as they are a source of live EBV, and should only be handled by personnel known to be EBV-immune.

2.8.2 **Preparation of human B-cell hybridoma**

This technique may be used on B lymphocytes isolated from spleen, peripheral blood or EBV-transformed lines (see above). It is a modification of the method described by Lu *et al.* (1993).

MATERIALS AND EQUIPMENT
EBV-transformed cells from the section above, or non-transformed B cells
RPMI 1640 containing 20% fetal calf serum (FCS)
Heterohybridoma cell line, e.g. K6H6/B5
Dulbecco's modified Eagle's medium
Polyethylene glycol 1500 (PEG-1500)
Dimethyl sulphoxide (DMSO)
Growth medium: RPMI 1640 containing 10% FCS, 1% non-essential amino acids, 1 mM sodium pyruvate, 10 mM HEPES buffer, 2 mM L-glutamine, 100 units/ml penicillin and 100 µg/ml streptomycin
Growth medium containing 16 µM thymidine, 100 µM hypoxanthine, 1 µg/ml azaserine
Culture plate, 96 microwells

METHOD

1 Prepare a culture of K6H6/B5 cells to around 2×10^6 cell/ml in an equal volume of modified RPMI 1640 culture medium and Dulbecco's modified Eagle's medium.
2 Mix 5×10^6 EBV-transformed cells with 2.5×10^6 K6H6/B5 cells in a conical flask, and centrifuge at 250 *g* and room temperature for 5 min.
3 Discard the supernatant and resuspend the cell pellet in 1 ml of RPMI 1640 containing 35% w/v PEG and 7.5% DMSO.
4 Slowly add an additional 3 ml of RPMI 1640, then make up to a volume of 120 ml with growth medium containing 16 µM thymidine, 100 µM hypoxanthine, 1 µg/ml azaserine.
5 Add 1×10^4 cells per well to 96-microwell culture plate.
   Place all the plates in a humidified 37°C incubator with 5% CO_2.

Continued

6   Feed the cells once a week with fresh medium (growth medium containing 16 μM thymidine, 100 μM hypoxanthine, 1 μg/ml azaserine).

7   At 2 weeks, microscopically examine the wells for the presence of hybrid colonies.

8   Test the tissue culture supernatant for the presence of antibodies of interest.

9   Clone positive wells by the same method as the mouse hybridomas.

TECHNICAL NOTES

- It is possible to expand the B-cell clones by growing in SCID mice. However, this technique has the same reservations as applied to growth of mouse hybridomas in whole animals and wherever possible *in vitro* cell culture should be used.
- To expand hybridomas it may be expedient to invest in a hollow fibre system that allows bulk production of monoclonal antibodies.

2.9 Monoclonal antibody purification

Methods include ammonium sulphate precipitation, gel filtration and ion-exchange chromatography, although a rapid and more convenient method is affinity chromatography. The use of protein G/protein A for mouse isotypes has previously been covered in Chapter 1. For IgM isotypes, alternative methods are now available (e.g. PROSEP®-Thiosorb-M©, Bioprocessing Ltd; rProtein L, Actigen Ltd), which can be followed according to manufacturer's instructions. In general immunoglobulins are preferable as monoclonal reagents, since IgM antibodies are prone to degradation, particularly following freezing and thawing.

2.9.1 Purification of murine IgM using PROSEP®-Thiosorb-M© (Bioprocessing Ltd)

PROSEP®-Thiosorb-M© is an affinity adsorbent which facilitates the purification for IgM by covalent attachment of a ligand with thiophilic properties, to PROSEP®. The matrix will bind IgM at high concentration of lyotropic (water-structuring) salt such as ammonium sulphate, or potassium sulphate, and release it at low concentration or in the absence of a lyotropic salt. Furthermore, standard chromatography columns are suitable for use with PROSEP®-Thiosorb-M©. A simple protocol (from Emma Waldron, Konstantinos University, Greece, and Wolverhampton University, UK) is provided for the culture supernatant known to contain IgM.

MATERIALS

PROSEP®-Thiosorb-M© (Bioprocessing Ltd)

Chromatography column, e.g. disposable syringe

Culture supernatant containing monoclonal antibody B35B

20 mM HEPES, 0.5 M NaCl, 7.5% $(NH_4)_2SO_4$, pH 7.5 (wash buffer)

20 mM HEPES, 2 M NaCl, pH 7.5 (elution buffer 2)

60% ethylene glycol (elution buffer 3)

6 M urea (regeneration solution)

BioLogic HR chromatography system (e.g. Bio-Rad) plus column

1.5-ml Eppendorf tubes

UV spectrophotometer and quartz cuvette (particularly if performing purification without a flow cell and chart recorder)

METHOD

1 Prepare a 50% slurry of the matrix in wash buffer (1 g swells to about 3.25 ml) and pour swelled slurry into column. Ensure the bed height is even and connect to a suitable chromatography system. (BioLogic HR, BioRad).

2 For a column containing 4–5 ml matrix, use 20 ml of wash buffer to flush out the tubing and wash the column. Check the absorbance of the flow-through.

3 Add 20 ml of culture supernatant (previously centrifuged at 1000 g for 5 min to remove any debris).

4 Add 20 ml of wash buffer (UV monitoring should ultimately indicate a zero base line).

5 Add 20 ml of elution buffer 2 and subsequently add 20 ml of elution buffer 3 to release IgM antibody. Check against UV monitor and test fractions for immunological reactivity. The absorbance of pooled fractions may also be analysed using a quartz cuvette and UV spectrophotometer set at 280 nm.

6 Aliquot antibody in Eppendorfs/dialyse against appropriate buffer/estimate protein concentration using extinction coefficient or bicinchroninic acid (BCA) system (see also Appendix B.5).

7 Regenerate column with 6 M urea, and then equilibrate with 10 column volumes of wash buffer.

2.9.2 Isotyping of murine monoclonal antibodies

Antibodies in hybridoma cell culture supernatant can be typed in a capture enzyme-linked immunosorbent assay (ELISA) using anti-isotype antibodies provided in a commercially available kit, e.g. Sigma. The following protocol provides a means of qualitatively determining the isotype of murine monoclonal antibodies IgG1, IgG2a, IgG2b, IgG3, IgM or IgA. A 200 µl system is used.

MATERIALS AND EQUIPMENT

Mouse monoclonal antibody isotyping reagents—kit Sigma ISO-2

Washing buffer (phosphate-buffered saline (PBS)–0.05% Tween 20)

PBS

Horseradish peroxidase (HRP) conjugate diluted in washing buffer

0.1 M citrate buffer

Hydrogen peroxide, 30% w/v solution

2,2′-azinobis(3′ethylbenzthiazoline sulphonic acid) (ABTS) tablets

0.1% sodium dodecyl sulphate

Flat-bottomed 96-well ELISA plate

Multichannel pipette plus tips

0.5–10-µl pipette

40–200-µl pipette

200–1000-µl pipette

Universal tubes

1.5-ml Eppendorfs
Petri dishes
Plate reader and printer (Labsystems Multiskan MS or equivalent)

METHOD

1 Dilute the isotype-specific antibodies to 10 µg/ml in PBS, 1600 µl per plate required for each solution (see kit information leaflet for protein concentration).

2 Pipette 200 µl of IgG_1 into each well of column 2, do the same for IgG_{2a} in column 3 and so on for all the antibodies. Incubate plate at 37°C for 1 h, or at 4°C overnight.

3 Remove coating solution and wash plate three times with washing buffer.

4 Add 200 µl of hybridoma supernatants to be tested to appropriate row of wells, i.e. into wells A2–A7. Also add 200 µl of HT or HAT medium (according to the medium the cells were grown up in) to a row of wells as a control. Incubate plate at 37°C for 2 h.

Note: Supernatants of known isotype should also be included as controls and to ensure that the system is functioning.

5 Wash plate three times with washing buffer.

6 Dilute HRP conjugate 1 : 1000 (or an optimal dilution) with washing buffer (20 µl HRP in 20 ml buffer).

7 Add 200 µl HRP to all wells and incubate plate for 1 h at 37°C.

8 Wash plate as in step 5.

9 Dissolve one ABTS tablet in 20 ml 0.1 M citrate buffer. Immediately prior to substrate use, add 12 µl of hydrogen peroxide to solution and mix well.

10 Add 200 µl of above substrate solution to each well and allow reaction to proceed for 30 min. A green colour will develop in the appropriate wells to indicate the MAb isotype. If preferred, the reaction can be stopped by adding to each well 200 µl of 0.1% sodium dodecyl sulphate.

11 The absorbances produced by the antibodies should be read on a plate reader at 414 nm and a printed record made to aid identification of sample isotype.

TECHNICAL NOTES

• Remove background noise by calculating the mean HT/HAT values and subtracting this from all other values produced.

• If more than one isotype is indicated, then the hybridoma may need recloning.

• It is advisable for the laboratory to have a stock of immunoglobulin isotypes to be used as controls in the experiments.

• Check the isotype of the monoclonal antibody regularly when purified and after cryopreservation as there have been occasional incidences where IgM antibodies have switched to another isotype after cryopreservation.

2.10 Antigen immunoadsorbents

Protein antigens (not necessarily in a pure form) may be linked to a support matrix, e.g. cyanogen bromide-activated Sepharose and packed into a column. Filter ascitic fluid or culture supernatant through the column, wash to remove unbound proteins and then elute the antibody under the most gentle conditions compatible with antibody release.

2.11 Isolation of monoclonal immunoglobulin

If purified antibody cannot be isolated directly by antigen binding, prepare an immunoglobulin fraction of the ascitic fluid using either affinity or ion-exchange chromatography (see Sections 1.3 and 1.4).

2.11.1 Problems and solutions

Purification of monoclonal antibodies follows the same general procedures outlined for poly-clonal antibodies. As each monoclonal antibody is unique, an individual determination will be required to establish the particular conditions for the isolation of each antibody.

Antibodies in tissue culture supernatants must first be concentrated either in a membrane concentrator or by ammonium sulphate precipitation before they can be isolated.

Ascitic fluids can be treated in a similar manner to serum immunoglobulins. However, they frequently contain appreciable quantities of lipid that should be removed at the beginning of the isolation procedure by treatment with Aerosil.

Hybridoma antibodies grown in serum-free medium contain little immunoglobulin other than that of hybridoma origin, but contain a lot of albumin. Thus, problems of antibody purification are essentially the same for serum-supplemented or serum-free media. Concentration and partial purification can be obtained by precipitation at a 50% saturation with ammonium sulphate, using solid ammonium sulphate to avoid excessive increase in volume. Excess albumin may be removed by affinity chromatography on Cibacron blue dye affinity gel before attempting ion-exchange chromatography.

Note: A combination of Cibacron blue with diethylaminoethyl (DEAE) is available from Biorad that allows albumin removal and ion-exchange in one step.

DEAE and quaternary aminoethyl (QAE) ion-exchangers are suitable for purification of IgG monoclonal antibodies. As monoclonal antibodies have a unique isoelectric point and charge density, use gradient elution from the ion exchanger.

Monoclonal IgA is more difficult to prepare but can be isolated by ammonium sulphate pre-cipitation, followed by ion-exchange chromatography. Using gradient elution, the IgA should elute after IgG but before the albumin fraction.

IgM antibodies are most readily prepared by gel filtration using a high-resolution gel such as Sephacryl S-300 HR.

2.11.2 Anti-immunoglobulin affinity columns

The IgG or antibody fraction of goat or rabbit anti-mouse immunoglobulin may be linked to Sepharose and the affinity column so formed used to isolate hybridoma immunoglobulin.

MATERIALS AND EQUIPMENT

As for Section 1.5.2 (Use of immunoadsorbent for antibody purification) but in addition:

Anti-mouse immunoglobulin, goat or rabbit
Mouse immunoglobulin
Hybridoma-derived antibody

TECHNICAL NOTES

- These columns are precycled with normal mouse IgG and eluted with acid buffer to saturate the high-affinity anti-immunoglobulin antibodies that would otherwise bind the precious monoclonal antibody virtually irreversibly. In any case, these columns should always be pre-eluted with acid buffer and re-equilibrated before use to remove any loosely bound material.
- To minimize denaturation, elution should be accomplished under the most gentle conditions compatible with the release of antibody.
- Mouse immunoglobulin may also be isolated by ion-exchange chromatography (see Section 1.3) or by affinity chromatography on staphylococcal protein A–Sepharose (subclass IgG_{2a}, IgG_{2b} and IgG_3—see Section 1.4). (Rat immunoglobulins, with the exception of the minor subclass IgG_{2c}, do not bind to protein A, but may be prepared by streptococcal protein G.)

2.12 Enzymic fragmentation of monoclonal antibodies

Removal of the Fc region of monoclonal antibodies, to leave a divalent fragment which is no longer able to bind to Fc receptors or to activate the complement pathway, is often desirable but, in practice, is often difficult or impossible to achieve. Amongst the IgG subclasses there is a differential sensitivity to proteolysis; with pepsin, for example, IgG_{2b} is most sensitive followed by $IgG_3 > IgG_{2a} > IgG_1$, while for papain, IgG_1 is most sensitive followed by $IgG_{2a} > IgG_3 > IgG_{2b}$.

There are individual sensitivities unique to each monoclonal antibody, so it is essential to perform a range of trial digests on each antibody preparation to optimize conditions. Each batch of the same monoclonal antibody will be structurally identical; once the digestion conditions are determined they will not need to be varied.

In the experiment described below, a batch of purified antibody is mixed with the enzyme, under digestion conditions and samples taken for fragment analysis by SDS-PAGE to determine the optimal time of incubation, i.e. that which gives maximum yield of the desired fragment with minimum subfragmentation to smaller peptides.

Note: Only small amounts of monoclonal IgG will be available; slightly lower concentrations are used than for rabbit or human IgG.

2.12.1 Pepsin digestion

MATERIALS AND EQUIPMENT
0.1 M citrate buffer, pH 3.5
IgG, monoclonal antibody
Pepsin (1 mg/ml) in 0.1 M citrate buffer, pH 3.5
SDS-PAGE (see Appendix B.2.1)

METHOD

1 Dissolve or dialyse the IgG in the citrate buffer and adjust concentration to 1 mg protein/ml.
2 Place 300 µl in a small tube and add 6 µl of a 1 mg/ml solution of pepsin in the same buffer and incubate at 37°C.
3 Immediately (time 0) and then at 5, 10, 15 and 30 min, 1, 2, 4, 8, 16 and 24 h, remove a 20 µl aliquot.
4 The pH of each aliquot should be adjusted to just above 7.0 to stop the reaction.
5 At the end of the time course, analyse the fractions by SDS-PAGE under reducing and non-reducing conditions (see Appendix B.2.1).

TECHNICAL NOTE
From an examination of these gels, for example Fig. 2.2, it should be possible to select a suitable set of conditions to apply to a bulk preparation of the monoclonal antibody. The fragments may then be separated by a combination of gel filtration and protein A chromatography.

2.12.2 Papain digestion

Papain needs activation by cysteine accomplished by either: (a) incorporating cysteine in the reaction mixture or (b) pre-activating the papain prior to addition to the digestion mixture.

Using pre-activated papain with mouse IgG sometimes gives a $F(ab')_2$ fragment similar to the pepsin $F(ab')_2$. If cysteine is present during the enzyme reaction the fragmentation proceeds to give Fab and Fc.

MATERIALS AND EQUIPMENT
Papain
Phosphate-buffered saline (PBS)
IgG monoclonal antibody (2 mg/ml in PBS)
0.002 M ethylene diamine tetra-acetic acid (EDTA) in PBS
0.5 M cysteine in PBS
0.1 M iodoacetamide
Sephadex G-25
Chromatography column, e.g. 10-ml disposable syringe plugged with glass wool (*Caution: Wear gloves when handling glass wool*)

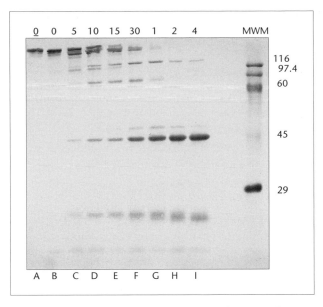

Fig. 2.2 Time course of papain digestion of monoclonal IgG. To determine the optimum conditions for the papain digestion of a monoclonal antibody a time course experiment was performed. Samples were taken, at intervals, and run on an SDS-PAGE system in non-reducing conditions.

0   Sample prior to digestion.
0   Reaction stopped immediately on addition of papain.
5   Reaction stopped 5 min after addition of papain.
10 Reaction stopped 10 min after addition of papain.
15 Reaction stopped 15 min after addition of papain.
30 Reaction stopped 30 min after addition of papain.
1   Reaction stopped 1 h after addition of papain.
2   Reaction stopped 2 h after addition of papain.
4   Reaction stopped 4 h after addition of papain.

Easily detectable digestion products are visible at first sampling at 5 min. The reaction proceeds through a number of intermediates, such as one Fab linked to Fc, before arriving at the 50 kDa products. With prolonged incubation small molecular weight degradation products begin to appear. Choosing an optimum time is a balance between efficient usage of starting material and not too much degradation.

METHOD

Pre-activation of papain

1   Place 100 μg papain in a small tube containing 50 μl 0.002 M EDTA in PBS and 10 μl 0.5 M cysteine in PBS.

2   Incubate at 37°C for 30 min.

3   Prepare a small Sephadex G-25 column. A disposable 10-ml disposable syringe plugged with glass wool at the bottom would be suitable. The column should be filled with Sephadex G-25 and equilibrated with PBS containing 0.002 M EDTA.

4   Apply the activated papain to the column and elute with PBS-EDTA. Collect 0.25 ml fractions and determine their protein content to locate the papain peak. Use the peak tube for the digestion; this should contain about half the total absorbance units of enzyme.

Continued on p. 66

Digestion of IgG

5 Add the papain to 1 mg IgG in 0.5 ml PBS containing 0.002 M EDTA.

6 Incubate at 37°C.

7 Immediately remove 20 µg IgG and mix with 0.1 M iodoacetamide to a final concentration of 0.025 M to stop the reaction.

8 Remove further 20 µg samples at 5, 10, 15 and 30 min, 1, 2, 4 and 8 h and each time stop the reaction with iodoacetamide.

9 Analyse the fractions by SDS-PAGE in both non-reducing and reducing conditions. As the samples contain iodoacetamide, add 2-mercaptoethanol to a concentration of 0.02 M before proceeding to the normal sample preparation conditions for the reducing gel (see Appendix B.2.1).

Having established the optimal conditions for digestion, proceed with the bulk preparation and isolate the resultant fragments by gel filtration and protein A affinity chromatography.

2.13 Characterization of monoclonal antibodies

Frequently, the isolation of a novel monoclonal antibody has been the first step in the identification of a minor, but functionally important, component within a complex mixture of antigens. Fortunately it is possible to determine many of the chemical properties and biological attributes of the molecule thus defined in advance of purification or gene cloning, even though the molecule might reside in a cell's surface membrane. The value is obvious: there would be little point in taking a DNA cloning route if the antibody defined a carbohydrate epitope on a glycoprotein.

2.13.1 Chemical nature of monoclonal antibody-defined epitopes

The advantages of monoclonal antibody technology include its ability to provide highly discriminatory ligands that are able to define and detect epitopes present in trace amounts in a complex mixture of antigens. Although the antigen might be present as a minor determinant on a minority cell population, it can still be regarded as a valid target for hybridoma production.

Conventional techniques may be used to characterize the antibody in terms of isotype, biological activity (complement fixation, agglutination, precipitation) or the subpopulations of cells.

Determination of apparent molecular weight and isoelectric point of the antigen (by immuno-precipitation or immunoblotting requires little advance purification as these determinations can be made using the discriminatory power of the antibody.

The use of immune affinity chromatography provides the definitive route to antigen isolation and its characterization by standard chemical means (structural, composition and sequence analysis).

Flow cytometry using monoclonal antibodies provides a reproducible means of measuring the relative amount of antigen (through antibody binding) in its native state and environment, often in heterogeneous cell mixtures (the cell population of interest need only be delineated at the time of analysis).

The use of techniques that modify antigen expression (enzymes, metabolic inhibitors, chemical treatment, etc.) is an indirect means of acquiring information on the chemical nature of the antigen carrying the monoclonal antibody-defined epitope.

2.14 **Practical applications of monoclonal antibodies**

The production, selection and maintenance of hybridoma clones synthesizing antibody of a required specificity is so time consuming. Is it the best way? For example, the monospecific antibody is a distinct disadvantage in the production of antibodies for class-specific precipitation of immunoglobulins or screening of recombinant DNA expression libraries. Monoclonal antibodies bind to only one determinant per molecule when used with non-polymeric antigens, thus precluding the formation of a matrix for precipitation.

The availability of monoclonal antibodies compared with conventional antisera has greatly improved existing technology and has been fundamental for the generation of new techniques in that:

(a) monospecific, hybridoma-derived antibodies can be used to estimate degree of structural homology between antigens. For example, with influenza virus, antibodies against chemically defined antigens have been used to investigate strains of virus for the presence of identical or closely related antigens;

(b) within solid-phase binding assays, these antibodies can be used at very low concentrations. These assays are essentially affinity independent and detect the very low-affinity non-specific protein–protein interactions often found with conventional sera. As the degree of non-specific binding shown by an unrelated monoclonal antibody is much less than would be found with a normal control serum or unrelated antiserum the results can be interpreted with greater confidence; and

(c) the production of hybridoma-derived antibody is highly reproducible. Thus, whenever a new batch of antibody is produced from the same cloned cell line, it will have the same specificity.

In general the use of monospecific antibody is limited to research and diagnostic applications. One obvious example is the definition of cell-surface markers for the investigation of specialized or abnormal cell function. This has given powerful diagnostic, and in some cases prognostic, tools for the study of tumours. Moreover, such techniques should continue to yield new information on the development and control of the immune system.

Potential applications of monospecific antibodies include:

(a) clinical diagnostic testing; and

(b) the production of therapeutic antisera with suitable human plasmacytoma parent line.

Monospecific antibodies produced by mouse fusion hybrids have many immediate applications in the clinical laboratory as diagnostic or immunoassay reagents.

(a) *Tissue typing*. Current typing techniques rely on antisera derived from multiparous women or from patients who have received multiple blood transfusions. They are of low titre and often possess several specificities. A research programme has been established in the USA for the production of typing reagents using hybridoma techniques, although it seems likely that this approach could be overtaken by the use of gene probes.

(b) *Blood group serology*. A range of standard reagents are available through the National Blood Service.

(c) *Immunoassay of hormones.* Fusions can be performed with spleen cells from mice immunized with relatively impure antigen. The need for antigen purification is circumvented by the selection of appropriate cell lines from cloned populations. This, and the monospecificity of the antibody thus obtained, has greatly enhanced the range and sensitivity of immunoassay techniques. For example, an improved pregnancy test has been introduced using hybridoma-derived antibody for the immunoenzymatic detection of human chorionic gonadotrophin (hCG). These tests are now sensitive, rapid, accurate and unequivocal in their interpretation. In one variant, the enzyme substrate develops a minus sign in the event of a negative test; the anti-hCG antibody is arranged so that it then adds an additional bar, to create a plus sign, in the event of a positive test. Monoclonal antibody technology has transformed this test from a highly specialized laboratory technique to a 'home-based' immunoassay.

(d) *Immunodiagnosis of infectious disease.* Sensitive immunoassays using monoclonal antibodies allow the diagnosis of infectious disease by the detection of microbial antigen rather than antibody. This is of much greater clinical value as it is a direct measure of the current state of the patient. Antibody detection has the disadvantage that it is practically impossible to distinguish between a past or present infection using a single blood sample. In addition these reagents avoid the diagnostic imprecision due to cross-reactivity between serologically related organisms.

Attempts to produce human monoclonal antibodies have met with only limited success. Major limitations are that: (a) peripheral blood is the only readily available source of lymphocytes (which must be activated *in vitro* as deliberate immunization *in vivo* would be unethical); and (b) there are really no human tumour parents equivalent to the MOPC 21 sublines used in the murine system. Attempts have been made to circumvent these deficiencies, e.g. EBV lines used both alone and fused with B-cell tumours, but no generally applicable technique has emerged.

Recombinant DNA techniques have helped to overcome the problem of antigenicity of murine antibodies destined for clinical use. The solution has been fusion of the DNA sequences encoding murine variable regions with the sequence encoding human constant regions, thus producing a minimally antigenic molecule. Although there is the problem of an anti-idiotypic response, there appears to be a sufficiently large time window in which to achieve therapeutic potential. Recombinant techniques may be applied to the production of novel hybrid molecules in which the combining site of antibody is used to target a secondary effector function; for example, an enzyme active site.

2.15 Generation of recombinant phage antibody

As an alternative approach to fusing B cells or perhaps modifying existing hybridomas, the recombinant phage antibody system may be used. Specific details of protocols and reagents are available commercially from Amersham Pharmacia Biotech. This company has produced the system as three components, i.e. mouse ScFv module, expression module and detection module. Obviously molecular biological technical expertise and equipment are required for polymerase chain reaction (PCR), submarine gel electrophoresis, gel visualization equipment and bacterial culture facilities.

Overview of the Protocol

1   The mRNA encoding the heavy chain and light chain variable regions of immunoglobulins are amplified using PCR, followed by re-amplification to include a linker moiety.

2   The assembled product is then ligated (using the appropriate restriction enzyme sites) into a phagemid vector which is used to transform competent TG1 *Escherichia coli* cells. Following phage rescue the recombinant phage contains a single-strand copy of DNA encoding the *ScFv* (single-chain variable fragment) gene and one or more copies of the recombinant antibody (as fusion proteins) on their tips.

3   Recombinant phage is utilized as an 'antibody molecule' for panning against a desired antigen in an ELISA system. Following selection, re-infection of the TG1 cells and enrichment, the recombinant phage is used to infect *E. coli* HB2151 cells to produce soluble ScFv antibodies.

2.16 **Further reading**

Aouama, K. & Chiba, J. (1993) Separation of different molecular forms of mouse IgA and IgM monoclonal antibodies by high performance liquid chromatography on spherical hydroxyapatite beads. *J Immunol Meth* **162**, 201–210.

Birch, J.R. & Lennox, E.S. (1995) *Monoclonal Antibodies—Principles and Applications*. John Wiley & Sons, Chichester.

Bonwick, G.A., Cresswell, J.E., Tyreman, A.L. *et al.* (1996) Production of murine monoclonal antibodies against sulcofuron and flucofuron by *in vitro* immunization. *J Immunol Meth* **196**, 163–173.

Borrebaeck, C.A.K. & Hagen, I. (1993) *Electromanipulation in Hybridoma Technology: A Laboratory Manual*. Oxford University Press, Oxford.

Burd, R.S., Raymond, C.S., Ratz, C.A. & Dunn, D.L. (1993) A rapid procedure for purifying IgM monoclonal antibodies from murine ascites using a DEAE-disk. *Hybridoma* **12**, 135–142.

Delves, P. (ed.) (1997) *Antibody Production: Essential Techniques*. John Wiley & Sons, Chichester.

Faguet, G.B. & Agee, J.F. (1993) A simple technique for the enrichment of class and subclass hybridoma switch variants. A 1000-fold enrichment in half the time, for half the cost. *J Immunol Meth* **165**, 217–224.

Falkenberg, F.W., Hengelage, T., Krane, M. *et al.* (1993) A simple and inexpensive high density dialysis tubing cell culture system for the *in vitro* production of monoclonal antibodies in high concentration. *J Immunol Meth* **165**, 193–206.

Food and Drugs Administration, Office of Biologics Research and Review, Center for Drugs and Biologics (1994) *Points to consider in the manufacture and testing of monocloncal antibody products for human use*. Food and Drugs Administration, Rockville Pike, Bethesda.

Gearing, A.J.H., Thorpe, R., Spitz, L. & Spitz, M. (1985) Use of 'single shot' intrasplenic immunization for production of monoclonal antibodies specific for human IgM. *J Immunol Meth* **76**, 337–343.

Goding, J.W. (1996) *Monoclonal Antibodies: Principles and Practice*, 3rd edn. Academic Press, New York.

Howard, G.C., Bethell, D.R. & Vilsaint, F. (2000) *Basic Methods in Antibody Production and Characterization*. Cambridge University Press, Cambridge.

King, D.J. (1999) *Applications and Engineering of Monoclonal Antibodies*. Taylor & Francis, London.

Köhler, G. & Milstein, C. (1975) Continuous culture of fused cells secreting antibody of predefined specificity. *Nature* **256**, 495–497.

Leickt, L., Grubb, A. & Ohlson, S. (1998) Affinity screening for weak monoclonal antibodies. *J Immunol Meth* **220**(1–2), 19–24.

Lennox, E.S. & Birch, J.R. (eds) (1995) *Monoclonal Antibodies: Principles and Applications*. John Wiley & Sons, Chichester.

Lu, E.W., Deftos, M., Olee, T. *et al.* (1993) Generation and molecular analyses of two rheumatoid synovial fluid-derived IgG rheumatoid factors. *Arthritis Rheum* **36**(7), 927–937.

Manzke, O., Tesch, H., Diehl, V. & Bohlen, H. (1997) Single-step purification of bispecific monoclonal antibodies for immunotherapeutic use by hydrophobic interaction chromatography. *J Immunol Meth* **208**(1), 65–73.

McCafferty, J., Hoogenboom, H. & Chiswell, D. (1996) *Antibody Engineering A Practical Approach*. IRL Press, Oxford.

Milstein, C. (2000) With the benefit of hindsight (Review). *Immunol Today* **21**(8), 359–364.

Ritter, M.A. & Ladyman, H.M. (1995) *Monoclonal Antibodies—Production, Engineering and Clinical Application*. Cambridge University Press, Cambridge.

Schwarz, A. (2000) Affinity purification of monoclonal antibodies. *Methods Mol Biol* **147**, 49–56.

Shepherd, P.S. & Dean, C. (eds) (2000) *Monoclonal Antibodies: A Practical Approach*. Oxford University Press, Oxford.

Siegel, D.L., Chang, T.Y., Russell, S.L. & Bunya, V.Y. (1997) Isolation of cell surface-specific human monoclonal antibodies using phage display and magnetically activated cell sorting: applications in immunohematology. *J Immunol Meth* **206**(1–2), 73–85.

Turner, D.J., Ritter, M.A. & George, A.J. (1997) Importance of the linker in expression of single-chain Fv antibody fragments: optimization of peptide sequence using phage display technology. *J Immunol Meth* **205**(1), 43–54.

de Wildt, R.M., Steenbakkers, P.G., Pennings, A.H., van den Hoogen, F.H., van Venrooij, W.J. & Hoet, R.M. (1997) A new method for the analysis and production of monoclonal antibody fragments originating from single human B cells. *J Immunol Meth* **207**(1), 61–7.

Williams, S., van der Logt, P. & Germaschewski, V. (2001) Phage display libraries. In: *Epitope Mapping: A Practical Approach* (eds O.M.R. Westwood & F.C. Hay), pp. 225–254. Oxford University Press, Oxford.

Zola, H. (2000) *Monoclonal Antibodies: Preparation and Use of Monoclonal Antibodies and Engineered Antibody Derivatives* (Basics: From Background to Bench). Springer-Verlag, New Jersey.

3 Antibody interactions with antigens

3.1 Determination of antibody affinity

Antibody–antigen interaction may be considered in terms of the quantity of antibody produced or able to bind to a specified amount of antigen. For each antigenic determinant a range of different antibodies is formed, some of which will 'fit' the antigen better than others. Those with a better 'fit' will bind the antigen more strongly than the poorer fitting molecules.

Avidity is concerned with the interaction of multivalent antigens and antibodies, which is more complex. The thermodynamic description of avidity may be thought of in simple terms as the increased strength of binding gained because of the interdependence of binding sites. The fact that one arm of an IgG antibody molecule has bound to a multivalent antigen greatly increases the chance that the second arm will also bind. Having bound, both arms will then be required to release simultaneously if the immune complex is to be broken. For example, the avidity of IgG is related to its affinity by the product of the two interacting binding forces. Consequently, it is easy to see why for the same affinity IgM has a much greater avidity than IgG.

Affinity is a measure of the strength of antibody–antigen combination. More correctly, affinity refers to the interaction between monovalent antigenic determinants, i.e. haptens, and single antibody-combining sites. Measuring antibody affinity used to be confined to specialized immunochemistry laboratories where dedicated researchers probed the significance of antigen–antibody interactions. More recently its importance has become much more widely appreciated, and kits to measure affinity are reaching the diagnostic laboratory.

For example, consider the diagnosis of an infection by detection of the specific antibody being produced by a patient. Knowledge of the class of antibody provides some guide for distinguishing between a recent infection and one which the patient has had in the past or is currently responding to, i.e. IgM is produced early in the response and other classes later. However, some IgM is produced in the secondary immune response and also IgG–antigen immune complexes frequently stimulate the formation of rheumatoid factors (an IgM autoantibody against complexed IgG), which then gives rise to a false positive result for IgM.

Most immune responses start with antibodies of an 'average' (low) affinity and then mature to higher affinity as somatic mutation and B-cell selection takes place in the germinal centres. The change in affinity can well be up to six orders of magnitude. This difference provides a useful tool for determining whether an immune response is new (low affinity) or long-standing (high affinity). This approach has been particularly helpful in detecting acute primary *Toxoplasma* infections during pregnancy (Holliman *et al.* 1994). The increase in IgG avidity that occurs with time after infection was sufficiently reliable to estimate the period that had elapsed after infecting bank voles with hantavirus (Gavrilovskaya *et al.* 1993).

3.1.1 Mathematical basis of affinity

The combination of antigen (*Ag*) and antibody (*Ab*) to form a complex is a reversible reaction:

$$Ab + Ag \underset{K_\mathrm{d}}{\overset{K_\mathrm{a}}{\rightleftharpoons}} Ab \cdot Ag$$

where K_a and K_d are the association and dissociation constants, respectively. The law of mass action can be applied to this reaction with the affinity being given by the equilibrium constant K. As mentioned at the beginning of the section, although the law of mass action is used in general here, strictly it applies only to homogeneous systems such as monoclonal antibodies, from hybridomas or plasmacytomas, reacting with monovalent haptens. In the real world, antibodies in serum are polyclonal and therefore heterogeneous.

By the law of mass action:

$$K = \frac{K_\mathrm{a}}{K_\mathrm{d}} = \frac{[Ab \cdot Ag]}{[Ag][Ab]}$$

where K, K_a and K_d are as defined above, $[Ab \cdot Ag]$ is moles of immune complex (products), $[Ab]$ is moles of antibody (reactant) and $[Ag]$ is moles of antigen (reactant).

Remember that *Ag* refers to monovalent antigenic determinants and *Ab* to independent antibody-combining sites. As can be seen the amount of complex formed is proportional to the value of K. As each reactant is expressed in mol/l the overall units of K are litre/mol.

If K is determined with respect to total antibody-binding sites, Ab_t, the following form of the Langmuir adsorption isotherm may be derived from the mass action equation:

$$Ab + Ag \leftrightarrow Ab \cdot Ag.$$

By the law of mass action:

$$\frac{[Ab \cdot Ag]}{[Ab][Ag]} = K \text{ (equilibrium constant)},$$

therefore

$$[Ab \cdot Ag] = K[Ab][Ag]. \tag{1}$$

Make

$$Ab_\mathrm{t} = [Ab \cdot Ag] + [Ab],$$

therefore

$$[Ab] = [Ab_t] - [Ab \cdot Ag]. \qquad (2)$$

Substituting (2) in (1):

$$[Ab \cdot Ag] = K[Ag]([Ab_t] - [Ab \cdot Ag]),$$

therefore

$$[Ab \cdot Ag] = K[Ag][Ab_t] - K[Ag][Ab \cdot Ag]$$

$$[Ab \cdot Ag] + K[Ag][Ab \cdot Ag] = K[Ag][Ab_t]$$

$$[Ab \cdot Ag](1 + K[Ag]) = K[Ag][Ab_t]$$

$$\frac{[Ab \cdot Ag]}{[Ab_t]} = \frac{K[Ag]}{1 + K[Ag]} \qquad (3)$$

Make $[Ab \cdot Ag] = b$, then (3) may be rewritten as:

$$\frac{b}{[Ab_t]} = \frac{K[Ag]}{1 + K[Ag]}$$

$$\frac{b(1 + K[Ag])}{[Ab_t]K[Ag]} = 1$$

$$\frac{1}{b} = \frac{1 + K[Ag]}{K[Ab_t][Ag]}$$

$$= \frac{1}{K[Ab_t][Ag]} + \frac{K[Ag]}{K[Ab_t][Ag]}$$

$$= \frac{1}{K[Ab_t][Ag]} + \frac{1}{[Ab_t]} \qquad (4)$$

when $\dfrac{1}{[Ag]} = 0$ in (4)

$$\frac{1}{b} = \frac{1}{[Ab_t]}$$

As $b = [Ab \cdot Ag]$ = bound Ag concentration and $[Ag]$ = free antigen concentration, then a plot of $1/b$ against $1/[Ag]$ can be extrapolated to obtain $[Ab_t]$. This is the total of antibody-combining sites.

Note: The concentrations expressed in the above equations are molar equivalents; hence, for example, when $[Ab \cdot Ag]$ = bound Ag concentration, this is a molar equivalence and not a weight equivalence.

The determination of the total antibody-combining sites, although theoretically straightforward, is often difficult to determine experimentally. With a monoclonal antibody of high affinity there will be no problem obtaining a straight line for the Langmuir plot experimentally; thus, the extrapolation back to the ordinate is valid and accurate. However, with a heterogeneous antiserum, there can be considerable deviation from linearity. This is often the case with a small amount that is predominantly composed of low-affinity antibody. Under these conditions the

Langmuir plot can curve upwards as it nears the ordinate. In these situations, it is essential to have the maximum possible number of points along the linear part of the curve so that the best estimate of the intercept of this linear portion on the ordinate can be made. It is possible to circumvent some of these practical problems by using an independent method for determining the total antibody, e.g. quantitative precipitation or elution from immunoadsorbants. Unfortunately these alternatives also present their own problems.

To return to the mass action equation:

$$K = \frac{[Ab \cdot Ag]}{[Ab][Ag]}$$

If increasing amounts of antigen are reacted with a fixed amount of antibody, a point is reached where half the antibody-combining sites are occupied by antigen. At this point

$$[Ab] = [Ab \cdot Ag],$$

therefore in the mass action equation,

$$K = \frac{[Ab \cdot Ag]}{[Ab][Ag]}$$

$$K = \frac{1}{[Ag]}$$

In other words, affinity is equal to the reciprocal of the free antigen concentration when half the antibody sites are occupied by antigen.

The value of K can be obtained from the plot in Fig. 3.1 by calculating the value of 50% Ab_t and reading off from the graph the value of K.

In experimental systems this value can also be obtained from a plot of the logarithmic transformation of the Sip's equation as follows. If:

$$\frac{r}{n} = \frac{(K[Ag])^a}{1 + (K[Ag])^a}$$

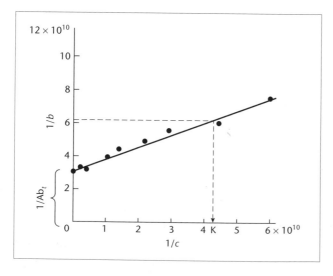

Fig. 3.1 Langmuir plot of reciprocal of bound (1/b) versus reciprocal of free antigen (1/c or 1/Ag) of a serum, from a baboon immunized with human chorionic gonadotrophin. The regression coefficient, $r = 0.98$. The value for Ab_t obtained by extrapolation to infinite antigen concentration is 3.21×10^{-11} mmol/l. Antibody affinity $K = 4.3 \times 10^{10}$ l/mol.

where r is moles of antigen bound per mole of antibody, n is antibody valency and a is heterogeneity index (see below), then:

$$\log \frac{r}{n-r} = a \cdot \log K + a \cdot \log[Ag] \qquad (5)$$

For IgG, $n = 2$, therefore:

$$\text{moles of antibody} = \frac{[Ab_t]}{2}$$

and

$$r = \frac{b}{[Ab_t]/2}$$

where $b = [Ab \cdot Ag]$.
Substituting for n and r in (5):

$$\log \frac{b}{[Ab_t]-b} = a \cdot \log K + a \cdot \log[Ag].$$

If:

$$\log \frac{b}{[Ab_t]-b} \text{ is plotted against } \log[Ag]$$

when:

$$\log \frac{b}{[Ab_t]-b} = 0$$

then:

$$K = \frac{1}{[Ag]}$$

The *heterogeneity index*, a, is a measure of the number of different molecular species of antibody. It can range from a value of 0 to 1. Low values represent a large degree of heterogeneity, whereas monoclonal antibody should theoretically have an index of 1. These relationships have been derived on the assumption that the distribution of antibody affinities in a polyclonal population is random and symmetrical about the mean. There is now good experimental evidence to suggest that the distribution of affinities is often skewed or even bimodal.

3.1.2 Equilibrium dialysis

This technique was devised in 1932 as a direct method for studying the primary interactions between antibody and hapten, and generally regarded as the standard method for affinity determination against which the other methods are judged. However, it is rather cumbersome to perform and uses up large amounts of antibody and antigen. Since many haptens (but not oligosaccharides) bind to albumin, it is necessary to work with antibody isolated by ammonium sulphate precipitation, though further purification is not usually required.

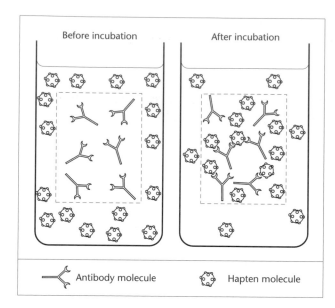

Before incubation   After incubation

Antibody molecule   Hapten molecule

Fig. 3.2 Equilibrium dialysis showing relative distribution of the antibody and hapten molecules at time zero and after the equilibrium is established. Cell to left shows distribution at the beginning of the experiment, cell to right shows distribution at equilibrium. There is a greater concentration of hapten molecules in the inner cell of the diagram on the right because of the hapten molecules bound to the antibody.

Constant amounts of antibody (approximately the reciprocal of the expected equilibrium constant) are placed in dialysis bags and allowed to equilibrate with various concentrations of hapten over an antigen excess of 1 to 40. Free hapten will enter the dialysis bag along its concentration gradient (Fig. 3.2). Some of the hapten will complex with antibody and so will not contribute to the free hapten concentration. At equilibrium, the free hapten concentration will be the same on either side of the dialysis membrane, but the total hapten concentration will be relatively greater inside the dialysis bag. For each experimental point on the binding curve the following samples, each in triplicate, are required:

(a) antibody immunoglobulin;
(b) irrelevant immunoglobulin of the same isotype for the determination of non-specific binding; and
(c) buffer alone, to check that equilibrium has in fact been established.

Outline of the technique

Typically each sample of protein or buffer solution (about 0.5 ml) is placed in a small dialysis bag. For each concentration of free hapten on the binding curve, nine sample bags can be equilibrated against a single pool of radioactive hapten (or hapten with alternative label), usually in a 50-ml bottle. Bottles are left in a water bath with mixing for 24–48 h and then triplicate volumetric samples are taken from each free hapten solution and each dialysis bag. The free hapten concentration at equilibrium may be determined directly from the counts per minute (c.p.m.) of the samples taken from the bottles. The bound hapten concentration may be calculated as follows:

Antibody-bound hapten, $Hb = (H_{Ab}) - (H_f + [H_N - H_f])$

where H_{Ab} is c.p.m. of sample from antibody bag, H_f is c.p.m. of free hapten in bottle and H_N is c.p.m. in bag containing irrelevant immunoglobulin.

Then allow for the specific activity of the hapten.

The association constant may then be calculated using the Langmuir plot as detailed in the following section.

3.1.3 Ammonium sulphate precipitation (Farr assay)

Determination of antibody affinity can be simplified and speeded up by using precipitation. Tests based on secondary mechanisms, such as precipitation, do not necessarily measure the degree of primary binding of antigen to antibody, as although antigen–antibody interactions occur for all proportions of antigen and antibody, in the region of antibody excess there is very little precipitate; the complexes form but remain soluble. Techniques such as the Farr assay were designed to overcome these problems and so are more direct measures of the primary binding reaction.

The basis of Farr assay is as follows: ammonium sulphate is added to diluted serum to 50% saturation, and most of the immunoglobulin is precipitated, while other serum proteins such as albumin, remain in solution. Antigen, e.g. albumin, is radiolabelled and allowed to react with antibody, generally in antigen excess, so that soluble complexes are formed. An equal volume of saturated ammonium sulphate is added and all the immunoglobulin is precipitated. Only antigen complexed with antibody is precipitated under these conditions. The precipitates are washed with 50% saturated ammonium sulphate solution to remove any free antigen and their radioactive content determined. The amount of radioactivity in the precipitate is proportional to the amount of antigen bound by the antibody, and so results are expressed in terms of the antigen-binding capacity per ml of serum.

For accurate determinations, the results need to be calculated to the same degree of antigen excess for each antiserum. Therefore, in the original form of the assay, constant amounts of antigen are added to a series of dilutions of serum and the antigen-binding capacity determined at each dilution. By convention, all results are calculated on the 33% end-point, i.e. the dilution of serum that binds 33% of the added antigen. For many purposes a simpler assay can be used at a single antiserum dilution.

Determination of antigen-binding capacity

MATERIALS AND EQUIPMENT
Radiolabelled ^{125}I-albumin (2 mg/ml), specific activity 5–30×10^5 Bq/mg protein
Test anti-albumin sera, diluted 1 : 10 with phosphate-buffered saline (PBS)
Control serum diluted 1 : 10, to determine background binding
Saturated ammonium sulphate solution (Section 1.1.2)
Gamma spectrometer

Protocol.

Solution to be added	Tube number (in duplicate)		
	1	2 . . . . *n*	
Serum diluted 1 : 10 with PBS	0	20 µl⸺⟶	
^{125}I-albumin, 2 mg/ml	100 µl⸺⟶		
	Incubate and then add:		
PBS	0	400 µl⸺⟶	
Saturated ammonium sulphate	0	520 µl⸺⟶	

Repeat for each test antiserum and normal serum control.
PBS, phosphate-buffered saline.

METHOD

1 Add 20 µl of each diluted serum to tubes, preferably in duplicate (see Protocol).
2 Add 100 µl of ^{125}I-albumin to each tube. Cap the duplicate tubes labelled number 1; these are for determining the c.p.m. in the original aliquot.
3 Incubate with occasional shaking at 37°C for 2 h, then 2 h in the cold at 4°C.
4 Add 400 µl PBS to each test tube.
5 Add an equal volume (520 µl) of saturated ammonium sulphate solution to each tube, mix rapidly and thoroughly. Allow to stand for 15 min.
6 Spin at 3000 *g* for 10 min.
7 Remove and discard the supernatant.
8 Wash precipitate twice with 50% saturated ammonium sulphate solution by centrifugation.
9 After removing final wash supernatant, count the precipitate and the tubes labelled 1 (containing ^{125}I-albumin alone) in a γ spectrometer.

Calculation of results

Specific activity of albumin c.p.m./µg $= \dfrac{\text{no. c.p.m. in 100 µl} \times 10}{\text{protein concentration (µg/ml)}}$

Antigen content of precipitate

$= \dfrac{\text{no. c.p.m. of antiserum precipitate} - \text{no. c.p.m. of normal serum precipitate}}{\text{specific activity of the albumin}}$

Antigen-binding capacity/ml of serum = antigen content of precipitate $\times 50 \times$ original serum dilution.

The antigen-binding capacity is expressed as µg albumin bound/ml original serum.

TECHNICAL NOTES

• Specific activity is quoted in Bq rather than c.p.m./mg as this enables standardization. Determination of c.p.m. depends upon the efficiency of the counting equipment and so would vary from laboratory to laboratory.

- For demonstration purposes, the incubation times in step 3 above may be reduced to 15 min at 37°C and 30 min on ice, and still yield useful data.
- With some antigens it is necessary to use precipitating agents other than ammonium sulphate to ensure that the antigen remains in solution unless bound to antibody. A mixture of ethanol and ammonium acetate has been found useful for several assays of antibody binding to hormones, and polyethylene glycol (PEG) for peptide and immunoglobulin antigens. A neat adaptation utilizes PEG, in which labelled C1q is soluble, to precipitate and detect immune complexes binding to the labelled C1q (see also June *et al.* 1979).
- The technique can be modified to yield qualitative as well as quantitative information. With ammonium sulphate each immunoglobulin isotype is precipitated; however, it is possible to induce selective precipitation by adding an excess of anti-isotype serum. For example, anti-IgG precipitation of IgG antibodies would allow the determination of the antigen-binding capacity of this isotype in a polyclonal serum. This can be repeated with specific antisera for each class and subclass. The response in the different classes is found to differ markedly with different immunization schedules.

Ammonium sulphate precipitation for determining antibody affinity

Determination of antibody affinity can be simplified by using a variation of the Farr assay. A constant amount of antibody is reacted with increasing concentrations of antigen and left to equilibrate. The concentration of bound antigen is detected in the complex after ammonium sulphate precipitation and the concentration of free antigen determined in the supernatant. If the reciprocal of bound antigen is plotted against the reciprocal of the free antigen concentration and the line extrapolated to $1/[Ag] = 0$, the reciprocal of the bound antigen will equal the reciprocal of the total antibody-combining sites.

MATERIALS AND EQUIPMENT

Radiolabelled antigen, e.g. ^{125}I human serum albumin (HSA)

Antiserum, e.g. anti-HSA

Normal serum, as control

Saturated ammonium sulphate solution

Conical centrifuge tubes, 0.4 ml capacity

Beckman 152 microfuge (or equivalent)

Gamma spectrometer

Protocol.

	Tube number							
	1	2	3	4	5	6	7	8
Antiserum or control serum	50 µl ————————————————————→							
PBS	50 µl ————————————————————→							
^{125}I Ag µg in 100 µl PBS	2.5	5.0	10	20	40	80	160	320

1 Set up 16 tubes (eight each for antiserum and normal control serum) as shown in the Protocol.
2 Mix the contents of the tubes thoroughly and incubate for 1 h at room temperature.
3 Add 0.2 ml saturated ammonium sulphate solution and mix immediately.
4 Incubate for 1 h at room temperature.
5 Spin the tubes at 10 000 g for 5 min.
6 Remove and keep 0.1 ml of supernatant.
7 Wash each precipitate twice with 50% saturated ammonium sulphate.
8 Determine the c.p.m. of radioactivity in the supernatant samples and precipitates using a γ spectrometer.

Data required

Free antigen concentration = total radioactivity (c.p.m.) in the supernatant, i.e. radioactivity in 100 µl sample from step 6 multiplied by 4. Bound antigen concentration = (c.p.m. antiserum precipitate – c.p.m. control precipitate), for each antigen concentration.

Calculation of results

All the values should be expressed as molar concentrations; 1 pmol HSA = 0.068 µg.
1 Record and calculate the results as in Table 3.1(a,b).
2 Plot $1/b$ (column 9) against $1/[Ag]$ (column 10). Extrapolate the graph line to $1/[Ag] = 0$, i.e. the intercept on the $1/b$ axis: this is the value of $1/[Ab_t]$.
3 Use the value for $[Ab_t]$ to calculate the values shown in Table 3.1(b).
4 From Table 3.1(b) plot:

$$\log \frac{b}{Ab_t - b} \text{ (column 3) against } \log[Ag] \text{ (column 4).}$$

The intercept on the $\log[Ag]$ axis, i.e. when

$$\log \frac{b}{[Ab_t] - b} = 0$$

equals $1/K$, therefore:

$$K = \frac{1}{[Ag]}$$

The units of K are litres per mole.

Low-affinity antibodies have K values around 10^5 l/mol, whereas high-affinity antibodies often have K values of 10^{12} l/mol or more.

TECHNICAL NOTES
• Errors always occur during the washing of precipitates, particularly as dissociation may take place on removal of the free antibody and free antigen. A procedure to avoid this has been introduced using radioactive sodium as a buffer tracer. This is described below.
• There has been discussion as to how quickly the addition of ammonium sulphate freezes the equilibrium. Most authors assume that this is immediate and so calculate the concentrations,

Table 3.1(a) Table for calculation of Ab_t

	Column number									
	1	2	3	4	5	6	7	8	9	10
Tube no.	µg albumin per tube	pmoles of albumin	c.p.m. in supernatant free [Ag]	c.p.m. antiserum precipitate	c.p.m. control precipitate	Bound antigen	Moles of Ag bound (b)	Moles of free Ag	$1/b$	$1/[Ag]$
						c.p.m. col. 4 – c.p.m. col. 5	c.p.m. col. 6 ÷ SA	c.p.m. col. 3 ÷ SA	Reciprocal of col. 7	Reciprocal of col. 8
1	2.5	1 pmole = 0.068 µg								
2	5									
3	10									
4	20									
5	40									
6	80									
7	160									
8	320									

* Specific activity (SA) of antigen $= \dfrac{\text{c.p.m.}}{\text{molar concentration of antigen}}$.

Table 3.1(b) Table for calculation of K

Tube no.	Column number			
	1	2	3	4
	pmoles of antigen	$\dfrac{b}{[Ab_t] - b}$	$\text{Log}\dfrac{b}{[Ab_t] - b}$	Log[Ag]
1			Log_{10} col. 2	Log_{10} free antigen
2				concentration, i.e.
3				log col. 8, Fig. 3.1a.
4				
5				
6				
7				
8				

at equilibrium, on the volumes prior to adding ammonium sulphate, but it has been suggested that calculating the concentration on the basis of the volume after adding the precipitating agent is more accurate.

- It must be recognized that the high salt concentrations used to precipitate the immunoglobulin may also dissociate some of the complexes, particularly those involving low-affinity antibodies. The use of polyethylene glycol as a precipitating agent avoids this problem.

3.1.4 Double isotope modification to avoid washing

A major problem with the ammonium sulphate method is the need to wash the precipitates, and thus the potential to lose precipitate or for some of the complex to dissociate. A useful development introduced by Steward (1997) was the incorporation of ^{22}NaCl as a marker of buffer volume. Most of the supernatant can then be removed, without accurate measurement, and the amount of free radioactive antigen remaining in the precipitate estimated from the ^{22}Na counts to indicate the amount of buffer solution remaining with the precipitate. The technique is possible as ^{22}Na and ^{125}I have substantially different radiation energy emission spectra and so can be counted separately in a two-channel γ counter.

There is some overlap of ^{22}Na counts into the ^{125}I channel; this is determined as part of the experimental design and is allowed for during the calculations. The method is as above (Ammonium sulphate precipitation for determining antibody affinity) except for the incorporation of ^{22}NaCl into the assay and the inclusion of tubes containing ^{22}NaCl alone, or ^{22}NaCl plus antigen, to estimate the spillover of ^{22}Na counts into the ^{125}I channel.

MATERIALS AND EQUIPMENT
These are as for the ammonium sulphate affinity determination but in addition:
^{22}NaCl
Two-channel γ spectrometer

Note: A single-channel counter may be used by resetting and counting the sample again.

1   Set up five microfuge tubes with the same amount of ^{22}NaCl in each tube (about 50 000 c.p.m. in 50 μl phosphate-buffered saline (PBS) should be sufficient) to provide replicate determinations of the total sodium counts.

2   Set up the 16 assay tubes for antiserum and control serum as in the Protocol above (see p. 79). In addition to adding varying amounts of ^{125}I-antigen also add the same amounts of ^{22}NaCl in 50 μl PBS to each tube as in step 1. This takes the place of the PBS mentioned in the Protocol.

3   Mix and incubate for 1 h at room temperature.

4   Add an equal volume of saturated ammonium sulphate solution and mix immediately.

5   Incubate for 1 h at room temperature.

6   Spin the tubes at 10 000 g for 5 min.

7   Aspirate the majority of the supernatant, taking great care not to disturb the precipitate.

8   Count the radioactivity of the ^{22}NaCl, ^{22}NaCl plus antigen, and precipitate tubes in a two-channel γ counter.

Calculation

For each antigen calculate the total ^{125}I counts added per tube (corrected for ^{22}Na spillover):

$$I = I' - \frac{Nx}{y}$$

where I' is total counts in ^{125}I channel including ^{22}Na spillover (for tubes containing ^{125}I antigen plus ^{22}Na), N is total counts in ^{22}Na channel (for tubes containing ^{125}I antigen plus ^{22}Na), x is counts in ^{125}I channel in tubes containing ^{22}Na only and y is counts in ^{22}Na channel in tubes containing ^{22}Na only.

Counts in ^{125}I channel of experimental tubes (corrected for spillover from ^{22}Na):

$$i = i' - \frac{nx}{y}$$

where i' is counts in ^{125}I channel of experimental tubes including spillover from ^{22}Na and n is counts in ^{22}Na channel of experimental tubes.

In the experimental tubes containing precipitate:

(a) the ^{22}Na counts allow a calculation of the carryover of free antigen (by determining the amount of buffer carried over); and

(b) the ^{125}I counts allow a calculation of the concentration of antigen, both free and bound to antibody.

Therefore, at each of the eight antigen concentrations:

$$\% \text{ antigen bound} = \frac{Ni - nI}{I(N - n)} \times 100$$

where terms of the equation are defined as above.

Antigen bound specifically to antibody =

$$\frac{100}{\% \text{ Ag bound by antiserum} - \% \text{ Ag bound by control serum}} \times \text{total Ag}$$

(thus correcting for non-specific uptake by the control serum).

Free antigen = total antigen − bound antigen.

Calculate antibody affinity graphically as in Section 3.1.1 above.

3.1.5 Determination of functional antibody affinity by ELISA

Absolute affinity determinations are complex and time consuming. Useful information on relative affinity can be obtained by performing ELISA assays in the presence and absence of diethylamine. This chaotropic agent has a much greater effect in inhibiting the binding of low-compared with high-affinity antibodies. Other reagents that can be used include 6 M urea (see Holliman *et al.* 1994).

Using a panel of monoclonal antibodies, diethylamine inhibition produced the same ranking of relative affinity as was seen with a full-affinity determination. This technique is especially useful for comparing the relative affinities of different immunoglobulin subclasses.

MATERIALS
As for ELISA (see Section 5.4.3)
Diethylamine
Phosphate-buffered saline (PBS) containing 0.25% gelatin and 0.05% Tween

---

METHOD

1 Prepare coated wells for the ELISA assay (see Section 5.4.3).
2 Instead of a single serum dilution, make serial dilutions of the antiserum in PBS/0.25% gelatin/0.05% Tween in the presence and absence of diethylamine. (A concentration of between 1 and 50 mM should be suitable depending on the affinity range of the antibody. A 20 mM solution is worth trying first.)
3 Proceed as for ELISA.
4 Plot the optical density (OD) on the ordinate against $\log_{10}$ serum dilution for the two curves.
5 Measure the degree of left displacement of the dose–response curve in the presence of diethylamine at 50% of the maximum OD.

Results are expressed as $\log_{10}$ of this displacement. The higher the value of the displacement the lower the functional affinity.

A simple ELISA technique for determining avidity has been based on the shift of end-point titre, in the presence of a dissociating agent, 6 M urea, following examination of serum dilution curves (Hedman *et al.* 1989; Lappalainen *et al.* 1993; Holliman *et al.* 1994).

The antibody is expressed as:

$$\frac{\text{End-point titre in the presence of 6 M urea}}{\text{End-point titre in the absence of 6 M urea}} \times 100\%$$

An extremely high-affinity antibody would bind just as well with urea as without, and so would have a value of 100%. However, low-affinity antibodies might have values nearing zero.

Antigen must be coated onto the plate in urea, or at least shown to be stably coated upon addition of the urea in order to avoid loss of antigen in the assay. A similar approach has been used for cellular antigens with hantavirus-infected cells. Virus-infected cells are dried down onto glass microscope slides, and serial dilutions of the antivirus antibody samples are allowed to bind, with and without urea. After detection by immunofluorescence, the end-point titre may be compared. The technique has been shown to produce useful results on estimating the time course of viral infections in bank voles (Gavrilovskaya *et al.* 1993).

3.2 Secondary interactions: precipitation

3.2.1 Quantitative precipitin test

Developed by Heidelberger and Kendall, this technique is the basis of all quantitative studies of antigen–antibody interaction. Increasing amounts of antigen are added to a constant amount of antibody and the weight of precipitate formed in each tube is determined. It is dependent on the presence of an intact Fc region in the antibody. Precipitation is far less efficient with F(ab')$_2$ fragments of antibody, even though they are divalent. The procedure outlined below is suitable for most antisera and antigens.

MATERIALS
Antiserum, e.g. anti-human serum albumin (aged or inactivated by heating at 56°C for 15 min)
Human serum albumin (HSA) (1 mg/ml)
Phosphate-buffered saline (PBS)
0.1 M sodium hydroxide

Note: One of the properties of complement is to maintain immune complexes in solution and to resolubilize insoluble complexes. Therefore, if fresh sera are used to produce the precipitin curve, little precipitation will occur unless they are heated to 56°C for 30 min to destroy complement prior to assay. Most stored or commercially obtained antisera have already lost this activity.

METHOD

1 Add antigen, PBS and antiserum to a series of numbered tubes (suitable for centrifugation), according to the Protocol. (For antisera with high or low antibody content it will be necessary to increase or decrease the range of antigen concentrations used.)

Protocol.

Reagent	1	2	3	4	5	6	7	8	9	10
Antigen (µl)	0	10	20	50	100	150	200	250	350	450
PBS	450	440	430	400	350	300	250	200	100	0
Antiserum (µl)	100———————————————————————————————→									

2 Mix the reactants thoroughly.
3 Incubate at 37°C for 1 h and then at 4°C overnight. (For accurate determinations, these incubations can be extended for up to 10 days at 4°C. However, for demonstration

Continued on p. 86

---

purposes using high-titred and high-avidity antisera, illustrative curves may be obtained with only 30 min incubation at 37°C and 30 min at 4°C.)

4 Spin at 3000 g for 5 min at 4°C and remove supernatant. An angle-head rotor should be used as the precipitate is then formed at the side of the tube, thus facilitating removal of the supernatant.

5 Check each supernatant for free antigen and antibody using a sensitive technique, e.g. single radial immunodiffusion.

6 Wash the precipitate twice by centrifugation with cold PBS.

7 Redissolve the final precipitate in 0.1 M sodium hydroxide (the volume to be used depends on the spectrophotometer cuvettes available, but should be about 1 ml for the amounts of reagents used here).

8 Measure the absorbance at 280 nm and plot a graph of the absorbance units of the redissolved precipitate against the amount of antigen added (see Fig. 3.3).

Calculations

1 Determine the antibody content per ml of antiserum.

2 Calculate the number of antigenic determinants on each antigen molecule (i.e. antigenic valency).

Theoretical basis of the calculations

Antibody content of the serum

If the supernatant from each tube is examined for the presence of excess antibody or antigen, there will be one point at which no free antibody or antigen can be detected. This is the point of *equivalence* which occurs just before maximum precipitation (Fig. 3.3). The amount of precipitate increases after the equivalence point because of continued incorporation of antigen into the complex. Eventually soluble complexes are formed in antigen excess and the amount of precipitate decreases.

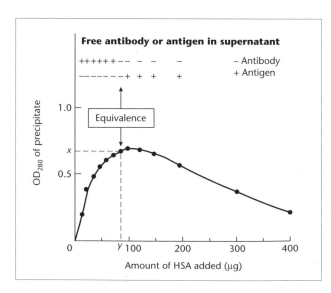

Fig. 3.3 **Precipitin curve of human serum albumin (HSA) with anti-HSA.** An increasing amount of antigen was added to a fixed concentration of antiserum and the optical density of the precipitate (in sodium hydroxide) determined. The supernatant was assayed for the presence of free antibody or antigen by single radial immunodiffusion. The equivalence point (arrowed), when all the antibody and antigen is complexed in the precipitate, occurs just before the point of maximum precipitation. To determine the equivalence point exactly, it is frequently necessary to repeat the assay using smaller steps in antigen concentrations around the concentration required to give maximum precipitation.

In Fig. 3.3, at equivalence, the precipitate contains x µg of total protein; if this includes y µg of antigen then there is $(x - y)$ µg of antibody. This is the total amount of antibody in the volume of serum used.

Specimen calculation (from Fig. 3.3)

The precipitate was dissolved in 1 ml of 0.1 M sodium hydroxide and absorbance measurements made in 1-cm light path cells.

IgG absorbance of 1.0 at 280 nm in 1-cm cell = 0.695 mg/ml.

HSA absorbance of 1.0 at 280 nm in 1-cm cell = 1.886 mg/ml.

From the graph, at equivalence absorbance of precipitate $x = 0.65$.

The precipitate contains 87.5 µg HSA which, if dissolved alone in 1.0 ml of sodium hydroxide, would give an absorbance of 0.004 (calculated from the extinction coefficient). Hence:

absorbance of antibody component of the precipitate = OD precipitate − OD due to HSA

$$= 0.65 - 0.04$$

$$= 0.61.$$

Hence,

$$\text{total antibody content of serum (mg/ml)} = \frac{\text{absorbance} \times \text{extinction coefficient}}{\text{sample volume}}$$

$$= \frac{0.61 \times 0.695}{0.1}$$

$$= 4.24 \text{ mg/ml.}$$

This antiserum has a relatively high antibody content.

Determination of antigenic valency

For this determination some theoretical aspects of the precipitation curve must be considered. When the antigen concentration is low there is a relative antibody excess (Fig. 3.3). At the other extreme, at high antigen concentrations, there is free antigen and so each combining site of the antibody is occupied. At either of these extremes the complexes are relatively small. At equivalence, however, there is much cross-linking between molecules and large complexes are formed.

Every antigenic determinant is likely to be covered by a separate antibody molecule at extreme antibody excess. If we calculate the amount of antibody in the precipitate at this point, in the same way as above, we can determine the ratio of antibody : antigen, and so the relative numbers of molecules of each in the precipitate, i.e.

$$\frac{\text{weight of antigen}}{\text{molecular weight antigen}} : \frac{\text{weight of antibody}}{\text{molecular weight antibody}}$$

In a hyperimmune serum the major proportion of antibody will be of the IgG class with a molecular weight of 150 000. The molecular weight of HSA (the antigen in this case) is 68 000.

To obtain the best estimate of antigenic valency, the ratio of antibody : antigen in the precipitate should be plotted against the amount of antigen added, as in Fig. 3.4. If the plot is extended to the antibody : antigen axis, the intercept will give the ratio at infinite antibody excess.

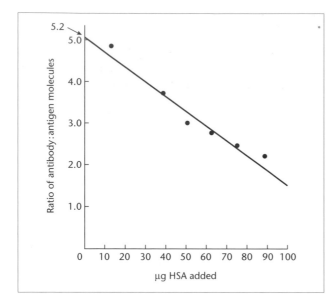

Fig. 3.4 Ratio of antibody : antigen molecules at different levels of antibody excess. The regression line calculated from the antibody : antigen ratios over a range of antigen concentrations, all in antigen excess, gives an intercept of 5.2 (arrow), indicating that there are five antigenic determinants detected on the HSA molecule by this antiserum. This antiserum differs from that used in Fig. 3.3.

Specimen calculation (from Fig. 3.4)

Absorbance of precipitate = 0.15.

Absorbance of HSA (calculated as above) = 0.005 (10 µg).

Hence absorbance of antibody in the precipitate = 0.145 which is equivalent to 101.5 µg/ml IgG. Therefore the molar ratios are:

$$\frac{10}{68\,000} : \frac{101.5}{150\,000} = 0.000147 : 0.000677.$$

Therefore the ratio of antibody : antigen molecules = 4.6 : 1. This antiserum recognizes between four and five determinants on the HSA molecule.

The quantitative precipitin test is particularly useful as it can be carried out without antibody standards; only known concentrations of antigen are required. The shape of the curve varies with different antigens: with protein antigens a sharp peak is usually obtained, but with polysaccharides there is usually a broader peak. In addition, the various antisera have different properties. Rabbit antisera give the typical curve shown in Fig. 3.3, whereas horse antisera give precipitates that have relatively greater solubility in both antigen and antibody excess. Both types of precipitin curve may be obtained with human antisera.

3.3 **Precipitation in gels**

The precipitin test gives a great deal of basic information, but it is lengthy to perform and requires relatively large quantities of reagents. In addition, it does not provide an easy basis for a qualitative comparison of antisera or antigens. Many gel precipitation techniques have been developed for qualitative analysis, based on the principle that if antigen and antibody are placed in two adjacent wells in agar, they will diffuse into the agar and set up two opposing concentration gradients between the wells; at a point of optimal proportions between these gradients a line of precipitation will form. Thus, the analysis will be carried out with the reactants at their equivalence point, without the need for empirical determination.

Buffered agar and agar-coated slides may be prepared as described below for use in the procedures described in this section. The simplicity of precipitin gel techniques should not decry their usefulness. They are robust and easy to perform and still form the basis of many commercial kits.

3.3.1 Buffered agar

MATERIALS AND EQUIPMENT
Barbitone buffer
Agar

> **METHOD**
>
> 1   Mix 2 g of agar with 50 ml of distilled water and dissolve by heating in a microwave oven.
> 2   Add 50 ml of hot barbitone buffer and mix well. The agar may be stored at 4°C for many weeks.
> *Note*: The agar must be bought specifically for electrophoresis; many of the culture agars are not suitable for this purpose.

3.3.2 Precoating glass slides

Gel precipitation techniques may be conveniently performed on glass microscope slides and the gel then dried down onto the glass for permanent storage. To ensure good adhesion of the gel to the slide it is necessary first to coat the slide with a thin layer of agar which is allowed to dry, before layering on the analytical agar gel.

MATERIALS AND EQUIPMENT
Glass microscope slides
Agar

> **METHOD**
>
> 1   Dissolve 0.5 g of agar in 100 ml of distilled water as above.
> 2   Pipette the agar solution onto clean, dry slides. Add enough to cover sparingly one surface of the slide.
> 3   Dry the slides and store at room temperature until required.

3.4 Single radial immunodiffusion (SRID)

Oudin originally used analytical techniques involving the diffusion of antigens into an antibody-containing gel (single diffusion in one direction). Feinberg and later Mancini, Carbonara and Heremans extended this technique by incorporating the antiserum into a thin layer of agar and placing the antigen in wells cut into the antibody-containing agar.

As the antigen diffuses radially a ring of precipitation forms around the well and moves outwards, eventually becoming stationary at equivalence. At equivalence, the diameter and area of the ring are related to the antigen concentration in the well. Using standard antigen concentrations a calibration curve may be constructed to determine unknown concentrations of the same antigen.

The optimal dilution for the antiserum will, of course, depend upon the strength of the antiserum and antigen as the diameter of the precipitation ring is inversely proportional to the antiserum concentration. In practice, with rabbit antisera to human IgG, a final dilution of approximately 1 : 40 in the agar is suitable for measuring IgG concentrations in the range of 50–200 µg/ml. However, this is only a guide; a standard curve should be determined for each antiserum.

MATERIALS AND EQUIPMENT

2% agar in barbitone buffer

Precoated slides

Antiserum, e.g. anti-human IgG

Standard antigen solution, e.g. human IgG

Phosphate-buffered saline (PBS)

Flat, level surface (use a spirit level)

Gel punch

Humid chamber (plastic box with damp filter paper)

Pasteur pipettes

Water vacuum pump

METHOD

1 Melt the agar in a microwave oven and transfer to a 56°C water bath. This temperature will keep the agar molten but is low enough to avoid denaturation of the antibody.

2 Dilute the antiserum with PBS. Typically, add 75 µl of an antiserum to 1.9 ml of PBS and warm to 56°C.

3 Add the diluted antiserum (~ 2 ml) from step 2 to 1 ml of agar at 56°C and mix well.

4 Layer the agar onto a precoated slide standing on a levelled surface and allow to set.

5 After the agar has set, use a gel punch to cut about eight wells per slide. The wells should be 2–3 mm in diameter, and must have vertical sides.

6 Remove the agar plug with a Pasteur pipette attached to a water vacuum pump.

7 Fill each of four wells with standard solutions of 50, 100, 150 and 200 µg/ml IgG. Use the other wells for the IgG solutions of unknown concentrations. Maintain a standard volume by filling the wells quickly until the meniscus just disappears. Alternatively a measured volume, such as 10 µl, may be accurately pipetted into each well.

8 Leave the slide in a humid box to equilibrate. (Although a satisfactory standard curve may be obtained by overnight equilibration, the points will better approximate to a straight line if the slide is allowed to equilibrate longer: IgG and IgA 48 h, IgM 72 h. IgG concentrations may also be determined by incubation at 37°C for 4 h.)

3.4.1 Measurement of precipitation rings

The diameter of each ring may be measured either directly using a magnifying glass with a µm scale or, after staining, with a plastic ruler.

Direct measurement

Hold the slide over a black background and illuminate it from the side. Measure the rings from the reverse side through the glass plate, do not rest the magnifying glass on the gel. If the rings are not distinct, soak the slides in 4% tannic acid for 1 min to increase resolution. (This is not a permanent preparation.)

Stained preparations

1 Wash the slide for 24 h in several changes of PBS to remove free protein from the agar.
2 Cover the slide with good-quality, lint-free, filter paper and dry overnight.
3 Remove the filter paper after dampening it slightly.
The slide may then be stained with any protein dye, but we suggest Coomassie blue R-250.

MIXTURE FOR STAINING SOLUTION
Coomassie brilliant blue R-250 (1.25 g)
Glacial acetic acid (50 ml)
Distilled water (185 ml)

METHOD

1 Dissolve the Coomassie dye in the glacial acetic acid and distilled water.
2 Stain the slide for 5 min and differentiate in the same solution without the dye. Staining with this dye is reversible so do not leave the slide too long in the destaining solution.
3 Place the dry, stained slides in a photographic enlarger and measure the diameter of the precipitation rings with a ruler.

The staining solution may be stored for several weeks in a stoppered bottle. The destaining solution can be regenerated by passing through powdered charcoal.

Calculation of results

Figure 3.5 shows a typical determination. The diameters of the rings were measured and plotted on a linear scale against the log of the antigen concentration. With a semilog transformation, the points should approximate to a straight line. If the assay has been allowed to reach equilibrium the areas of the rings should be calculated and plotted against the antigen concentration on a linear scale.

TECHNICAL NOTES
- The assay can be made more sensitive by incorporating from 2 to 4% polyethylene glycol in the agar to enhance precipitation.
- If chicken antisera are used, 7–8% NaCl should be added to the agar to improve precipitation.
- Although single radial immunodiffusion is now used as a quantitative technique, its first use was to compare the identities of different antigen solutions. If two antigens, placed in neighbouring wells close together, are identical in terms of their antigenic determinants then the two rings of precipitation fuse completely. If the antigens share no determinants recognized by the antiserum then each ring forms independently. Since the work of Ouchterlony, simpler procedures have been introduced to test the relationships between antigens or antibodies.

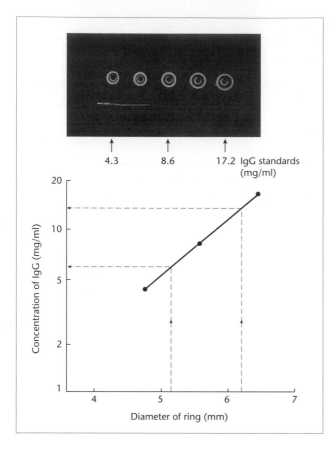

Fig. 3.5 Measurement of IgG concentration by single radial immunodiffusion. A calibration curve is constructed from the diameter of the precipitation rings formed at equilibrium by IgG standards of known concentration. The concentration of unknown samples can then be determined with reference to the standard curve.

3.5 **Double diffusion in two dimensions**

In this technique the antigen and antibody are allowed to migrate towards each other in a gel and a line of precipitation is formed where the two reactants meet. As this precipitate is soluble in excess antigen, a sharp line is produced at equivalence, its relative position being determined by the concentration of the antigen and antibody in the agar. The local concentration of each react-ant depends on: (a) absolute concentration in the well; (b) its molecular size; and (c) the rate at which it is able to diffuse through the gel. Multiple lines of precipitation will be present if the antigen and antibody contain several molecular species.

The particular advantage of the technique is that several antigens or antisera can be compared around a single well of antibody or antigen.

MATERIALS AND EQUIPMENT
2% agar in barbitone buffer
Antigen and antibody solutions (see procedure for details)
Gel punch
Pasteur pipettes
Water vacuum pump

Antigen concentration: initially use 1 mg/ml, but vary the concentration to obtain optimal results

Antiserum: use whole anti-IgG, non-absorbed. Specific anti-IgG sera available commercially are often absorbed with light chains to render them class specific

METHOD

1 Melt the agar in a microwave oven.

2 Pour agar onto precoated slides; use a levelled surface.

3 Punch pattern required.

4 Suck out agar plugs with a Pasteur pipette connected to a water vacuum pump.

5 Fill the wells with antibody or antigen until the meniscus just disappears.

6 Place the slide in a humid chamber and incubate overnight at a constant temperature.

Suggested antibody and antigen patterns

A straightforward demonstration of identity and non-identity can be shown using the antigen mixtures as in Fig. 3.6. In addition, this technique may be used to show the relationships between IgG molecules and their enzymic digests prepared in Chapter 2. Arrange the wells as shown in Fig. 3.7.

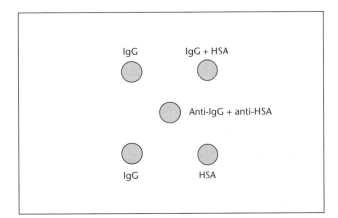

Fig. 3.6 Design of Ouchterlony plate to show reactions of identity and non-identity IgG and albumin (HSA) with their respective antisera.

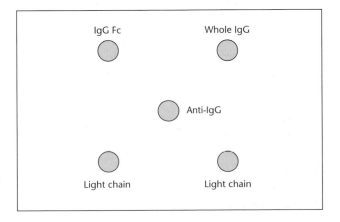

Fig. 3.7 Well arrangement to demonstrate spur formation, lines of identity and lines of non-identity. IgG Fc prepared by papain digestion of IgG (Section 1.7). Light chains prepared by reduction and alkylation of IgG (Section 1.6).

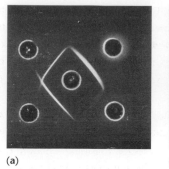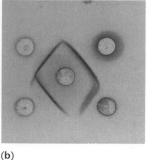

(a)　　　　　　　　　　　　　(b)

Fig. 3.8 The relationship of human IgG subclasses. In (**a**) and (**b**) wells 1–4 contain human IgG_1, IgG_2, IgG_3 and IgG_4, respectively, and the central well contains rabbit anti-human IgG. (Antisera prepared by immunizing rabbits with IgG obtained from normal human serum and isolated by ion-exchange chromatography.) Antiserum (**a**) recognized subclass differences between IgG_1 and IgG_4, hence the double spur, but failed to recognize IgG_3. Antiserum (**b**) recognized subclass differences associated with IgG_1 alone and so produced a single spur. Both antisera were raised against the same pool of antigen, the variation is due to the rabbits used for immunization.

TECHNICAL NOTE

The rate of diffusion is temperature dependent. Precipitin lines can often be seen within 3 h at 37°C.

Interpretation of results

The basic patterns of precipitation as shown in Fig. 3.8.

(a) *Reaction of identity.* This occurs between identical antigenic determinants; the lines of precipitation fuse to give one continuous arc.

(b) *Reaction of non-identity.* Where two antigens do not contain any common antigenic determinants the two lines are formed independently and cross without any interaction.

(c) *Reaction of partial identity.* This has two components: (i) those antigenic determinants which are common to both antigens give a continuous line of identity; (ii) the unique determinant(s) recognized on one of the antigens give(s), in addition, a line of non-identity so that a spur is formed. Of course, the antiserum may recognize unique determinants in both antigens: this would give rise to two spurs.

All these concepts of identity and non-identity are in terms of recognition by the antiserum. An antiserum recognizing many determinants on the antigen molecules is necessary for the demonstration of all these features.

3.6 Turbidimetry and nephelometry

Many laboratories quantify immune complexes formed by the interaction of antigen and antibody using the techniques of turbidimetry or nephelometry. In these techniques monochromatic light is used to illuminate a cuvette containing a suspension of the immune complex. Light is both absorbed and deflected by the complexes.

In turbidimetry the amount of light absorbed is measured in a spectrophotometer. In nephelometry the amount of light scattered is measured by a detector mounted at an angle to the original light path. In both cases the measurements are proportional to the quantity of complex. The most sensitive instruments, incorporating laser light sources, are able to detect nanogram quantities of complex. Many of the machines are automated so that many hundreds of samples may be processed each day.

Both turbidimetry and nephelometry measure the same immune complexes, only the detection equipment is different. The apparatus is usually automated and great care must be taken to establish the standard curve to work out only within the standard range. The precipitin curve (Fig. 3.3) clearly shows that in antigen excess, the complexes become more soluble as they become smaller; the phenomenon can lead to erroneously low values being obtained from the instrument.

3.7 Immunoelectrophoretic analysis

Studying antibody–antigen interaction solely by simple diffusion is possible if there are only a few components in the system but, if there are multiple antigens reacting with several antibodies, the precipitin lines become difficult to resolve and impossible to interpret.

Increased resolution can be obtained by combining electrophoresis with immunodiffusion in gels, in the technique known as immunoelectrophoresis. This is useful in the immunological examination of serum proteins: Serum proteins separate in agar gels, under the influence of an electric field, into albumin and α1-, α2-, β- and γ-globulins. If you are not familiar with this electrophoretic separation of serum proteins, it is advisable to perform a simple agar gel electrophoresis as this will aid your understanding of the patterns obtained with the later techniques.

3.7.1 Agar gel electrophoresis

MATERIALS AND EQUIPMENT
2% agar in barbitone buffer
Barbitone buffer
Precoated microscope slides
Normal and myeloma sera
10% v/v glacial acetic acid in water
Electrophoresis tank and power pack, e.g. BioRad; Shandon Scientific Ltd
Gel punch

METHOD
1 Melt the agar in a microwave oven.
2 Mark the end of the slide that will be positive during the electrophoresis. If required, number the slides.
3 Pour 3–5 ml of agar onto the slide on a levelled surface.

Continued on p. 96

4 When the agar has set, punch the pattern. (Smaller wells than used for immunodiffusion are required. A fine Pasteur pipette or a hypodermic needle with a square cut end may be used.)

5 Suck out the agar plugs.

6 Fill the wells with serum to which a small amount of bromophenol blue dye has been added.

7 Fill the electrophoresis tank with full-strength barbitone buffer.

8 Place the slide in the electrophoresis tank and connect each end of the slide to the buffer chambers with rayon or filter paper wicks. Close the tank.

9 Apply a current of about 8 mA/slide. The voltage drop will be about 5–7 V/cm.

Note: The bromophenol blue dye binds to the serum albumin and as this is the fastest migrating band it serves as a marker throughout the electrophoresis. If excess dye has been added, however, a bright blue band of free dye will run in front of the albumin towards the anode.

10 When the albumin band (blue) nears the end of the slide—after about 60 min—remove the slide and fix the proteins by immersing the slide in 10% glacial acetic acid.

11 Cover the slide with fine filter paper and leave to dry.

12 Dampen the paper and remove, then stain the slide with Coomassie brilliant blue.

Suggested design

One well should contain normal serum and the other serum from a patient with multiple myelomatosis (a disease in which a single clone of antibody-forming cells becomes malignant and produces large amounts of monoclonal antibody). If you are using mouse reagents, then ascitic fluid or serum from a hybridoma-bearing animal will do equally well.

Results

The main serum proteins should show clearly as oval bands. Identify each band (albumin, α1-, α2-, β- and γ-globulins), and assign the abnormal monoclonal band to one of these (see Fig. 3.9).

TECHNICAL NOTE

The negative charge on the agar generates an electroendosmotic flow of water through the gel. This flow, and not the potential difference, is responsible for most of the separation seen with some of the globulins, which are near their isoelectric point under the conditions used. This is discussed in more detail later (see Section 3.7.2).

3.7.2 Immunoelectrophoresis

This is a powerful analytical technique with great resolving power, combining prior separation of antigens by electrophoresis with immunodiffusion against an antiserum (see Fig. 3.10).

MATERIALS AND EQUIPMENT

As for agar gel electrophoresis but in addition:

Anti-human whole serum

Fig. 3.9 Electrophoresis of serum samples. (a) Agar gel electrophoresis. Well 1, normal serum; well 2, serum from patient with multiple myeloma. Myeloma patients show an overproduction of antibody, usually of a single clone, in this case running in the γ-globulin region. You can see by inspection that there is an apparent decrease in the albumin content of the myeloma serum. (b) Electrophoresis on cellulose acetate membranes. Sample 1, normal serum as in (a); sample 2, myeloma serum as in (a); sample 3, serum from another patient with multiple myeloma. The principle of this separation of serum proteins is basically similar to that described for agar gel electrophoresis, except that the sample is applied onto the membrane as a band rather than via a well. The advantages of this technique are: (i) it is easier to discern the individual protein bands; and (ii) it is possible to clear the membrane with either glycerol or one of the commercially available clearing oils. Thus, the protein content of each band can be determined by scanning photometry. The 'hawk-shaped' band seen in sample 3 is often observed with myeloma protein and is probably caused by overloading of this band. (c) The traces obtained from scanning samples 1 and 2 of (b) are shown here. By integrating the area under each peak (this is usually done automatically by the scanner) it is possible to determine the total protein content of each band, and so confirm the observation made in (a), that there is indeed an albumin : γ-globulin reversal in the myeloma serum. Sample 1: normal serum, above albumin : globulin ratio 4.5. Sample 2: myeloma serum, below albumin : globulin ratio 0.7.

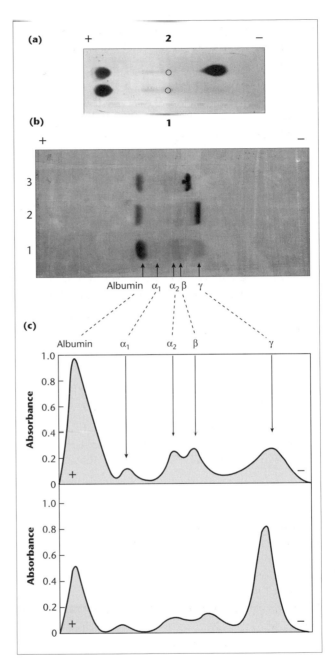

METHOD

1 Prepare slide as for agar gel electrophoresis.
2 Cut the pattern shown in Fig. 3.11. (Although cutters and moulds are available commercially for many different patterns, the holes can be made with hypodermic needles (cut square and sharpened) and the trough with razor blades.)

Continued on p. 98

3 Suck out the agar wells but do not remove the agar from the trough as this may cause abnormalities in protein banding during electrophoresis.
4 Fill one well with normal human serum and the other with myeloma serum.
5 Electrophorese as before.
6 Remove the agar trough and fill with anti-whole human serum.
7 Leave the slide to incubate overnight in a humid chamber at a constant temperature. (Again, lines will appear within 2–3 h if the slide is incubated at 37°C.)
8 Examine the lines produced and identify the IgG, IgA and IgM bands, and the bump in the precipitation arc typical of monoclonal immunoglobulin in the myeloma serum. The result obtained should be similar to that shown in Fig. 3.11.

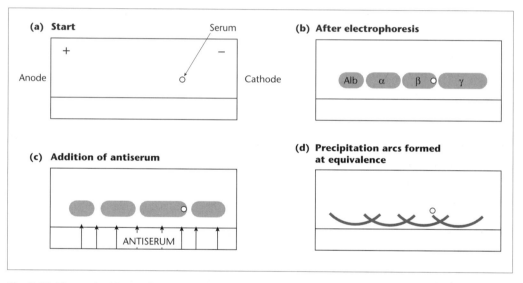

Fig. 3.10 Theoretical basis of immunoelectrophoresis. The antigen diffuses from a point source after the initial electrophoresis and interacts with the antiserum advancing on a plane front thus producing an arc of precipitation at equivalence.

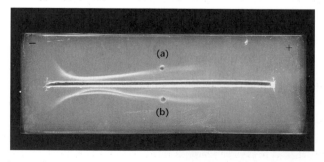

Fig. 3.11 Immunoelectrophoresis of human serum. Sample (**a**): normal human serum showing normal IgG precipitation arc. Sample (**b**): serum of a patient with multiple myeloma. In this case the monoclonal protein is identified as IgG because of the 'bump' in the IgG precipitation arc towards the antiserum well. Antiserum in central trough: rabbit anti-human immunoglobulin. (Photograph of unstained preparation.)

Although the relative distribution of the bands will depend on the batch of agar used and the initial electrophoresis distance, at the pH of the barbitone buffer (pH 8.2) the γ-globulins are close to their isoelectric point and so would not migrate appreciably in the applied electric field. However, as mentioned earlier, the negative charge on the agar generates an electroendosmotic flow of water in the gel which sweeps the γ-globulins towards the cathode. Often agarose is used as a supporting medium. This has less charge and so generates a lesser electroendosmotic flow.

3.7.3 Counterimmunoelectrophoresis

Gamma-globulins are exceptional in their cathodic migration; most other proteins move to the anode. The technique is similar to a one-dimensional Ouchterlony immunodiffusion but much faster as it is electrically driven, and more sensitive as all the antigen and antibody are driven towards each other. This property is used to advantage to cause antibody and antigen to migrate towards each other in the gel and form lines of precipitation.

MATERIALS AND EQUIPMENT
As for agar electrophoresis plus
Human serum albumin (HSA)
Anti-HSA serum

METHOD

1 Prepare slide as for agar gel electrophoresis.
2 Punch two wells (5–10 mm apart).
3 Place anti-HSA in the anodal well and HSA in the cathodal well.
4 Run the slide in an electrophoresis tank as before.
5 After 10–15 min, examine for a line of precipitation.

This technique lends itself to the rapid processing of many antisera or antigens.

3.8 Electrophoresis in antibody-containing media

Electrophoresis in antibody-containing media is related to the single radial immunodiffusion (SRID) test. Again, the speed of counterimmunoelectrophoresis is utilized to provide a fast quantitative assay. As in SRID the antiserum is incorporated into agar and wells are cut into the agar to hold the antigen. When an electric current is applied, the antigen migrates anodally into the agar while the antibody migrates cathodally. At first, soluble complexes are formed in antigen excess. As the antigen migrates further, it becomes more dilute, because antigen is held back in complexes; eventually equivalence is reached and an insoluble precipitate is formed. The precipitate redissolves and moves forward as more antigen reaches it. When no more antigen remains to enter the precipitate, a stable arc is formed which becomes stationary. Rocket shapes of precipitation are usually formed. The area under the rockets is proportional to the concentration of antigen (see Fig. 3.12).

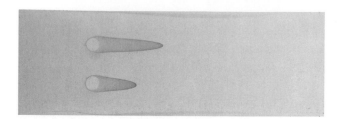

Fig. 3.12 Electrophoresis of human serum albumin (HSA) into agar containing anti-HSA. At equilibrium the height of the precipitation arc is proportional to the antigen concentration.

MATERIALS AND EQUIPMENT
2% agar in barbitone buffer
Human serum albumin (HSA)
Anti-HSA
Phosphate-buffered saline (PBS)
Agar precoated slides
Levelling table
Gel punch
56°C water bath
Electrophoresis tank and power pack, e.g. BioRad; Shandon Scientific Ltd.

METHOD

1 Melt agar in a microwave oven and allow to cool to 56°C.
2 Add antiserum to test tube and dilute for use (as a guide, use 0.1 ml of antiserum and add 0.9 ml PBS).
3 Mix and warm to 56°C.
4 Add 2 ml agar to the diluted antiserum and mix.
5 Pour onto precoated slides on the levelling table.
6 Punch wells.
7 Fill the wells with antigen solutions—in the range 50–500 µg/ml should be suitable.
8 Electrophorese at about 8 mA/slide, 5–10 V/cm.
9 Run for at least 2 h.
10 The peaks may be measured immediately, but this is easier after staining (see Section 3.4.1 for staining protocol).
11 Plot the height of the peaks against the antigen concentration if a full standard curve has been determined.

If the slide was run until the precipitin arcs became stationary, the relationship of peak height to antigen concentration is linear.

TECHNICAL NOTE
The assay cannot be used directly to quantify IgG as both the antigen and antibody would be moving in the same direction in the electrophoretic field. However, the electrophoretic mobility of the IgG antigen may be altered by carbamylation.

3.8.1 Carbamylation of IgG

MATERIALS

IgG samples (concentration around 1 mg/ml)

2 M KCNO (freshly prepared)

METHOD

1 Mix equal volumes of IgG sample and 2 M KCNO.
2 Incubate at 45°C for 30 min.
3 Cool mixture to 10–15°C and dilute appropriately (50–500 µg/ml) with electrophoresis buffer.
4 Electrophorese as above.

3.9 Two-dimensional or crossed immunoelectrophoresis

This technique combines the benefits of electrophoretic separation of antigens with their quantification by electrophoresis into an antibody-containing gel. It was originally introduced for the analysis of serum proteins but it has now been used in many systems. One application that is of particular interest is the analysis of C3 activation. The active and inactive forms of C3 share many antigenic determinants and so are detected simultaneously in simple immunodiffusion assays. C3 in its inactive state has a β_{1C} electrophoretic mobility which changes to a β_{1A} mobility after activation. Thus it is possible to show the appearance of activated C3 and the disappearance of inactive C3. The two forms of C3 are first separated by electrophoresis in agarose. Rockets of immune precipitates are formed by a second electrophoretic step, at right angles to the first, into a gel containing anti-C3.

MATERIALS AND EQUIPMENT

Barbitone buffer containing 0.01 M ethylene diamine tetra-acetic acid (EDTA, disodium salt)

Agarose

Anti-C3 serum

Serum samples for C3 quantification

Glass microscope slide (not precoated)

8 × 8 cm glass plate (precoated with agar)

Electrophoresis tank and power pack, e.g. Bio Rad, Shandon Scientific Ltd.

METHOD

First dimension
1 Prepare a 2% agarose solution in the barbitone buffer containing EDTA.
2 Layer 3 ml of agarose solution onto the uncoated microscope slide and allow to set. Use a levelled surface.
3 Cut a 1-mm well in the centre of the slide, remove the agarose plug, and fill the well with the serum sample.

Continued on p. 102

(a) Fresh human serum

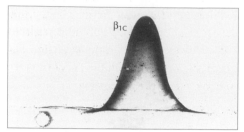

(b) Serum treated with heat-aggregated IgG

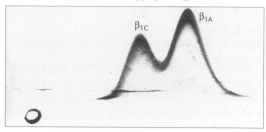

Fig. 3.13 Quantification of C3 activation. Although the inactive and active forms of C3 share many antigenic determinants, the activation of C3 is accompanied by a change in electrophoretic mobility from β_{1C} to β_{1A}. It is therefore possible to quantify C3 activation by combining electrophoresis in one dimension with 'rocket' immunoelectrophoresis in the second dimension. Activation of C3: C1q, C1r, and C1s are linked, probably through calcium, to form a trimolecular complex. The binding of C1q to the Fc of the immune complex (in this case we have substituted heat-aggregated IgG) initiates the esterase activity of the C1s component which activates C4 and C2. (The complement components were numbered before their order in the activation sequence was known.) The resulting C4b2a complex has 'C3 convertase' activity and so splits C3 (β_{1C} mobility) to C3a and C3b (β_{1A} mobility). The two rocket arcs of C3a and C3b are fused because of shared antigenic determinants.

4 Apply a potential difference of 150 V (constant voltage setting on power pack) for 2–3 h.
5 Cut and remove a 5-mm wide longitudinal strip of agarose from the centre portion of the slide, along its complete length. It must, of course, include the sample.

Second dimension
1 Prepare 12 ml of a 1 : 50–1 : 100 dilution of anti-C3 in 2% agarose solution at 56°C; the precise dilution of the antiserum to be used must be determined empirically.
2 Place the agarose strip at one end of the square glass plate (precoated) and cover the whole slide with 12 ml of agarose containing anti-C3.
3 Place the plate in the electrophoresis tank. The cathode must be at the end of the plate with the agarose strip, i.e. the electric field will cause the separated complement components to enter the antibody-containing gel at right angles to the first electrophoresis. Electrophorese at 40–50 V overnight (if cooling apparatus is available a higher voltage may be used for a shorter time).
4 Wash and stain the precipitin arcs (see Section 3.4.1).

Fresh serum should give a pattern similar to Fig. 3.13(a), while aged serum or serum with immune complexes should give a pattern more like Fig. 3.13(b).

3.10 Secondary interactions: agglutination

Particulate antigens may be cross-linked by antibody to give visible agglutination in a manner analogous to the formation of precipitates with soluble antigens.

The agglutination reaction has principally been exploited using erythrocytes as the particles and has been exploited in blood group serological techniques. Latex and bentonite suspensions have also proved useful. Antisera may be compared semiquantitatively by determining the end-points of their respective titration curves. The sera are diluted until they no longer give a visible reaction with antigen by agglutination. This is a measure of the relative antigen-binding capacity of a serum and can only be used to compare antisera when they are tested at the same time and with the same antigen. Conversely, the concentration of an antigen in solution may be determined by the degree of inhibition of a standard, homologous agglutination system.

3.11 **Haemagglutination**

The simplest form of this test involves the agglutination of erythrocytes (as antigens) by increasing dilutions of anti-erythrocyte sera.

MATERIALS AND EQUIPMENT
Anti-sheep erythrocyte sera (anti-SRBC)
Normal serum, as control
SRBC in phosphate-buffered saline (PBS), 2% v/v
0.1 M 2-mercaptoethanol in PBS
Microhaemagglutination trays (V-shaped)
Diluting loops or tulips (25 μl)
Standard dropping pipettes (25 μl) or multichannel automatic pipette
Sealer strip

Preparation in advance

Aged sera may be used directly but fresh sera must first be incubated at 56°C for 15 min to inactivate complement.

METHOD

For each antiserum and control serum prepare two rows of dilutions as follows:
1 Add 25 μl of PBS to all the test wells with the dropping or multichannel pipette. (Hold the dropping pipette vertically to deliver precisely 25 μl.)
2 Using a positive displacement pipette, make a 1 : 2 dilution of the antisera (in duplicate).
3 Add 25 μl of PBS to each well of the left-hand row of each replicate pair of dilutions.
4 Add 25 μl of 0.1 M 2-mercaptoethanol in PBS to each well of the right-hand dilutions. (*This reagent is toxic, and so this and all subsequent steps must be carried out in a fume cupboard.*)
5 Add 25 μl of SRBC suspension to all the wells used, and 25 μl to an empty well, as control. (Add 50 μl of PBS to this control well.)
6 Cover the tray with a sealer strip and mix the contents of the wells by gentle shaking.
7 Leave the tray at room temperature for 1 h.

Assessment of results

Read the plate either on a white surface or using a magnifying mirror. A typical pattern of agglutination is shown in Fig. 3.14.

Positive agglutination is seen when the cells form a continuous carpet on the base of the cup. If no agglutination has occurred the cells fall as a tight button to the bottom of the V-shaped cup.

If round-bottomed wells are used the non-agglutinated cells form a ring around the bottom. The 2-mercaptoethanol in each right-hand row of the duplicate dilutions reduces the disulphide bonds holding together the subunits of the IgM pentamer so that it is no longer able to agglutinate the cells.

The titre of the 2-mercaptoethanol-resistant antibody is roughly equivalent to that of the IgG in the serum, and so the greater titre obtained without 2-mercaptoethanol is due to the IgM.

A more exact estimate of the IgG and IgM agglutination titres may be determined using indirect haemagglutination with specific anticlass sera.

TECHNICAL NOTES

- Many antisera or normal human sera contain spontaneous anti-SRBC antibodies (heterophile antibodies). These are usually of low titre (< 1 : 10).
- The final concentration of SRBC in the trays may be varied from 0.5 to 1.5%. If the cells are valuable, e.g. red blood cells (RBC) coupled with a soluble antigen, a lower concentration may be used for reasons of economy.
- The haemagglutination test detects IgM antibodies preferentially not only because of the multivalency of this antibody, but also because of the relatively large size of IgM. Hence, as

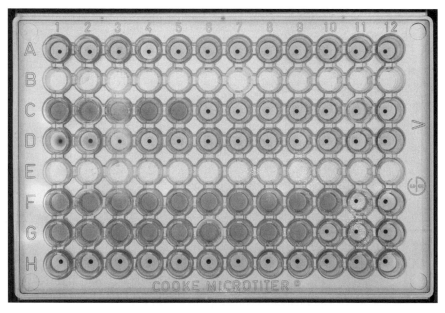

Fig. 3.14 Haemagglutination test on primary and secondary response antisera. Doubling dilutions left to right along the plate starting at 1 : 2, antigen : sheep erythrocytes.
Well A: normal mouse serum, preimmunization bleed.
Well C: mouse serum from an animal 5 days after one intraperitoneal injection of 10^5 sheep erythrocytes.
Well D: as for C but with 1 drop of 2-mercaptoethanol (0.1 M).
Well F: mouse serum from an animal 7 days after third injection of 10^8 sheep erythrocytes (previous injections given at 0, 10 and 29 days).
Well G: as for F but with 1 drop of 0.1 M 2-mercaptoethanol.
Well H: sheep erythrocytes alone.
(Note: In wells not receiving 2-mercaptoethanol, 1 drop of saline was added to equalize the dilution effect.)

erythrocytes are further apart when agglutinated by IgM compared with IgG, the repulsive force that is due to the cell's ζ potential is less.

- You should not see any spontaneous agglutination of erythrocytes in the control well. This is seldom a problem with fresh cells as they have a high negative ζ potential which causes the cells to repel each other. When erythrocytes are coupled to soluble antigens, however, the surface charge is often reduced and so spontaneous agglutination may occur. This is discussed in the Technical notes of Section 3.11.3.

- Greater sensitivity may be obtained with U-shaped wells if the cells are allowed to sediment in the normal way and the plate is then tilted to an angle of 45 degrees. Unagglutinated cells stream to the edge, whereas cross-linked cells are fixed in place by antibody.

- Agglutinated and unagglutinated erythrocytes have different light-scattering properties; this may be quantified using an ELISA reader (see Section 5.4.3).

- As an alternative, avian RBC may be used that are denser than mammalian RBC since they are nucleated.

3.11.1 Primary versus secondary antibody response

In the primary response there is an early production of IgM antibody which soon declines and is replaced by IgG. In contrast, IgG production is greatly accelerated in the secondary response (Fig. 3.14), the peak titre is attained rapidly and declines slowly. There appears to be no accelerated IgM production; the kinetics are essentially that of the primary response.

The differences between these two responses can be conveniently demonstrated using haemagglutination, comparing the total and 2-mercaptoethanol-resistant antibody titres of sera taken from mice immunized with sheep erythrocytes (SRBC) as follows:

(a) 2×10^8 SRBC given i.p., bleed 3–4 days later;

(b) 2×10^8 SRBC given i.p. on day 0 and day 7, bleed 7 days later.

3.11.2 Agglutination of antigen-coated erythrocytes

Erythrocytes may be coupled to soluble antigens by various methods and agglutinated by antisera to the coupled antigens.

(a) Spontaneous uptake: erythrocytes will adsorb polysaccharides to their surface during incubation. Although this is a non-covalent binding, there is very little leaching off of the antigen during the assay.

(b) Coupling to chemically modified erythrocytes.

3.11.3 Tanned erythrocytes

This procedure is suitable for many protein antigens; in the method below human serum albumin is used.

MATERIALS
Sheep erythrocytes (SRBC) in Alsever's solution
0.2 M phosphate–saline buffer, pH 7.2
0.15 M borate–succinate buffer, pH 7.5
0.14 M saline

Tannic acid

Human serum albumin (HSA)

40% (v/v) aqueous formaldehyde

METHOD

Tanning of RBC

1 Wash SRBC three times with 40 volumes of saline by centrifugation (300 g for 10 min).

2 Adjust SRBC suspension to 40% v/v in phosphate–saline buffer, pH 7.5.

3 Add 2.5 mg of tannic acid to 50 ml of phosphate–saline buffer and mix with 50 ml of 4% SRBC suspension.

4 Incubate at 37°C for 15 min.

5 Spin down cells very gently (100 g for 20 min). If the cells are pelleted too quickly they will agglutinate.

6 Divide the cells into two aliquots, and wash each with 50 ml phosphate–saline buffer by centrifugation (100 g for 20 min). One aliquot will be used for antigen coating and the other as control cells.

Agglutination of RBC

7 Resuspend one aliquot of cells in 50 ml phosphate–saline buffer and add 50 ml of HSA solution (2 mg/ml initial concentration).

8 Incubate at 37°C for 30 min.

9 Wash in phosphate–saline buffer by gentle centrifugation and resuspend in 100 ml of borate–succinate buffer.

10 Resuspend the second aliquot of cells in 100 ml of borate–succinate buffer. The control cells are not coated and are used both to absorb the test antisera and as control cells in the assay.

11 Add 10 ml of 40% formalin to both cell suspensions while stirring. The formalin must be added dropwise over 20–30 min.

12 Leave overnight at 4°C and add a further 10 ml of formalin to both suspensions.

13 Leave the cells to settle (24 h) and pour off the supernatant.

14 Add a large volume of borate–succinate buffer and resuspend the cells by vigorous shaking.

15 Allow cells to settle (24 h) and wash again by sedimentation in borate–succinate buffer.

16 Adjust both cell suspensions to 1% v/v and add 0.2% formalin (final concentration) as a preservative.

The cells can be stored at 4°C for up to 2 years.

Assay procedure

MATERIALS AND EQUIPMENT

Agglutination as above (Section 3.11), but use antigen (HSA)-coated erythrocytes (SRBC) and control erythrocytes as prepared above together with appropriate antiserum.

METHOD

1 Titrate the antiserum as described in Section 3.11, but use an initial dilution of 1 : 5 (100 μl of buffer to the first well) (omit the 2-mercaptoethanol from the left-hand row and the 25 μl of buffer from the right-hand row).

Continued

> **2** Add 25 μl of the 1% suspension of HSA-coated SRBC to the right-hand row of dilutions.
> **3** Add 25 μl of 1% control (uncoated but tanned) SRBC to the left-hand row of dilutions.
> **4** Place 25 μl of coated and uncoated cells in two separate empty wells to test for spontaneous agglutination. (Add 25 μl of buffer to each of these control wells.)
> **5** Gently shake and leave to stand for 1 h.

Again, positive agglutination is seen when the cells form a continuous carpet on the base of the cup.

TECHNICAL NOTES

- If agglutination occurs with control cells the antiserum must be absorbed to remove heterophile antibodies as follows:
  (a) Add 0.1 ml of serum to 1 ml of packed control cells.
  (b) Incubate at 37°C for 10 min and spin off the erythrocytes.
  (c) Repeat the agglutination assay and re-absorb if necessary.
- If the coated or control cells agglutinate spontaneously, add 1% normal serum to the buffers used in the assay.

Antigens may also be coupled to erythrocytes using bisdiazotized benzidine, glutaraldehyde and chromic chloride. The basic principles are similar to those described above (technical details may be found in the references cited in Section 3.14). Other particles such as bentonite or latex may be used as antigen carriers for agglutination tests. They have the advantage of not being antigenic but have a more limited range of applications than the antigen-coated erythrocyte assay described above.

3.11.4 Indirect agglutination

IgG antibodies are less efficient at agglutinating red cells. Addition of 25 μl of 1% bovine serum albumin to each well can sometimes enhance the agglutination. Otherwise the addition of a second antibody can be used. The erythrocytes should be gently centrifuged down, the supernatant removed, and the erythrocytes gently resuspended in 50 μl of suitably diluted anti-IgG.

3.11.5 Latex agglutination

Latex beads are a convenient carrier for antigens in agglutination tests. Sophisticated equipment has been developed to quantify the degree of agglutination of the latex beads very accurately. This apparatus has led to a whole new field of immunoassay known as particle-counting immunoassay that has a sensitivity approaching that of radioimmunoassay. It is, however, simple to set up basic slide agglutination tests without any expensive equipment.

Coating the beads with antigen is not difficult, especially when using IgG or albumin as these antigens adsorb readily to polystyrene latex. However, many proteins, including immunoglobulin isotypes other than IgG, bind less well and require covalent coupling with carbodiimide. A specialist company, Bangs Laboratories, produces a quarterly newsletter *Painless Particles* with a bewildering range of immunological assays based on latex particles (Bangs Laboratories Inc., 9025 Technology Drive, Fisher, IN 46038–2886, USA).

Latex coating

MATERIALS
Latex suspension, 10% w/v
Antigen, e.g. IgG
0.25 M and 0.05 M glycine–saline buffer, pH 8.2 (prepared from the 0.5 M stock solution, see
Appendix A)

METHOD

1 Wash 800 µl latex suspension twice by adding 40 ml 0.054 M glycine–saline; mix and centrifuge at 12 500 g for 15 min.
2 Resuspend the latex in 20 ml 0.05 M glycine–saline and add 300 µl of a 10 mg/ml solution of antigen.
3 Mix the suspension for 30 min at room temperature.
4 Wash the latex twice by adding 40 ml 0.05 M glycine–saline; mix and centrifuge the latex at 12 500 g for 15 min.
5 Resuspend the latex in 20 ml 0.25 M glycine–saline containing 0.1% of an irrelevant protein to block any remaining protein-binding sites and store at 4°C.

Slide agglutination

MATERIALS
Antigen-coated latex (as above)
Specific antiserum
0.25 M glycine–saline buffer, pH 8.2

METHOD

1 Prepare doubling dilutions of the test antiserum.
2 Mix 25 µl of each antiserum dilution with 25 µl coated latex on a glass slide.
3 Rock gently for 2 min and read agglutination visually, illuminating the slide from the side, against a dark background.

TECHNICAL NOTE
It is advisable to dilute the sera for use, as a prozone effect (where no agglutination is seen at the highest concentrations of serum) can easily occur.

Applications

Several commercial latex agglutination tests are available; one of the most widely used is the detection of autoantibodies in rheumatoid arthritis. Patients with rheumatoid arthritis often develop antibodies to 'self-IgG'. This antiglobulin antibody, known as rheumatoid factor, is readily detected by its ability to agglutinate latex particles coated with IgG.

3.12 Use of antibody for purification of cellular antigens

Much of our knowledge of the chemistry of the important antigens and receptors on cell surfaces has been gained by the purification of membrane molecules from detergent-solubilized cells by immune affinity chromatography.

The sheer specificity of the reversible binding reaction between antibody and its antigen permits impressive gains in purity in a single-step procedure. The general technique described can be applied to monoclonal antibodies or polyclonal sera, whether raised against a whole molecule or a partial sequence.

MATERIALS

Cells carrying the antigen of interest, solubilized in a non-ionic detergent

Monoclonal antibody, purified or IgG fraction coupled to Sepharose CL-4B

Irrelevant monoclonal antibody, purified or normal mouse IgG coupled to Sepharose CL-4B

0.05 M diethylamine–HCl buffer, pH 11.5

10 mM tris(hydroxymethyl)-aminomethane (Tris)–HCl buffer, pH 8.2

Sodium deoxycholate (for incorporation into buffers)

Bovine serum albumin (BSA)

Glycine, solid

Absolute ethanol

10-ml disposable syringe plugged with glass wool (*Caution: Wear gloves when handling glass wool*)

METHOD

1 Before use, elute each column with 3 times its bed volume of diethylamine buffer.

2 Re-equilibrate with three times its bed volume of 10 mM Tris–HCl buffer, pH 8.2, containing 0.5% w/v sodium deoxycholate.

3 Saturate the non-specific protein-binding sites by treating each column with Tris–HCl buffer containing 1 mg/ml BSA, and wash through with Tris–HCl–deoxycholate buffer.

4 Apply the detergent-solubilized cells to the control column, collect the effluent and apply it immediately to the monoclonal antibody column (see also Section 1.5).

5 Wash the monoclonal antibody column with 3 times its bed volume of Tris–HCl–deoxycholate buffer.

6 Elute the bound material by treating the monoclonal antibody column with 0.05 M diethylamine–HCl buffer, pH 11.5, containing 0.5% w/v deoxycholate.

7 Titrate the eluate back to pH 8.5 with solid glycine and dialyse against Tris–HCl–deoxycholate buffer.

8 If a further purification cycle is required the sample may be applied to the monoclonal antibody column after re-equilibration, as in steps 1–7.

9 Concentrate the final product by precipitation with ethanol; mix the effluent with 3 volumes of cold absolute ethanol and leave at –20°C overnight.

10 Recover the precipitate by high-speed centrifugation at 4°C and 5000 g for 10 min, redissolve in a minimum volume of 1% v/v non-ionic detergent (see Appendix B.3) and compare its purity with that of the starting material using SDS-PAGE.

TECHNICAL NOTES

- When choosing a non-ionic detergent, Renex 30, an aliphatic polyoxyethylene isoalcohol may be used, but Nonidet P-40 or Triton X-100 are preferred as they do not absorb at 280 nm.
- The detergent deoxycholate precipitates out of solution at high salt concentrations.
- For maximum solubility after purification, the cell-derived proteins should be handled in slightly alkaline buffers.

3.13 **Immunoprecipitation**

This technique may be used to analyse antigens in complex protein mixtures. The combination of antibody specificity and the discrimination of SDS-PAGE fractionation of proteins by molecular weight permits an impressive resolution of antigen moieties. There are many analytical applications that have exploited this because of its relative ease of use and wide applicability, e.g. to determine the molecular weight and distribution of an antigen in various cell populations using a monoclonal antibody. The range of antigens recognized during the development of a humoral immune response may be determined by carrying out an immunoprecipitation reaction between the immunizing antigen and timed sample bleeds.

Immunoprecipitation is usually used to gain quantitative information about the apparent size of polypeptides (Fig. 3.15a) but rarely about their relative abundance. The resolution of the analysis of antigen in the immune complex can be greatly increased by the combination of isoelectric focusing and SDS-PAGE separation as illustrated in Fig. 3.15(d).

Fig. 3.15 (*opposite*) **SDS-PAGE fractionation of immunoprecipitated cell-surface polypeptides in one- and two-dimensional gels.** (**a**–**c**) show the use of different autoradiograph exposure times to gain maximum information from the powerful combination of immunoprecipitation, polyacrylamide gel electrophoresis under denaturing conditions (SDS-PAGE) and autoradiography. In the experiment, a single antiserum and its control were reacted with detergent-solubilized, ^{125}I-labelled polypeptides from three different cell types. After 24 h exposure there was a clear image of the distribution of the polypeptides in the track containing the original mixtures—photograph (**a**)—but virtually nothing else visible. After 3 days' exposure the photographic images of labelled polypeptides were visible in the other lanes—photograph (**b**)—but the starting material was then overexposed. Photograph (**c**) shows the result of a collage of both exposures, labelled to identify the tracks and sizes of the molecular weight (MW) standard proteins. It is remarkably difficult to balance the initial loading of each lane in the SDS-PAGE gel, even using c.p.m. per sample. It is not usually possible to predict in advance whether the radioactivity will be associated with few or many polypeptide bands. (**d**) The combination of isoelectric focusing and SDS-PAGE results in an analytical technique with exquisite discrimination between polypeptide chains separated on the basis of both their size and their charge. In photograph (**d**) radioactive polypeptides were precipitated by a polyclonal antiserum against the blood stage of the malaria parasite, *Plasmodium yoelii*, and electrofocused under non-reducing conditions in a pH 4.0–7.0 gradient. A strip from this first gel was sealed onto an 12.5% SDS-polyacrylamide gel under denaturing conditions and separated by size. This combined technique resolves mixtures of polypeptide chains which otherwise would run at the same isoelectric point or migrate to the same position in a sizing gel.

Although the tremendous complexity of the protozoan antigens shown in this figure might seem bewildering and unnerving at first sight, remarkable advances in the characterization of functionally important molecules have been made by the combination of molecular biological techniques with monoclonal antibodies and also the analysis of the antigen specificity of T-lymphocyte cloned lines and hybridomas. In this way, a spot on two-dimensional gel can be related not only to the functional protein in the intact organism but also to its DNA sequence.

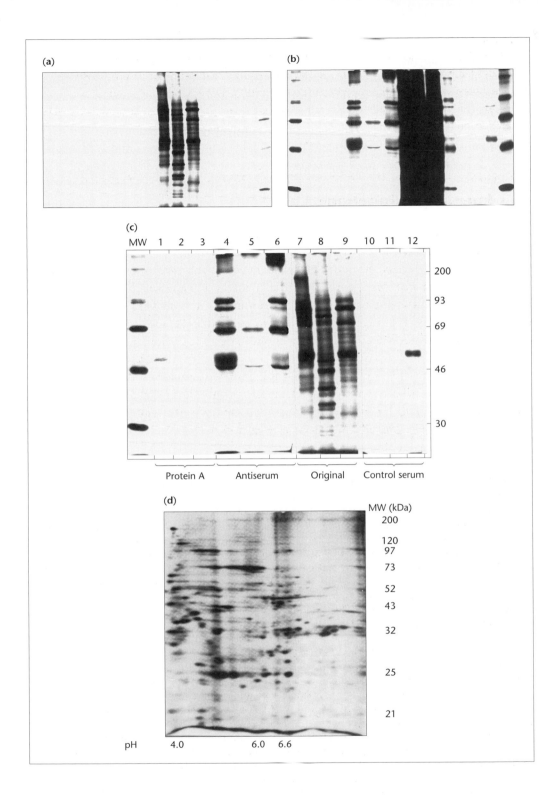

Briefly, the antigen mixture of interest is usually radioactively labelled, by either exogenous or endogenous (biosynthetic) labelling and, if cell associated, is solubilized by the addition of a non-ionic detergent. After high-speed centrifugation to remove aggregates and insoluble material, the antigen of interest may be delineated by the addition of a specific antiserum or monoclonal antibody.

Although immune complexes are formed, there is usually no precipitation because of the low concentration of the reactants. Isolation of the complex is achieved by the addition of an affinity particle or bead (e.g. whole fixed *Staphylococcus aureus* (Cowan strain) or protein A or anti-immunoglobulin antibody covalently bound to Sepharose 4B followed by centrifugation). After thorough washing, the immune complexes are released by denaturation induced by boiling in the presence of sodium dodecyl sulphate (SDS) and a reducing agent, e.g. dithiothreitol.

Preparation in advance

1   Radiolabel the antigen mixture or cells using one of the techniques described in Section 4.9.
2   If the antigen is cell associated, solubilize the cell pellet in a non-ionic detergent, e.g. 1% w/v Renex 30 (alternatively Triton X-100 or Nonidet P-40), in the presence of a cocktail of proteinase inhibitors (see Appendix B.4).
3   Centrifuge at high speed (100 000 *g* for 20 min) to remove aggregated and insoluble material.
4   Recover the supernatant and determine its content of protein-bound radioisotope.
5   Store at –80°C until used.

MATERIALS AND EQUIPMENT
Radiolabelled antigen mixture
Affinity beads, e.g. protein A–Sepharose
Poly- or monoclonal antibody, with relevant control
Affinity-purified anti-immunoglobulin and control antibodies, if required
Sodium dodecyl sulphate (SDS) in water, 20% w/v
Non-ionic detergent, e.g. Renex 30
Phosphate-buffered saline (PBS)
Ethylene diamine tetra-acetic acid (EDTA)
Sodium hydroxide 0.1 M
Sodium chloride
Bovine serum albumin (BSA)
Microcentrifuge tubes, 1.5 ml
Microcentrifuge, e.g. Microcentaur
Mixing rotor for microcentrifuge tubes

METHOD

1   Dissolve 220 mg of EDTA in a minimum volume of water and adjust the pH of the solution to neutrality with 0.1 M sodium hydroxide.
2   Weigh 8.7 g of sodium chloride into a 500-ml measuring cylinder, add 30 ml of 10-fold concentrated PBS and 3 ml of Renex 30. Wash the EDTA solution into this mixture and adjust the final volume of the solution to 300 ml (high-salt buffer).
3   Dissolve 100 mg of BSA in 100 ml of high-salt buffer (BSA buffer).

Continued

4 Add 0.25 ml of 20% w/v SDS to 100 ml of high-salt buffer (SDS buffer).

5 Mix the detergent-solubilized radiolabelled antigens with a half-packed volume of Sephadex immunoadsorbent (previously washed with PBS containing 2% w/v Renex and 2 mg/ml BSA) and mix for 30 min at 4°C on a rotor.

6 Recover the supernatant by microcentrifugation and dispense aliquots containing approximately 10^6 c.p.m. into each assay tube to be used.

7 Add an aliquot of the first antibody (5 μl of a polyclonal antiserum or ascitic fluid containing a monoclonal antibody, alternatively 100 μl of tissue culture supernatant from a hybridoma line) and incubate on ice (5 min for a monoclonal antibody or 15 min for an antiserum).

8 If required, add 2 μl of affinity-purified anti-immunoglobulin antibody (10 mg/ml) and incubate on ice for 5 min.

9 Add 30 μl of 50% v/v protein A–Sepharose to each tube, mix by vortexing and incubate for 30 min at 4°C on a mixing rotor.

10 Wash the Sepharose free of unbound proteins by two cycles of centrifugation and resuspension in each of the following buffers: BSA buffer, high-salt buffer, SDS buffer and finally PBS alone.

11 The dry pellet may be stored at −80°C or processed immediately for SDS-PAGE analysis.

TECHNICAL NOTES

- It is essential to include appropriate controls for each antibody used in this assay. Although normal serum is acceptable as a control for unfractionated polyclonal serum, it is essential to match a monoclonal antibody with an irrelevant monoclonal antibody of the same isotype. Similarly, the appropriate control for affinity-purified anti-immunoglobulin antibodies is affinity-purified irrelevant antibodies.

- If the first antibody used in this reaction binds directly to the affinity bead or particle, then an anti-immunoglobulin second antibody is not required.

- Three main parameters influence the apparent difference between specific and non-specific adsorption: the length of the incubation period with antibody; the amount of total protein present (purified antibody versus whole serum, or whether a second anti-immunoglobulin is used or not); and the stringency of the washing procedure. If the antisera used are weak, incubation periods may be extended up to 24 h. The washing cycle needs to be particularly thorough because of the fine point of the microcentrifuge tube; it is advisable to resuspend the dry cell pellet prior to the addition of washing buffer.

- Renex is often semisolid at room temperature, so warm in a 60°C water bath prior to dispensing.

- If *Staphylococcus aureus* is used as the affinity particle, it is important to note that some proteins react directly with the bacterial cell wall. Consequently, preabsorption of the radiolabelled proteins with a strain of the bacterium not producing protein A is necessary.

- No matter what affinity particle is used, it is good practice to wash a portion of the preabsorption pellet in parallel with the rest of the assay and analyse any bound protein in the same SDS-PAGE (see Appendix B.2.1) as the antibody-treated samples. The results do not necessarily merit publication, but might save embarrassment.

3.14 Further reading

Boldicke T., Struck F., Schaper F. *et al.* (2000) A new peptide-affinity tag for the detection and affinity purification of recombinant proteins with a monoclonal antibody. *J Immunol Meth* **240**(1–2), 165–83.

Gavrilovskaya, I., Apekina, N., Okulova N., Demina V., Bernshtein A. & Myasnikov, Y. (1993) IgG avidity assay for estimation of the time after onset of hantavirus infection in clonized and wild bank voles. *Arch Virol* **132**, 359–367.

Hames, B.D. (1998) *Gel Electrophoresis of Proteins—A Practical Approach*, 3rd edn. Oxford University Press, Oxford.

Hedman, K., Lappalainen, M., Seppäiä, I. & Mäkelä, O. (1989) Recent primary toxoplasma infection indicated by a low avidity of specific IgG. *J Infect Dis* **159**(4), 734–740.

Holliman, R.E., Raymond, R., Renton, N. & Johnson, J.D. (1994) The diagnosis of toxoplasmosis using IgG avidity. *Epidemiol Infect* **112**(2), 399–408.

June, C.H., Contreras, C.E., Perrin, L.H. & Lambert, P. (1979) Improved detection of immune complexes in human and mouse serum using a microassay adaptation of the C1q binding test. *J Immunol Meth* **31**(1–2), 23–29.

Lappalainen, M., Koskela, P., Koskiniemi, M. *et al.* (1993) Toxoplasmosis acquired during pregnancy: improved serodiagnosis based on avidity of IgG. *J Infect Dis* **167**(3), 691–697.

Layer, A., Tissot J.D., Schneider, P. & Duchosal, M.A. (1999) Micropurification and two-dimensional polyacrylamide gel electrophoresis of immunoglobulins for studying the clonal diversity of antigen-specific antibodies. *J Immunol Meth* **227**(1–2), 137–48.

McCloskey, N., Turner, M.W. & Goldblatt, D. (1997) Correlation between the avidity of mouse-human chimeric IgG subclass monoclonal antibodies measured by solid-phase elution ELISA and biospecific interaction analysis (BIA). *J Immunol Meth* **205**, 67–72.

Metus, P., Ruzzante, N., Bonvicini, P., Meneghetti, M., Zaninotto, M. & Plebani, M. (1999) Immunoturbidimetric assay of glycated haemoglobin. *J Clin Lab Anal* **13**(1), 5–8.

Nezlin, R. (2000) A quantitative approach to the determination of antigen in immune complexes [Review]. *J Immunol Meth* **237**, 1–17.

Ouchterlony, O. & Nilsson L.A. (1997) Immunodiffusion and immunoelectrophoresis. In *Weir's Handbook of Experimental Immunology* (eds L.A. Herzenberg, D.M. Weir, L.A. Herzenberg & C. Blackwell), 5th edn. Blackwell Science Ltd, Oxford.

Pokric, B. (2000) Precipitation at equivalence and equilibrium: a method for the determination of equilibrium constants of reaction between multideterminant antigen and specific polyclonal antibodies. *J Chem Inf Comput Sci* **40**(3), 524–9.

Polak, J.M. & Van Noorden S. (1997). *Introduction to Immunocytochemistry*, 2nd edn. Springer Verlag, New York.

Pound, J.D. (1998) Immunochemical Protocols. *Methods Enzymol* **80**. Academic Press, London.

Rabilloud T. (2000) *Proteome Research: Two-Dimensional Gel Electrophoresis and Identification Methods (Principles and Practice)*. Springer Verlag, New York.

Rose, N.R., (1997) *Manual of Clinical Laboratory Immunology*, 5th edn. ASM Press, .

Steward, M.W. (1997) Introduction to methods used to study the affinity and kinetics of antibody/antigen reactions. In: *Weir's Handbook of Experimental Immunology* (eds L.A. Herzenberg, D.M. Weir, L.A. Herzenberg & C. Blackwell), 5th edn. Blackwell Science Ltd, Oxford.

Vunakis, H.V. & Langonc J.J. (eds) (1986 onwards) Immunochemical Techniques. In: *The Methods in Enzymology Series*, volumes 70, 73, 74, 84, 92 and 93. Academic Press, New York.

Westermeier, R., Barnes, N., Gronau-Czybulka, S., Habeck C (1997) *Electrophoresis in Practice: A Guide to Methods and Applications of DNA and Protein Separations*. John Wiley & Sons, Chichester.

4 Antibodies as probes

Antibodies are widely used as biospecific probes to identify other molecules. To detect the binding of probe to its target molecule, the antibody must be labelled.

- Radioisotope labels, e.g. ^{125}I, have been used extensively. However, there may be problems with safety, and the relatively short half-life of this isotope has meant that other labels have taken precedence.

   Refer to the following websites for comprehensive details on radioisotope health and safety procedures as well as useful information regarding detection and half-life:

   http://www.practicingsafescience.org

   http://www.hse.gov.uk

- Fluorescent labels are frequently used for cellular applications.
- Enzyme labels are common in immunoassay and immunoblotting. They were originally used to generate coloured products, e.g. to visualize antigen using a light microscope, or soluble products which could be quantified using a spectrophotometer. Recently, enzymes have been used to generate light, providing incredibly sensitive assays systems.
- Hapten labels such as dinitrophenol (DNP) and penicilloyl groups may be coupled to antibodies, then detected with labelled antibodies to the appropriate hapten. For example, there is a commercially prepared assay system which uses digoxygenin-labelled antibodies. Another uses binding of labelled avidin to biotin-coupled antibodies which provides a very flexible system for detecting antibody probes.
- Gold labels allow fine structural detail to be revealed using antibodies labelled with ultrasmall gold particles.

Where an antibody to a receptor is not available, immunoprobes are possible by using the idiotypic network to produce surrogate anti-idiotypic antibodies that bind to the receptor in the same way as the original ligand.

4.1 Immunohistochemistry

Specific labelled antibodies raised against cellular membrane-bound or intracellular antigens may be used for the *in situ* localization of membrane-bound or intracellular antigens on tissue sections by light or electron microscopy. But a word of caution: whilst antibodies may effectively bind to the native antigen, certain fixatives employed for the preservation of the integrity of tissues and cells may denature the protein, with a resultant loss of antigenicity.

4.1.1 Preparation of tissues or cells

Solid tissue may either be immobilized as frozen sections (see below) or embedded in paraffin for effective cutting of sections (5–10 μm thickness) using a microtome.

Cell suspensions may be visualized by preparing a thin smear of cells on a microscope slide. With respect to blood cells, plasma is very viscous, so it protects the cells from damage as they are smeared.

Cytocentrifugation is useful for visualizing single-cell suspensions.

Frozen sections

MATERIALS AND EQUIPMENT

Tissue to be analysed

Frozen section

Liquid nitrogen cooled isopentane

Dewar flask

Cryostat microtome

METHOD

1   Tissue should be collected into tissue culture media or normal saline solution to prevent drying out of the specimen.
2   Tissue section should then be flash frozen in liquid nitrogen cooled isopentane contained in a Dewar flask.
3   Frozen section may now be cut into 5–8 μm sections using a cryostat microtome and applied to individual glass microscope slides (see Technical note).

TECHNICAL NOTE

Frozen sections may be stored at 4°C for up to 1 week, but to preserve DNA long-term, it is advisable to store the sections on slides in a suitable box at −70°C.

4.1.2 Fixatives

Fixatives are used to preserve cellular morphology, protect constituents from autodigestion, inhibit microbial growth and achieve structural stabilization. Some fixatives chemically cross-link to proteins, e.g. glutaraldehyde, formaldehyde, paraformaldehyde. Other fixatives precipitate and thus immobilize protein, e.g. methanol, ethanol.

Formalin is a frequently used irreversible fixative and is made up of 4% w/v formaldehyde in buffer such as phosphate-buffered saline (PBS), pH 7.4. It is often the preservative used by clinical diagnostic laboratories as it is good for long-term preservation of cellular morphology. The aldehyde-based fixatives are commercially prepared as aqueous solutions. Such fixatives cross-link and alter protein structure and this can result in loss of epitopes. Glutaraldehyde is often the fixative of choice for electron microscopic investigations, but where immunofluorescent techniques are performed it may result in less clear results due to a high degree of autofluorescence.

The alcohol-based fixatives are reversible, and they do not generally affect the antigenicity. However, dehydration and rehydration of tissues is necessary and this generally results in loss of cellular constituents.

Detergents e.g. saponin (0.1% w/v) may be added to fixatives in order to visualize intracellular antigens, e.g. cytoplasmic or nuclear antigens.

Dehydration and fixation of solid tissue for paraffin embedding

This is an example of dehydration and fixation of solid tissue for paraffin embedding.

MATERIALS AND EQUIPMENT
Tris-buffered saline (TBS) (see Appendix A)
Ethanol solutions: absolute, 95%, 70%, 50% v/v
Xylene
Acetone
Acetone containing 1% Necol
Acetone containing 5% Necol
Chloroform
Coplin jars or use of automated system for fixation and paraffin embedding
Poly L-lysine or vector-bond coated microscope slides
Tissue or cells of interest

METHOD

1 Immerse the tissue overnight in 4% w/v formaldehyde in PBS.
2 Serially immerse tissue in the following solutions at 4°C:
    50% ethanol for 2 h
    70% ethanol for 2 h
    95% ethanol for 2 h.
3 Serially immerse tissue in the following solutions at room temperature:
    absolute ethanol for 3 × 1 h
    xylene for 2 × 30 min.
4 Embed in paraffin wax (melting point 50–55°C) overnight.
5 Cut tissue sections using a microtome, then transfer onto the surface of water maintained at 37°C to straighten out the section.
6 Insert the glass slide into the warm water to pick up the tissue section.
7 Serially incubate the slides in Coplin jars:
    xylene for 3 × 4 min
    absolute ethanol for 2 × 2 min.

Continued on p. 118

8 Rehydrate the tissue sections by serially dipping slides into:

100% ethanol for 1 min

95% ethanol for 1 min

70% ethanol for 1 min

distilled water for 3×5 min.

9 Wash the slides in TBS for 2×5 min.

10 Tissue is now prepared for immunostaining.

Immunohistochemical staining (see Section 4.2)

Generally suppliers of antisera provide information on the suggested dilution and incubation times. Where the antibody is 'in house', usually 1–30 µg/ml of monoclonal antibody is used, but here again antibody concentration should be optimized for each system.

With direct immunohistochemical staining, a labelled antibody is used to detect the antigen being investigated. Conversely, in indirect immunohistochemical staining the primary antibody is not labelled but visualized by the binding of a second labelled antibody, e.g. with a fluorochrome, or horseradish peroxidase, i.e. a secondary antibody.

TECHNICAL NOTES

- A monoclonal antiserum may not be useful for the visualization of antigens by immunohistochemistry if its specific epitope has been destroyed. Instead a polyclonal antiserum is generally the preferred option, as this will bind more antigenic epitopes and thus have an increased likelihood of success.

- Epitopes may be exposed or destroyed by fixatives; hence antibodies work in some systems but not in others. Therefore when employing immunohistochemical techniques, it is necessary to ensure that the antigenicity is not affected by fixatives that denature the antigen. Immunization in order to obtain antisera against the fixed antigen is a definite consideration as this will reduce the risk of such problems.

4.2 Preparation of fluorochrome-conjugated antisera

Although a wide diversity of good quality conjugates is commercially available, the techniques in the following sections will be invaluable if you have to prepare and standardize your own conjugates for specialist applications.

4.2.1 Fluorescein conjugation technique

MATERIALS AND EQUIPMENT

Antiserum (monoclonal or polyclonal)

Saturated ammonium sulphate, pH 7.2

0.25 M carbonate buffer, pH 9.0

Sephadex G-25 column

UV spectrophotometer
Fluorescein isothiocyanate
Phosphate-buffered saline (PBS)

METHOD

1 Precipitate the antiserum with 40% saturated ammonium sulphate.
2 Dialyse the γ-globulin fraction of the antiserum against 0.25 M carbonate buffer, pH 9.0, using a Sephadex G-25 column (see Appendix B.1.4–B.1.5).
3 Determine the protein concentration of the solution and adjust to 20 mg/ml (see Appendix B.5.1–B.5.3).
4 Add 0.05 mg fluorescein isothiocyanate per mg of total protein.
5 Mix overnight at 4°C.
6 Separate the conjugated protein from the free fluorochrome by passing the mixture down a Sephadex G-25 column equilibrated with PBS.

Conjugation with tetramethylrhodamine isothiocyanate is done under the same conditions but it is necessary to separate rhodamine-conjugated antisera from free rhodamine on a DEAE (diethylaminoethyl) ion-exchange column (see Section 1.3 and Appendix B.1).

4.2.2 Calculation of fluorochrome : protein ratio

This should be done routinely every time a new conjugate is made. The presence of the fluorochrome interferes with the absorbance of the protein at 280 nm; this is allowed for in the formula.

$$\text{Fluorescein : protein ratio} = \frac{2.87 \times \text{abs}_{495\,\text{nm}}}{\text{abs}_{280\,\text{nm}} - 0.35 \times \text{abs}_{495\,\text{nm}}}$$

Unless you use crystalline rhodamine for conjugation, which we do not recommend, it is not possible to make the same correction when calculating the rhodamine : protein ratio.

$$\text{Rhodamine : protein ratio} = \frac{\text{abs}_{515\,\text{nm}}}{\text{abs}_{280\,\text{nm}}}$$

If you intend to use the conjugate to stain fixed material the fluorochrome : protein ratio should be low (2 : 1); however, antisera used to stain viable cells, where the specific and non-specific fluorescence is much weaker, should have a higher conjugation ratio (2–4 : 1).

4.2.3 Conjugation with phycoerythrin

Phycoerythrin is one of a family of phycobiliproteins which are crucial to the light-harvesting apparatus of blue-green algae, red algae and the cryptomonads. It contains multiple bilin chromophores, so can absorb efficiently over a relatively wide spectral range and emits with a high quantum yield of fluorescence. It can be conjugated to immunoglobulin and protein A using the heterobifunctional cross-linking agent N-succinimidyl-3-(2-pyridylthio) propionate (SPDP) (see Section 4.6.3).

Comparison of the useful absorption and emission wavelengths of fluorescein and phycoerythrin illustrates the advantages of this dye combination, particularly for flow cytometry:

	Fluorescein	Phycoerythrin
Excitation	488	488
Emission	515	576

Wavelengths shown in nm.

The two dyes may be excited at the same wavelength and their emissions resolved by the appropriate combination of long- and short-pass filters.

Phycoerythrin may be conjugated to immunoglobulin and protein A using the heterobifunctional cross-linking agent N-succinimidyl-3-(2-pyridylthio) propionate (SPDP). Although it is commercially available in crystalline form, the chemistry of derivatization and purification is sufficiently arduous to strongly recommend the purchase of commercial conjugates.

4.2.4 Fractionation of fluorochrome-conjugated antisera

The fluorochrome : protein ratio calculated above is only an average determination; some protein molecules will have more fluorochrome and others less.

As each fluorochrome molecule is added to the protein molecule there is a net decrease in charge. Consequently, conjugated antisera may be fractionated according to their substitution ratio by ion-exchange chromatography using an elution gradient of increasing ionic strength.

For fluorescein-conjugated proteins, adsorb the conjugate to a DEAE ion exchanger in 0.005 M phosphate buffer, pH 8.0, and elute with a linear gradient (limit 0.2 M) phosphate buffer, pH 8.0 (see Section 1.3).

4.2.5 Indirect versus direct immunofluorescence

Indirect immunofluorescence using an unlabelled antiserum detected by a second, fluorochrome-conjugated antiserum is much more sensitive than direct immunofluorescence where one antiserum alone is used. The direct technique gives excellent results with an incident light UV microscope or flow cytometric analysis and can save a lot of time. With the indirect technique, binding of a single first antibody can act as a target for up to eight secondary antibodies. This amplification is not always all gain, as the background due to non-specific binding can also increase.

The techniques of fluorochrome conjugation can be used with human, goat, sheep and rabbit antisera. They are, however, unsatisfactory for the conjugation of mouse antisera because of excessive denaturation of the antibody molecules.

Biotinylation offers better prospects for 'in-house' labelling of mouse antibodies, especially as the same biotin-derived antibody can then be detected with avidin molecules conjugated with fluorochrome, radioisotope or enzyme labels.

Mouse alloantisera and monoclonal antibodies can only be used as direct conjugates when staining mouse lymphocytes, as the anti-immunoglobulin second antibody would react directly with the B-cell receptors for antigen. To overcome this problem, it is advised that you use hapten sandwich labelling, whereby monoclonal antibodies required for single- or double-fluorochrome immunofluorescence may be chemically derived with different haptens and antibody binding visualized using antihapten sera conjugated with different fluorochromes.

4.2.6 Standardization of conjugated antisera

This should be done before attempting to use immunoconjugates in detection systems, even if you are using a commercially prepared conjugate. Determine the titration range over which the antiserum gives a plateau of staining values and then work within this titration range.

Protocol for rabbit anti-mouse Ig indirect immunofluorescent staining

Details of the staining technique are found in Section 8.2.1. A similar protocol may be used for standardization of any immunoconjugate provided the appropriate substrates are used.

MATERIALS AND EQUIPMENT
Mouse thymocytes and lymph node cells
Unconjugated antiserum
Fluorescein-coated second antibody

METHOD

1 Incubate mouse thymocytes and lymph node cells with a series of dilutions of the unconjugated antiserum starting at 1 : 5 (Fig. 4.1).
2 Detect the antibody with fluorescein-labelled goat or sheep anti-rabbit γ-globulin (1 mg/ml).

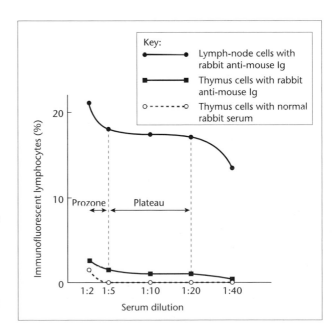

Fig. 4.1 Indirect immunofluorescent staining of mouse thymus and lymph-node lymphocytes. Lymph-node cells showed no prozone with normal rabbit serum. The binding of the rabbit antiserum was detected by a fluorescein-conjugated goat anti-rabbit IgG serum.

Remember to include a preimmunization bleed or pooled normal serum as control (normal rabbit serum—NRS). If you are using a monoclonal as the first antibody then it is essential to use a monoclonal with an unrelated antigen-binding specificity, but the same isotype, as a negative control.

Evaluation of results

Plot a graph of percentage staining for each antiserum dilution as shown in Fig. 4.1. As can be seen from Fig. 4.1, at low dilutions there is an elevated percentage staining, or prozone, before the plateau. This is probably caused by non-specific sticking of serum proteins at high concentration (cf. staining with NRS). Obviously the best dilution at which to use this antiserum would be between 1 : 10 and 1 : 15. One can be sure that the immunoconjugate is not limiting, but still economize in the use of antiserum.

4.2.7 Specificity of immunofluorescent staining

Antisera, their subfractions and even purified monoclonal antibodies are biological materials and not chemical reagents. Many antibodies do not behave as expected so be aware of the limitation on the use of these conjugates, especially in a sensitive system such as immunofluorescence. We list below some pitfalls of this technique and their correction. For maximum sensitivity you should use an epifluorescent microscope in the dark *and* ensure that the microscope has the correct filter combinations for the fluorochrome in use.

Everything staining everywhere

It is probable that one of the antisera is recognizing species or cell-surface determinants other than immunoglobulin. If both control and anti-Ig slides show total staining then the lack of specificity is probably due to the conjugate. If only one of the slides shows high staining it is probably one of the unconjugated sera. We suggest that you absorb the offending serum with liver membranes as follows.

Absorbing serum with liver

MATERIALS AND EQUIPMENT
Mouse liver
Tea-strainer or 63-μm steel sampling sieve
Ice-cold tissue culture medium

METHOD

1   Force chopped mouse liver through a tea-strainer or a 63-μm steel sampling sieve into tissue culture medium on ice.
2   Wash the membrane suspension 10–15 times by centrifugation (500 g for 20 min at 4°C) until the absorbance of the supernatant is below 0.1 ($E^{1\,cm}_{280\,nm}$).
3   Mix a volume of the packed cell membranes with an equal volume of the serum to be absorbed.

Continued

4 Leave the suspension to mix at 4°C overnight.

5 Spin off the cell membranes (500 g for 20 min at 4°C) and retest the antiserum.

TECHNICAL NOTE

If problems of non-specific staining are encountered these can be due either to non-specific adsorption (due to the forces which can cause any two protein molecules to interact) or to inappropriate antibody binding. Inappropriate binding can apply to the first or second (conjugated) antibody but only in the case of a polyclonal serum can this be removed by absorption. Similar absorption of a purified monoclonal antibody might leave only phosphate-buffered saline! Non-specific absorption is more frequently a problem with the fluorochrome-conjugated antibody, not only because it is usually used at higher concentration than the first (these forces of non-specific interaction are concentration dependent, as determined by the law of mass action) but also because it is more highly charged than a native molecule.

No staining anywhere

Almost certainly you have forgotten to add the conjugate. If you are sure you added the conjugate, then you have forgotten the positive unconjugated antibody or it does not bind in any case. It is rare for conjugates to become completely inactive during storage. This may also be due to the UV microscope—a transmitted light microscope is acceptable for stained sections but epi-illumination is essential for cell-surface immunofluorescence. Finally, ensure that the eye-pieces are of the correct magnification for the lens system; the intensity loss with × 12.5 compared with × 6.3 eye-pieces often makes the difference between nothing and superb fluorescence.

Everything staining with bright stars

Your conjugated antiserum is either contaminated with bacteria, or has been frozen or thawed too many times thus producing immune complexes. Ultracentrifuge the conjugate to remove the contamination. Whenever possible, store antisera at 4°C with a preservative (either 0.02% w/v sodium azide or 0.01% merthiolate, final concentration). If it is not desirable to use a preservative, store at −20°C in small aliquots.

Note: Azide is a dangerous chemical—do not discard down the sink.

Negative control serum giving positive staining

Strictly, the negative control serum must be taken from the animal before immunization. Staining indicates either non-specific binding (perhaps due to a high protein concentration, see Technical note above) or the presence of antibodies not elicited by immunization. It is not valid to attempt to absorb out this reactivity. You must purchase or prepare another serum and review the specificity of the whole system with care.

Uptake of exogenous proteins onto cell surfaces

In later sections, cells will be cultured in medium containing a serum supplement. Serum supplements can absorb to the surface of cultured cells and as a consequence might give rise to spurious staining reactions. If required, we suggest that you ensure that your conjugates stain specifically by absorbing them in the manner described below.

4.2.8 Absorption of antisera with insolubilized antigens

MATERIALS

Saturated ammonium sulphate, pH 7.2

Phosphate-buffered saline (PBS)

Fetal bovine, human or rat serum (whichever serum supplement is giving problems)

0.14 M sodium chloride (saline)

2.5% v/v glutaraldehyde in aqueous solution (*Caution: use protective glasses*)

METHOD

1 Precipitate the serum with 50% saturated ammonium sulphate and redissolve the precipitate in a minimum volume of PBS.

2 Dialyse against PBS to remove ammonium sulphate.

3 Measure the protein concentration of the sample and adjust to 20 mg/ml (see Appendix B.5.1–B.5.4).

4 Add glutaraldehyde dropwise to the protein solution while stirring (use 0.5 ml of a 2.5% aqueous solution of glutaraldehyde for each 100 mg of protein to be insolubilized). A gel should form almost immediately.

5 Allow the gel to stand for 3 h at room temperature and then disperse in PBS using a Potter homogenizer.

6 Wash the gel with PBS by centrifugation (500 g for 20 min) until protein cannot be detected in the undiluted supernatant by UV spectroscopy (absorbance less than 0.01, $E_{280\,nm}^{1\,cm}$).

7 Mix an equal volume of this immunoadsorbent gel with the anti-Ig serum. Mix at 4°C overnight.

8 Spin off this immunoadsorbent (500 g for 20 min) and store the antiserum at −20°C until used.

It is obviously necessary to ensure specificity of the antiserum under these conditions as one may simply be examining the uptake of proteins from the serum supplement of the tissue culture medium. It is important to use an insoluble immunoabsorbent to avoid the formation of soluble complexes in the absorbed antiserum.

4.3 Preparation of pig-liver powder

MATERIALS AND EQUIPMENT

Pig liver

0.14 M saline

Acetone

Waring blender

Glass wool (Caution: wear gloves)

METHOD

1 Remove blood from the isolated liver by an intravenous infusion of saline.

2 Chop liver into pieces and homogenize with 4 volumes of saline using a Waring blender.

Continued

---

3 Concentrate and wash in saline by centrifugation (600 g for 45 min at 4°C).

4 Remove large aggregates by filtering through a pad of glass wool or muslin.

5 Centrifuge filter effluent at 600 g for 45 min at 4°C and resuspend pellet in acetone.

6 Filter through a Buchner funnel and wash filtrate with acetone until the preparation is white on drying.

7 Grind up into a powder and store at 4°C under desiccation.

4.4 Detection of intracellular immunoglobulin

MATERIALS AND EQUIPMENT

Absorbed antiserum (see Section 4.2.8)

(Fluorescein isothiocyanate (FITC)-conjugate)

Phosphate-buffered saline (PBS)

Spleen sections or cytosmears

Magnetic stirrer

Mounting medium

UV microscope

Coverslip

METHOD

1 Dilute an aliquot of the absorbed antiserum to final dilutions of 1 : 10, 1 : 20 and 1 : 40 with PBS.

2 Apply 1 drop of each FITC-conjugate dilution to separate spleen sections or cytosmears.

3 Incubate for 20 min at room temperature.

4 Wash off the excess antiserum. This can be done by putting the slides in a tray (face up!) and flooding them with PBS. Washing can be made more effective by placing the tray over a magnetic stirring platform with the mixing bar at the extreme end of the tray from the slides. Mix slowly for 5 min.

5 Change the PBS and mix for a further 5 min.

6 Add 1 drop of mounting medium and add a coverslip. Ring with nail varnish.

7 Examine the slides under a UV microscope.

Plasma cells should be easily visualized, as shown in Fig. 4.2.

TECHNICAL NOTES

- You may see a high background reaction when staining spleen sections for immunoglobulin because of secreted antibody entrapment. This should not be a problem with cytosmears.
- Slides of tissue sections may be stored at –20°C for several weeks after drying. Remove from the deep freeze and dry before use.
- The antigen detected above (immunoglobulin) is relatively insensitive to drying-induced denaturation. For long-term storage, cells may be fixed after smearing.
- Sometimes antigen reactivity can be lost if cells are allowed to dry out before or after fixation (Fig. 4.3a,b). In this case, apply a concentrated suspension of cells to a slide pretreated with

(a) 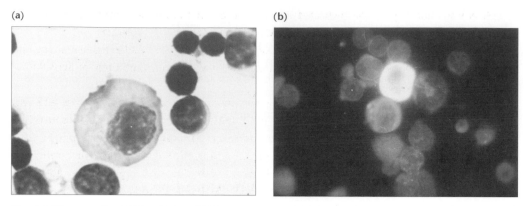 (b)

Fig. 4.2 Plasma cells. (a) May–Grünwald/Giemsa staining of a cytocentrifuge preparation, viewed under transmitted light. (b) Plasma cell stained with fluorescein-conjugated anti-mouse IgG and visualized under a UV microscope. The single stained plasma cell is seen slightly above centre.

(a) 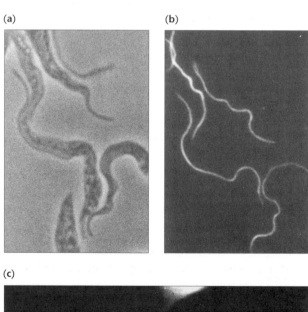 (b)

(c)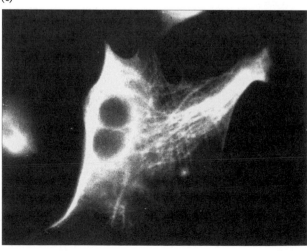

Fig. 4.3 Immunofluorescent staining of cells for intracytoplasmic epitopes. (a) and (b) show the flagellate *Trypanosoma cruzi* stained with a monoclonal antibody against an epitope in the paraxial rod (a structure associated with the flagellum), viewed under (a) transmitted light and (b) UV light. The staining reaction is completely lost if the preparation is allowed to dry out after fixation. Photograph (c) shows a Swiss 3T3 cell treated with the detergent Triton X-100 to remove the majority of the cell cytoplasm prior to staining with an antimicrotubule monoclonal antibody.

1% w/v solution of poly L-lysine (to aid adhesion), allow them to settle at room temperature in a humid chamber for 5–10 min and then add an aqueous fixative.

- An essentially similar technique can be used for staining paraffin-embedded tissue sections with monoclonal antibodies, thus gaining additional information from the better preservation of histological structure.

We have described a direct immunofluorescence technique here as this usually gives sufficient sensitivity to detect the relatively large amount of immunoglobulin in the average plasma cell. It is often more convenient, and sometimes essential, to use an indirect staining technique if the antigen to be detected is scarce or if it was poorly immunogenic when the detecting antiserum was raised. In the indirect technique the first antibody (in this case rabbit anti-mouse immunoglobulin) is unconjugated. Its binding is visualized by a second antibody; for example, FITC-conjugated goat anti-rabbit immunoglobulin (as illustrated in Fig. 4.2). The indirect technique gives a significant gain in sensitivity (up to eight second antibodies may bind for each first antibody), with only a marginal increase in the background of non-specific fluorescence, and can offer the convenience of having to prepare only a single conjugate of an antiserum from a large animal rather than a series of direct conjugates. For example, an FITC-conjugated IgG fraction of goat or sheep anti-rabbit immunoglobulin may be used to visualize a range of rabbit antisera to different antigens. However, the indirect technique takes more time and can be cumbersome if used for the simultaneous detection of different antigenic determinants in two-colour immunofluorescence. If you use indirect immunofluorescence to stain tissue sections, only the fluorescent conjugate need be absorbed with liver powder.

4.5 Cell fixation and permeabilization

A careful control of the procedures for cell fixation and permeabilization by removal of some or all of the membrane lipid is critical, particularly with monoclonal antisera. In the past a fixative might have destroyed the majority of epitopes recognized by a polyclonal antiserum; however, sufficient might remain to allow a visible antigen–antibody interaction still to take place.

For general use, fix cells with 4% paraformaldehyde in 0.1 M phosphate buffer, pH 7.4, for 20 min at room temperature followed by treatment with an organic solvent (methanol, acetone, etc.), as a way of optimizing structure preservation and permitting good permeabilization for antibody penetration for most mammalian cell types. The serological reactivity of surface H-2 immunoglobulin-receptor molecules and Thy-1 antigens is retained after fixation if the buffered paraformaldehyde solution is supplemented with paraperiodic acid (9 mg/ml) and 0.1 M L-lysine. Some antigenic determinants are destroyed by this procedure; in this case we recommend fixation directly in acetone for 5 min at −20°C.

Effective permeabilization can also be achieved by treating cells with a detergent solution (1% v/v Triton X-100 or Nonidet P-40) after formaldehyde fixation. Highly insoluble cellular proteins, such as those found in the cytoskeleton, may be prepared for immunofluorescent staining by detergent treatment without fixation (Fig. 4.3c).

It should be emphasized that time spent in optimizing fixation, permeabilization and staining techniques for each individual monoclonal antibody will usually yield dividends in the quality of the final result.

4.5.1 Permeabilization of cells, for example in preparation for flow cytometry (adapted from Lan *et al.* 1996)

To probe the contents of a cell, it is necessary to render the cell membrane permeable whilst still endeavouring (as much as possible) to maintain the antigenicity and structure of the cell. A variety of techniques are available and it is advisable for the researcher to identify the best method for the particular preparation of cells being investigated.

MATERIALS AND EQUIPMENT
Cultured cells
Phosphate-buffered saline (PBS)
Absolute methanol
Paraformaldehyde
0.5% v/v Nonidet P-40 (NP-40) in PBS
0.1% w/v saponin in PBS
0.01 M sodium citrate buffer, pH 6.0, containing 0.5% w/v bovine serum albumin (BSA)
Microwave oven (800 W; 2450 MHz)
50-μm filter
Polypropylene tubes

METHOD

1   Wash cells twice in PBS.
2   Resuspend the cells at a concentration of 10^6 cells/ml.
3   Fix the cells using either:
   (a) absolute methanol at –20°C for 15 min. Spin the cells at 1000 g for 5 min at room temperature and remove the methanol. Add an equal volume of 0.5% NP-40 in PBS for 5 min to permeabilize cells then resuspend in PBS; or
   (b) 2% paraformaldehyde on ice for 30 min. Spin cells at 1000 g for 5 min at room temperature to remove the paraformaldehyde solution. Permeabilize the cells with 0.1% saponin in PBS for 5 min, then resuspend in PBS; or
   (c) 2% paraformaldehyde on ice for 30 min. Remove the paraformaldehyde solution. Resuspend in PBS.
Microwave the cells (see below).

Microwave treatment of cells

4   Suspend cells in 15 ml 0.01 M sodium citrate buffer, pH 6.0, containing 0.5% w/v BSA in unsealed 50-ml polypropylene tube.
5   Put the tube in a 1-litre pyrex beaker and cover with cling film wrapping, then place in the microwave oven.
6   Heat the cell suspension at maximum power (800 W) for 30–60 s.
7   Recover any straying cells from around the beaker and add to the cells that remained in the polypropylene tube.
8   Chill the cell suspension on ice for 10 min. Wash in PBS.
9   Filter through a 50-μm filter (this step helps to remove aggregated cell debris). Cells are now prepared for labelling with antibody.

- Advantages of microwaving cells include:
  - (i) Better preservation of cell morphology compared with other methods of permeabilization.
  - (ii) Adequate permeabilization, thereby allowing large molecules into the cell for detection of intracellular contents.
  - (III) Production of a distinct DNA profile for the analysis of DNA content.
- Disadvantages of microwaving cells include:
  - (i) Antigens are denatured by microwave treatment.
  - (ii) Reduction of the microwave treatment time in order to limit the extent of denaturation may mean a reduced level of detection of intracellular antigens.

4.6 Enzyme labelling of immunoglobulins

Improvements in the technology of derivatization and detection of enzymes are such that their sensitivity has come to match that of radioisotopes for many applications. Moreover, their safety has been greatly improved, beyond that of radioisotopes, by the replacement of the commonly used carcinogenic substrates. Technically, enzyme labels compare favourably with fluorescent probes in that they do not require special microscopes and darkened rooms for visualization, and offer both speed and simplicity in detection compared with radioisotopes.

4.6.1 Conjugation of horseradish peroxidase

Peroxidase is a glycoprotein with about 18% carbohydrate that is not necessary for its enzymic activity. This carbohydrate can be converted to aldehyde groups by oxidation with sodium periodate. The periodate aldehyde can then form Schiff bases with immunoglobulin.

MATERIALS
Horseradish peroxidase
IgG fraction of antiserum or monoclonal antibody (8 mg/ml in carbonate buffer)
0.1 M sodium periodate
0.001 M acetate acetic buffer, pH 4.4
0.1 M sodium carbonate buffer, pH 9.5
Sodium borohydride (4 mg/ml in distilled water)
0.1 M borate buffer, pH 7.4
Glycerol
Bovine serum albumin (BSA)

METHOD

1 Dissolve 4 mg horseradish peroxidase in 1 ml distilled water.
2 Add 200 μl freshly prepared sodium periodate solution and stir gently for 20 min at room temperature. The mixture should turn greenish brown.
3 Dialyse overnight at 4°C against sodium acetate buffer.

Continued on p. 130

4 Add 20 μl of sodium carbonate buffer to raise the pH to approximately 9–9.5 and immediately add 1 ml (8 mg) of the protein to be conjugated.

5 Leave at room temperature for 2 h with occasional stirring.

6 Add 100 μl of freshly prepared sodium borohydride solution (4 mg/ml in distilled water) and leave for 2 h at 4°C. This reduces any free enzyme.

7 Dialyse against borate buffer.

8 To store, add an equal volume of 60% glycerol in borate buffer and store at 4°C. (Carrier protein such as BSA may be added to 1% w/v if required.)

TECHNICAL NOTES

- This conjugate should be stable for at least 1 year.
- Although it is not usually necessary to separate conjugated immunoglobulin from unconjugated immunoglobulin or enzyme, this may be done by gel filtration on Sephacryl S-200.

4.6.2 Conjugation of alkaline phosphatase

Alkaline phosphatase can generally be successfully conjugated to immunoglobulin with glutaraldehyde.

MATERIALS AND EQUIPMENT

Alkaline phosphatase suspension in ammonium sulphate

Phosphate-buffered saline (PBS)

IgG fraction of antiserum (minimum initial concentration 2 mg/ml in PBS)

Glutaraldehyde, 25% v/v in PBS (Caution: Wear protective glasses)

0.1 M tris(hydroxymethyl)-aminomethane (Tris)–HCl buffer, pH 7.4

Bovine serum albumin (BSA)

Sodium azide

Dialysis tubing

Note: Azide is a dangerous chemical—do not discard down the sink.

Alkaline phosphatase is supplied in various formats. This method assumes that the enzyme was purchased as an ammonium sulphate precipitate and the salt must be removed by dialysis. The method is easily adapted for use of dried or PBS solution of the enzyme by omitting the dialysis step.

METHOD

1 Place 5 mg alkaline phosphatase in a test tube, centrifuge and discard supernatant.

2 Add 2 mg of the IgG fraction of antiserum to the enzyme pellet.

3 Dialyse overnight at 4°C against PBS.

4 Adjust to 1.25 ml with PBS.

5 Add 10 μl of 25% v/v glutaraldehyde. Mix and allow to stand for 2 h at room temperature.

6 Dialyse exhaustively against PBS; five changes of 1 litre at 4°C.

7 Dialyse for 8 h against two changes of Tris–HCl buffer.

8 Adjust volume to 4 ml with Tris–HCl buffer containing 1% BSA and 0.02% sodium azide.

4.6.3 SPDP conjugation of enzymes

Very effective conjugates between antibody and enzymes can be made using the heterobifunctional cross-linking reagent N-succinimidyl-3-(2-pyridylthio) propionate (SPDP). This reagent can be coupled separately to both antibody and enzyme through free amino groups on the proteins. The resultant antibody–pyridyldithio groups can then be reduced to thiol groups and disulphide linked to the enzyme–pyridyldithio groups with the release of 2-pyridinethione (Fig. 4.4).

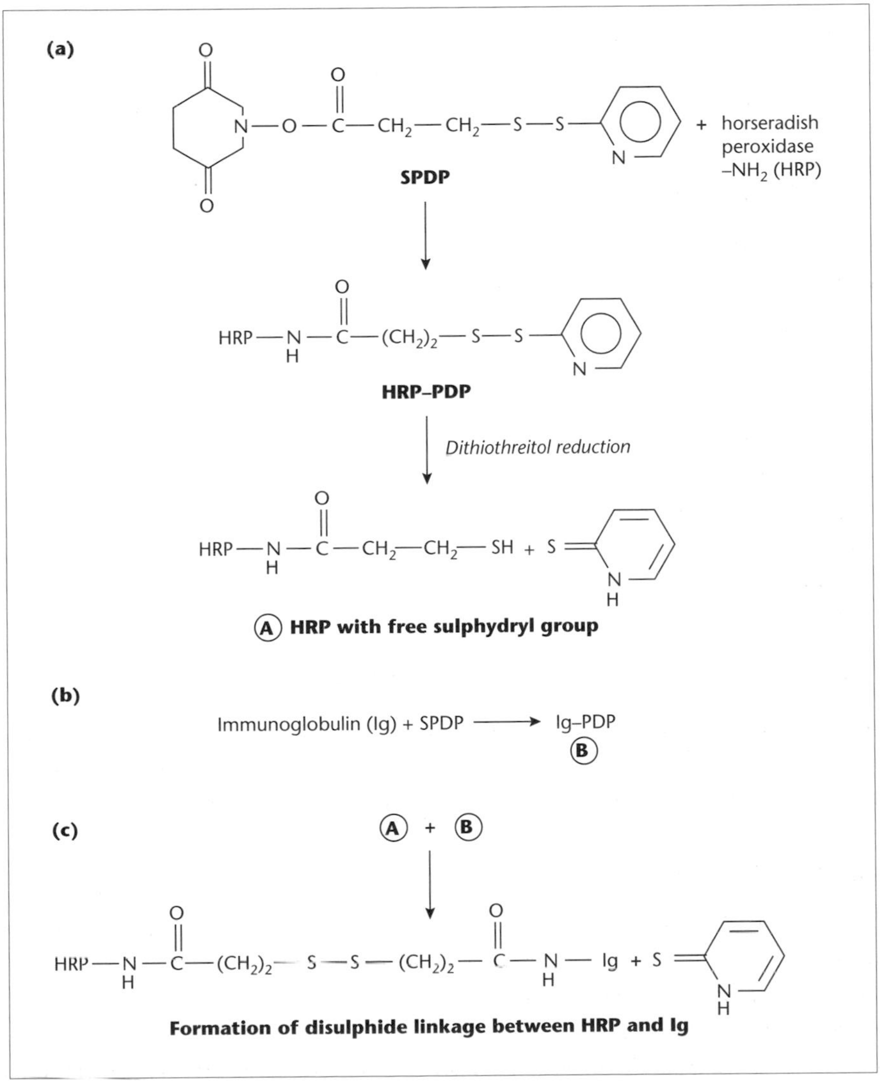

Fig. 4.4 Disulphide coupling of enzyme–immunoglobulin conjugates. The amino groups of a protein may be reacted with N-succinimidyl-3-(2-pyridylthio) propionate (SPDP) to form a PDP derivative, which in turn may be reduced with dithiothreitol to form sulphydryl groups. This modified protein may be reacted with other PDP-bearing proteins and coupled via disulphide linkages.

0.2 M phosphate–saline coupling buffer, pH 7.5

IgG fraction of antiserum (2 mg/ml in coupling buffer)

Horseradish peroxidase (1.0 mg/ml in coupling buffer)

N-succinimidyl-3-(2-pyridylthio) propionate (SPDP)

Methanol

1 M dithiothreitol

0.1 M iodoacetamide (stock)

Sephadex G-25 column for rapid buffer exchange

Rotator

Bovine serum albumin (BSA)

METHOD

1 Dissolve 3 mg of SPDP in 0.3 ml methanol. This solution must be prepared freshly each time.

Carry out steps 2–4 A and B in parallel.

A

2 Add 50 µl SPDP solution to the horseradish peroxidase (0.5 mg in 0.5 ml coupling buffer).

3 Rotate gently for 1 h at room temperature.

4 Isolate the labelled enzyme on the Sephadex G-25 buffer-exchange column equilibrated with coupling buffer.

B

2 Add 8 µl of SPDP solution to the antibody (1 mg in coupling buffer).

3 Rotate for 1 h at room temperature.

4 Isolate the labelled antibody on the Sephadex G-25 buffer-exchange column equilibrated in coupling buffer (see Appendix B.1).

5 Measure the volume of antibody solution and add 1 M dithiothreitol to a final concentration of 50 mM.

6 Incubate at room temperature for 15 min.

7 Re-equilibrate one of the Sephadex G-25 columns with coupling buffer.

8 Remove the dithiothreitol by passing sample down the Sephadex buffer-exchange column equilibrated in coupling buffer.

9 Mix the labelled enzyme with the reduced labelled antibody.

10 Rotate gently for 5–8 h.

11 Measure volume and alkylate any remaining thiol groups by adding iodoacetamide to a final concentration of 30 mM.

12 Incubate at room temperature for 15 min.

13 Isolate protein by passing down the Sephadex buffer-exchange column in coupling buffer. Store at 4°C with BSA added to 1% w/v.

4.7 The biotin–avidin system

Biotin is synthesized by plants and many microorganisms; in particular, large amounts are formed by the intestinal flora. It is essential for warm-blooded animals and acts as a coenzyme in CO_2 fixation and transcarboxylation reactions.

Avidin, found in egg white, has an extremely high affinity ($> 10^{15}$/mol) for biotin, and binding is so strong that for most purposes the binding can be treated as though it is covalent. There are four sites on the avidin molecule at which biotin may be bound. Biotin is a small molecule that can be easily coupled to proteins, including antibodies, enzymes and many antigens, without significant loss of the protein's biological activity. The loss of activity is much less than the damage done by coupling a large enzyme directly or following exposure to oxidizing agents, as in radiolabelling. Sandwich assays may then be performed in which antibodies bound to solid-phase antigen may be revealed by adding, in sequence, biotinylated anti-immunoglobulin, avidin and then biotinylated enzyme.

Avidin may be conjugated with enzyme, thus eliminating one step in the assay. Considerable amplification of the resultant signal can be obtained by use of preformed complexes of avidin and biotinylated enzyme—formed such that a few biotin-binding sites are still free on the avidin molecules. An advantage of the avidin–biotin system is that avidin may be labelled with enzyme, fluorochromes, radiolabels, ferritin, etc., so that the same biotinylated antibody may be used with the different avidin conjugates in enzyme immunoassay, radioimmunoassay, immunofluorescence and electron microscopy, without the need for preparing separate labelled antibodies.

Streptavidin from *Streptomyces avidinii* is also used. Although there are no problems with non-specific binding, the biotin-binding site is thought to be less accessible which sometimes necessitates coupling the biotin via a spacer arm. The technique described below may be used with proteins and carbohydrates. The biotinylated proteins tend to retain more of their activity after conjugation. Many different biotin-linked antibodies are commercially available. Similarly, avidin may be purchased already substituted with a wide variety of fluorochrome, enzyme or radioisotope labels.

4.7.1 Biotinylation

MATERIALS
Biotin-O-succinimide ester
IgG fraction of antiserum (see Section 1.3)
Enzyme; for example, horseradish peroxidase
Sephadex G-25 buffer-exchange column (see Appendix B.1) or dialysis tubing
0.1 M bicarbonate buffer, pH 8.4
Dimethyl sulphoxide (DMSO)
0.1 M tris(hydroxymethyl)-aminomethane (Tris)–HCl buffer, pH 8.4

1. Equilibrate IgG and enzyme separately in bicarbonate buffer using the Sephadex G-25 column or by dialysis.
2. Adjust each protein concentration to 1 mg/ml in bicarbonate buffer (see Appendix B.5.1–B.5.4).
3. Dissolve 1 mg biotin ester in 1 ml DMSO just before use.
4. Add 75 μl biotin solution to each 1 ml of protein solution.
5. Mix immediately and rotate for 4 h at room temperature.
6. Re-equilibrate the column with 0.1 M Tris–HCl buffer, pH 7.4, and buffer exchange the two samples on this column (or dialyse against this buffer).

TECHNICAL NOTE

The coupling reaction must be performed in a buffer lacking Tris or other primary amines as these will compete with amino groups on the protein. Hence the reason for switching to Tris *after* coupling.

4.8 Hapten sandwich labelling

Two monoclonal antibodies from the same species, e.g. two mouse antibodies, can be used in the same binding reaction as direct conjugates, e.g. with one labelled with fluorescein and the other with rhodamine. Frequently direct fluoresence is too insensitive and the indirect technique is necessary. This presents difficulties since both mouse antibodies would look alike to the secondary (mouse-revealing) reagent. However, indirect fluorescence can be achieved by modifying each monoclonal antibody to make it antigenically distinct.

If two monoclonal antibodies are derivatized, one with dinitrophenol (DNP) and the other with penicilloyl (Pen), they may be detected independently using, for example, fluorescein-conjugated anti-DNP and rhodamine- or phycoerythrin-conjugated anti-Pen.

To obtain reliable results from this system, considerable time and care is required for standardization; however, the method can yield considerable amplification in systems where the epitopes to be detected by the first antibodies are at low density. These techniques are also useful for coupling haptens to carrier molecules for use in experiments on the immune response.

Entirely synthetic antigens and chemically modified proteins have been used to investigate the nature of the lymphocyte surface receptor for antigen and to uncover the intricacies of T- and B-lymphocyte cooperation.

The techniques described in this section have had wide application in immunology.

4.8.1 Dinitrophenylation of immunoglobulin or protein antigen

A hapten is a small molecule that will bind to B cells or preformed antibody. One of the potential problems is that a hapten alone is too small to cross-link lymphocyte cell-surface receptors and so will not stimulate B-cell differentiation to plasma cells and antibody production. The B-cell response to antigen, in the majority of cases, requires cooperation by T cells. Again because of its

Fig. 4.5 Chemicals used for dinitrophenyl derivatization of protein carriers. 2,4-Dinitro-1-fluorobenzene (DNFB) is much more highly reactive than dinitrobenzene sulphonate (DNBS) and is used when rapid and higher molar substitution ratios are required. Both chemicals are extremely potent skin sensitizers so avoid personal contamination.

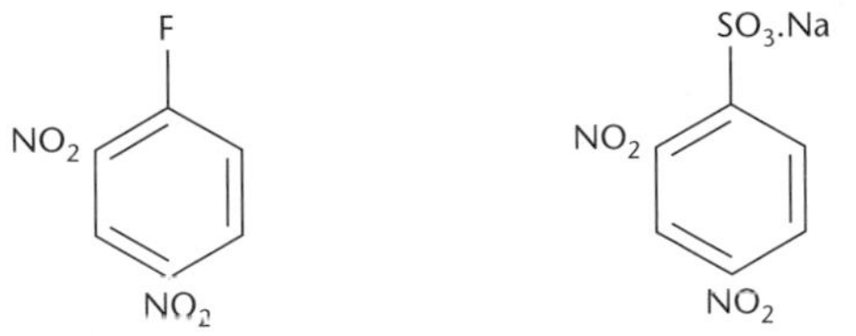

2,4-dinitro-1-fluorobenzene (DNFB)

2,4-dinitrobenzenesulphonate.Na (DNBS)

small size, around 400–800 Da, the hapten cannot stimulate two lymphocytes simultaneously. This may be overcome by hapten conjugated to an immunogenic protein. The T cells will recognize this protein, or carrier molecule, and so cooperate with B cells to produce antihapten antibody (anticarrier antibody is also produced). These defined antigens are powerful tools for investigating cell interactions in the immune response. Probably the most commonly used hapten is dinitrophenyl (DNP) which is conjugated to protein via one of its two reactive forms shown in Fig. 4.5.

Dinitrofluorobenzene is highly reactive with the amino groups of proteins under alkaline conditions where the peptide bond is quite stable. It is used when high substitution ratios are required.

High substitution ratios

MATERIALS AND EQUIPMENT
Protein antigen, e.g. keyhole limpet haemocyanin (KLH)
1 M sodium bicarbonate
2,4-dinitrofluorobenzene (DNFB) (Caution: an extremely potent skin-sensitizing agent)
Sephadex G-25 column (see Appendix B.1)
UV spectrophotometer

METHOD

1   Dissolve 100 mg KLH in 1 M sodium bicarbonate (minimum initial concentration 10–20 mg/ml).
2   Add 0.5 ml DNFB (*take care as DNFB is an extremely potent skin-sensitizing agent*).
3   Mix vigorously on a magnetic stirring platform for 45 min at 37°C.
4   Separate the DNP–KLH conjugate from the free DNFB on a Sephadex G-25 column (see Appendix B.1).
5   Determine the number of DNP groups per KLH molecule using the conversion:
    DNP: at 360 nm, absorbance of 1.0 (1-cm cuvette) is equivalent to 0.067 mmol DNP;
    KLH: at 278 nm, absorbance of 1.0 (1-cm cuvette) is equivalent to 0.00018 mmol KLH.
    The presence of dinitrophenyl groups on the protein accounts for approximately 40% of the absorbance at 278 nm. This is allowed for in the conversion.

TECHNICAL NOTES
• KLH tends to self-associate so it is not possible to assign an accurate molecular weight. The above calculations assume an average molecular weight of 3×10^6.
• Removal of KLH molecular complexes by ultracentrifugation tends to reduce its immunogenicity.

Low substitution ratios

MATERIALS AND EQUIPMENT
Immunoglobulin, e.g. fowl γ-globulin (FγG)
0.15 M potassium carbonate
Dinitrobenzene sulphonate (DNBS), sodium salt recrystallized
Sephadex G-25 column (see Appendix B.1)
UV spectrophotometer

METHOD

1 Dissolve 100 mg FγG in 5 ml 0.15 M potassium carbonate.

2 Add 20 mg Na DNBS and mix overnight at 4°C.

3 Prepare a column of Sephadex G-25 and equilibrate against phosphate-buffered saline (PBS) (see Appendix B.1.5).

4 Add the DNP–FγG mixture to the column and pump through, adding more PBS when required.

5 Collect the first visible band to elute from the column. This is the DNP–FγG conjugate. The free DNP is retained at the top of the column.

6 Collect 1.5 times the original sample volume.

7 Dilute DNP–FγG solution 1 : 20 with PBS, and read absorbance in the spectrophotometer at 280 and 360 nm.

Calculation of DNP : FγG ratio

DNP: at 360 nm, absorbance of 1.0 (1-cm cuvette) is equivalent to 0.067 mmol DNP.

FγG: at 280 nm, absorbance of 1.0 (1-cm cuvette) is equivalent to 0.0029 mmol FγG. (The DNP interferes with the absorbance reading at 280 nm. This is allowed for in the conversion factor.)

The chemical and antigenic properties of carrier proteins are often altered after hapten substitution. FγG, for example, is irreversibly denatured and becomes insoluble at ratios greater than DNP_{40} FγG. With the method described for dinitrophenylation of FγG you should obtain DNP_{3-4} FγG. There is good hapten and carrier priming when mice are immunized with conjugates with these molar ratios. With DNP_{15-20} FγG, carrier priming is greatly reduced, whereas with DNP_{30-35} FγG, direct (IgM) plaques alone are detected; there is no switching to indirect (IgG) plaque formation in the antibody response to the hapten.

The KLH molecule can accept up to 100 hapten groups before carrier priming is affected.

4.8.2 Penicilloylation of protein

MATERIALS
Penicillic acid
95% ethanol
Protein solution (5–10 mg/ml)
0.1 M phosphate buffer, pH 7.5
Phosphate-buffered saline (PBS)

METHOD

1 Prepare a 1 mM solution of penicillic acid in 95% ethanol and add 1 ml to 7 ml of protein solution.
2 Leave to mix overnight at room temperature.
3 Dialyse against five changes of PBS to remove unreacted penicillic acid or by desalting using Sephadex G-25 (see Appendix B.1.4–B.1.5).

Estimation of penicilloyl substitution

MATERIALS AND EQUIPMENT

p-(hydroxymercuri) benzoate
0.1 M sodium hydroxide
0.1 M carbonate buffer, pH 7.0
Derivatized protein solution
UV spectrophotometer

METHOD

1 Dissolve 0.5 g *p*-(hydroxymercuri) benzoate in minimum volume of 0.1 M sodium hydroxide.
2 Dilute with 0.1 M carbonate buffer, pH 7.0, to obtain a stock solution of approximately 1.5×10^{-2} M.
3 Determine the precise concentration of this solution spectrophotometrically (molar extinction coefficient, $E^{1\ cm}{}_{M}$, through a 1-cm light path at 232 nm is 1.69×10^{4}).

This solution will keep for months if stored in the dark at 4°C.

Titration of penicilloyl groups

1 Dilute the stock solution of *p*-(hydroxymercuri) benzoate with carbonate buffer, to obtain a 2×10^{-3} M solution.
2 Dilute the derivatized protein solution 1 : 10 with carbonate buffer and add 1.0 ml to a spectrophotometer cuvette.
3 Read absorbance at 280 nm.
4 Add 0.1 ml of diluted *p*-(hydroxymercuri) benzoate solution to the same cuvette, mix and leave at room temperature for 10 min. Determine the new absorbance value.

The difference in the two spectrophotometer readings is due to the *p*-(hydroxymercuri) benzoate reacting with the penicilloyl groups to form a penamaldate derivative which absorbs at 280 nm. The molar extinction coefficient of penamaldate at 280 nm, 1 cm light path, is 2.38×10^{4}.

Calculation of substitution ratio

Protein: the interference of the penicilloyl groups with the estimation of protein absorbance at 280 nm is insignificant. The extinction coefficients given for underivatized proteins in the Appendix may be used without correction.

Penicilloyl: at 280 nm, absorbance of 1.0 (1-cm cuvette) is equivalent to 0.0526 mM penamaldate. (An average molar extinction coefficient of 1.9×10^3 has been used for this calculation as the relationship between an increase in the molar substitution ratio and absorbance is not linear.)

TECHNICAL NOTES

- The p-(hydroxymercuri) benzoate stock solution may form a slight precipitate when carbonate buffer is added to the original solution in sodium hydroxide. This should be removed by centrifugation.
- Remember to allow for both the original dilution of the derivatized protein solution and the dilution due to benzoate addition when calculating the final penamaldate absorbance value.
- The rate of substitution varies with pH and protein concentration. At pH 11.0 and a 30–50 molar excess of penicillic acid with respect to the free amino groups on the protein, there is an almost quantitative substitution of the protein lysyl groups.

4.8.3 Chemical derivatization of first antibodies

MATERIALS

Monoclonal antibodies
Materials for DNP labelling (see Section 4.8.1)
Materials for Pen labelling (see Section 4.8.2)
Sephadex G-25 mini-columns (packed in Pasteur pipettes)
Mini-concentrator for multiple samples

METHOD

1 Isolate the antibody protein either by ammonium sulphate precipitation (see Section 1.1.2), or by protein A affinity chromatography (see Section 1.4.2).
2 Prepare the derivatization mixture for DNP or Pen (as above) labelling using 20 mg antibody protein in a total volume of 2 ml, and the other chemicals pro rata.
3 Remove 0.2 ml of sample at each of the following time points: 0, 0.25, 0.5, 1.0, 1.5 and 2.0 h and re-isolate the antibody by chromatography through a Sephadex G-25 column. (Use a fresh equilibrated column for each sample.)
4 At the end of the time course determine the molar substitution ratios for DNP or Pen as above.
5 Plot a graph of molar substitution ratio against time, as in Fig. 4.6.

The hapten-conjugated antibodies tend to work best at a substitution ratio of between 15 and 25 mol/mol. Having determined the time and conditions for optimum substitution, repeat the derivatizations for a single time point using sufficient antibody protein for the intended use.

TECHNICAL NOTES

- These chemically modified antibodies are very stable if stored at −20°C in the dark.
- The rate of reaction is temperature dependent. If greater control over derivatization is required, perform the reaction at 4°C. It will take about 16 h to obtain the maximum values shown in Fig. 4.6.
- If the antibodies are against pure antigens, it is possible to carry out the derivatization reactions while the antibody is bound to an affinity column, thus protecting the binding site. Subsequent

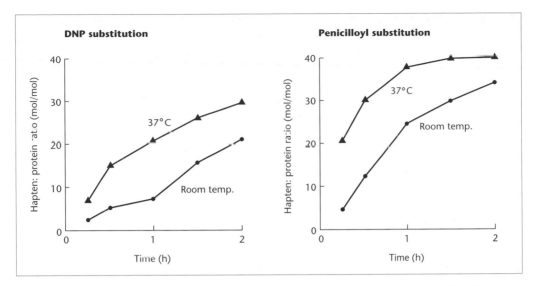

Fig. 4.6 Time course of dinitrophenyl and penicilloyl substitution of mouse IgG$_1$ monoclonal antibodies. Each time point shows the hapten : protein molar ratio determined for derivatization reactions carried out at room temperature or 37°C.

washing of the column with buffer prior to elution of the bound antibody eliminates the need for dialysis to remove unreacted hapten.

4.8.4 Preparation of anti-DNP and anti-Pen fluorescent conjugates

MATERIALS
Two cheap proteins, available in pure form; for example, ovalbumin and bovine serum albumin (BSA)
Materials for DNP and Pen labelling (see Sections 4.8.1 and 4.8.2)
Materials for fluorochrome conjugation (see Section 4.2)

METHOD

1 Prepare two hapten-carrier conjugates; for example, DNP–ovalbumin and Pen–BSA.
2 Immunize rabbits, or larger animals, with the conjugates independently, to obtain good antisera.
3 Isolate the IgG fraction of each antiserum (see Section 1.3) and conjugate one with fluorescein isothiocyanate (FITC), and the other with rhodamine isothiocyanate (RITC) or phycoerythrin (PE).

4.8.5 Determination of optimum reaction conditions

MATERIALS
DNP- and Pen-labelled monoclonal antibodies (see Section 4.8.3)
Fluorochrome-labelled anti-DNP and anti-Pen (see Section 4.8.4)
Target cells or tissues carrying antigens of interest

It is necessary to determine the optimum reaction conditions for the most intense specific staining and the lowest non-specific background. The major variables will be: (a) molar substitution ratio of hapten : antibody; (b) concentration of antibody protein; and (c) dilution of fluorescent conjugates. In practice, a molar substitution ratio of 20 : 1 (hapten : antibody protein) and a dilution of 1 : 20–1 : 40 of fluorescent conjugate has been found to give generally acceptable results. More precise refinements can be introduced as experience with the system increases. The concentration of first antibody will vary widely, both with the quality of the monoclonal and with the epitopes to be detected.

Carry out standardization as described in Section 4.2.6 according to the Protocol below. Remember to use a concentration range of haptenated antibodies to obtain optimum results.

Protocol.

Tube number	1	2	3	4	5	6	7
Cells carrying antigens A and B	+	+	+	+	+	+	+
DNP20 anti-A monoclonal	+	−	+	−	−	−	+
Pen20 anti-B monoclonal	−	+	−	+	−	−	+
FITC anti-DNP (1 : 30 dil.)	+	−	−	+	+	−	+
RITC (or PE) anti-Pen (1 : 30 dil.)	−	+	+	−	−	+	+

FITC, fluorescein isothiocyanate; RITC, rhodamine isothiocyanate; PE, phycoerythrin.

TECHNICAL NOTES

- As a guide, use 5–50 µg DNP or Pen antibody protein as an initial concentration range.
- Tubes 3–6 are specificity controls; 3 and 4 to ensure that the haptens and conjugates do not cross-react, 5 and 6 to ensure that the fluorescent conjugates do not react directly with the target cells.
- Tube 7 contains the full set of reactants—add the first antibodies as a mixture, but then wash thoroughly before adding the fluorescent conjugates. Remember to increase the volume of reactants to maintain the same protein concentration throughout. An increase in the protein concentration (as opposed to total protein) in tube 7 could give a higher non-specific background than with tubes 1–6.

This method can work well when sensitive double labelling is required either for microscopy or flow cytometry. The same general approach can be used with other detection systems, e.g. enzyme immunoconjugates.

4.9 Radiolabelling of soluble proteins

The methods in this section vary in the harshness (potential for alteration of the conformation of the labelled material) of the reaction required to achieve the desired result.

Chloramine T and Iodogen labelling involve tyrosyl residues predominantly; if they inactivate antibody binding then try labelling onto lysyl residues. It is essential that use of radiolabels is recorded appropriately and safety advice regarding the handling of radioisotopes is followed in accordance with the local guidelines of the institution where the work is carried out.

4.9.1 Chloramine T method

In alkaline conditions, chloramine T is slowly converted to hypochlorous acid which acts as an oxidizing agent. At pH < 8.0, oxidation results in iodine incorporation into tyrosine residues, but at a higher pH histidine also becomes labelled. The method is the best one to try first for labelling antigens or antibodies, either in solution or bound to a solid-phase immunoadsorbent to protect the active site.

MATERIALS AND EQUIPMENT
All reagents should be prepared just before labelling.
0.1 M tris(hydroxymethyl)-aminomethane (Tris)–HCl buffer, pH 7.4
Protein for iodination (500 µg/ml in Tris–HCl buffer)
Chloramine T (1 mg/ml in Tris–HCl buffer)
Sodium metabisulphite (2 mg/ml in Tris–HCl buffer)
Potassium iodide (5×10^{-5} M in Tris–HCl buffer)
Sodium ^{125}I, carrier free
Phosphate-buffered saline (PBS), containing 0.25% w/v gelatin
Sephadex G-25
Disposable chromatography column (e.g. a disposable pipette plugged with glass wool)
Gamma spectrometer
Caution: Wear gloves when handling glass wool.

METHOD

1 Mix 100 µl of protein (500 µg/ml initial concentration) with 18.5×10^6 Bq ^{125}I and 10 µl of chloramine T (1 mg/ml initial concentration).
2 Incubate for 2–4 min at room temperature.
3 Add 10 µl of sodium metabisulphite solution (2 mg/ml initial concentration) and mix thoroughly.
4 After 2 min, add 10 µl of potassium iodide solution.
5 Separate the labelled protein from the free iodine using a column of Sephadex G-25 equilibrated with PBS containing 0.25% gelatin.
6 Elute the column with PBS containing gelatin and collect 0.5-ml fractions.
7 Determine the c.p.m. of each fraction using a γ spectrometer. Identify the first peak of radioactivity—this contains the labelled protein.
8 Store at 4°C for use.

TECHNICAL NOTES
• Proteins denature readily at low concentration, therefore gelatin or bovine serum albumin (BSA) should be incorporated in the elution buffer. The gelatin or BSA is also necessary to prevent non-specific binding of protein to the Sephadex. If labelled proteins without carrier protein are needed, the column can be precycled with gelatin or BSA to block non-specific uptake and the column used with buffer alone.

- Although the Sephadex G-25 column is adequate to rapidly separate the protein from the harmful reaction reagents and the free iodine, the labelled protein often needs further purification. Frequently, labelled proteins show some non-specific 'stickiness' due to protein aggregates. These can be removed by gel filtration on Sephadex with an appropriate fractionation range. The nascent formation of unrelated immune complexes at equivalence within the labelled protein solution is also an effective way of removing non-specific binding, but must be used with care in case the complex components interfere with the subsequent assay.
- This labelling technique may be used to iodinate antibodies attached to an antigen immunoadsorbent (this protects the antigen-binding site). The free iodide is removed by washing with buffer, and the labelled antibody is recovered by acid elution (see Section 1.4.2).

4.9.2 Determination of specific activity of radiolabelled protein

The protein concentration of the labelled material changes during radiolabelling and one cannot assume that all of the radioactive iodine is covalently bound to the protein.

Total radioactivity (in c.p.m.) is a less useful measure of the efficiency of labelling than specific activity (c.p.m./mg protein). It is necessary therefore to determine the new protein concentration, either by its UV absorbance if it is a pure protein (see Appendix B for extinction coefficients of common immunochemicals), or by the Bradford method if it is a mixture of proteins (see Appendix B.5.1 and B.5.2).

MATERIALS AND EQUIPMENT
Radioiodinated sample
Glass-fibre filter discs, e.g. Whatman GF/A
Large mapping pins in a cork board
Automatic pipette, 1–5 µl
10-ml glass test tubes
Ice-cold 10% w/v trichloroacetic acid (TCA)
Absolute ethanol
Gamma spectrometer

METHOD

1 Mount each filter on a map pin (or hypodermic syringe needle) so that it is held clear of the cork board.
2 Dispense between 1 and 5 µl of each sample (this should correspond to approximately 10–50 000 c.p.m. of the total radioactivity) onto two separate filter discs and transfer one into a 10-ml test tube.
3 Add 2 ml of ice-cold TCA to the tube, mix by vortexing and leave for 10 min.
4 Decant the TCA and replace with 2 ml of ethanol.
5 Mix by vortexing and leave for 10 min.
6 Transfer each pair of TCA-treated and -untreated filters to separate small plastic tubes and determine their radioactive content in a gamma spectrometer.

Calculation of labelling efficiency

$$\% \text{ Protein-bound radioactivity} = \frac{\text{c.p.m. in TCA-treated sample}}{\text{total c.p.m. in untreated sample}} \times 100$$

$$\text{Specific activity (c.p.m./mg)} = \frac{\text{c.p.m. in TCA-treated sample}}{\text{volume of treated sample (µl)}} \times \frac{1000}{\text{protein concentration (µg/ml)}}$$

TECHNICAL NOTES

- Proteins labelled to a very high specific activity (e.g. for autoradiography or immunoprecipitation) can give problems in this procedure: often it is not possible to measure accurately a sufficiently small aliquot to obtain a c.p.m. within the spectrometer range and the protein concentration can be too low for efficient TCA precipitation. Both these problems can be overcome by prior dilution of an aliquot of the labelled protein in bovine serum albumin (1 mg/ml) dissolved in phosphate-buffered saline.
- The same principles apply for the measurement of any radioactive label bound to a protein molecule, with modifications to take account of the nature of the isotope. Clearly, if the radioisotope is a low-energy emitter (^{3}H, ^{14}C or ^{35}S) then a β spectrometer should be substituted for the γ spectrometer.
- Treating the filter with ethanol not only aids the removal of TCA-soluble material but also speeds drying. Low-energy emitters need liquid scintillants, many of which will not tolerate water.

4.9.3 Iodination of proteins with Iodogen

The main damaging reaction in the chloramine T method is the exposure of proteins to the oxidizing agent. The use of the insoluble chloroamide 1,3,4,6-tetrachloro-3a, 6a-diphenylglycoluril (Iodogen) coated onto the surface of the reaction tube, or a plastic bead, reduces denaturation of antigen or antibodies during iodination.

Preparation in advance

MATERIALS AND EQUIPMENT
Iodogen
Dichloromethane
Test tube, 10 × 75 mm solvent-resistant plastic (e.g. polypropylene)
Water bath
Nitrogen cylinder

METHOD

1   Prepare a solution of Iodogen (0.1 mg/ml) in dichloromethane.
2   Add 0.2 ml of this solution (20 µg Iodogen) to a test tube.
3   Evaporate the methylene chloride in a stream of nitrogen, while rotating the tube slowly in a water bath at 37°C, to leave a thin film of Iodogen in the bottom of the tube.
4   Store in the dark at –20°C. The stored tubes may be used for several weeks.

Iodination technique

Protein for iodination (1 mg/ml) in borate–saline buffer, pH 8.3, ionic strength 0.1
Sodium ^{125}I, carrier free
Iodogen-coated tubes, prepared as above

METHOD

1   Place the Iodogen-coated tube on ice and add 0.2 ml of protein solution (1 mg/ml initial concentration).
2   Initiate the reaction by the addition of 10 µl of sodium ^{125}I solution (37×10^6 Bq ^{125}I).
3   Incubate for 5 min with gentle stirring.
4   Terminate the reaction by decanting the protein solution and leave for 10 min to allow reactive iodine to decay.
5   Separate the labelled protein from the free iodine by gel filtration as for the chloramine T method.
6   Determine the protein-bound radioactivity and specific activity.

TECHNICAL NOTES

- This method has been found to be more efficient than the chloramine T reaction for some proteins but is inferior for others. The labelling technique of choice must be determined by experimentation.
- A similar method may be used for the iodination of cells. Typically, use 4×10^6 cells, 6.6 µg of potassium iodide and 3.7×10^6 Bq ^{125}I in a total volume of 400 µl of phosphate-buffered saline (PBS). Add mixture to a tube coated with 50 µg Iodogen. Incubate for 15 min on ice with gentle stirring. Terminate the reaction by decanting the cells and wash three times in PBS by centrifugation (150 g for 10 min at 4°C). This technique does not alter cell viability, as assessed by the uptake of trypan blue.

4.9.4 Biosynthetic labelling of hybridoma-derived antibody

Secreted proteins, as well as cellular components, can be labelled biosynthetically by incorporating labelled amino acids into a culture medium. Immunoglobulins, and many cell-surface and secreted molecules, are glycoproteins; therefore, radioactive sugars, as well as amino acids, can be used as labelled precursors. A culture medium deficient in the particular amino acid must be used to support cell culture during the incorporation of the labelled residue. Culture medium normally contains glucose as the sole sugar as cells biosynthesize the other sugars. If another sugar such as labelled galactose is added, little conversion to other sugars occurs. To optimize the utilization of the labelled sugar the level of glucose may be lowered, but cannot be omitted completely as cell viability and therefore incorporation of the label will be adversely affected.

Hybridoma cells (or other cells in tissue culture)

Horse or fetal bovine serum, dialysed against phosphate-buffered saline (PBS)

Selective culture medium deficient in leucine (selectamine is ideal) containing either ^{3}H-leucine
(74–740 × 10^3 Bq/ml) or ^{14}C-leucine (37–185 × 10^3 Bq/ml), and/or ^{14}C-galactose
(37–185 × 10^3 Bq/ml), in each case with 5% dialysed serum

Plastic culture tubes, sterile

METHOD

1 Count the cell suspension.

2 Add 2 × 10^5 cells to a sterile culture tube and centrifuge at 150 g for 10 min at room
temperature.

3 Remove the supernatant and add 0.2 ml of the labelling medium.

4 Incubate overnight at 37°C in a humid incubator gassed with 5% CO_2 in air.

5 After incubation, centrifuge (150 g for 10 min at room temperature) and remove the
supernatant.

6 Determine the protein-bound radioactivity and specific activity.

7 Store at –20°C.

TECHNICAL NOTES

- ^{14}C-leucine gives a higher energy emission than ^{3}H-leucine and so is counted more efficiently in
a scintillation counter, but ^{14}C-amino acids are produced at a lower specific activity than the ^{3}H
form and they are more expensive.

- ^{14}C and ^{3}H have far longer half-lives than ^{125}I; therefore, antibodies labelled with these radioisotopes have a longer potential lifetime for use.

- ^{35}S-methionine is another amino acid frequently used for biosynthetic labelling of proteins. It is
available at very high specific activity and has a higher energy of emission than ^{14}C or ^{3}H, but a
shorter half-life. This amino acid is less frequent in the average protein, about one in 20 residues,
so the protein is usually labelled to a lesser specific activity. The higher energy of emission is an
advantage when this label is used in fluorography (see below in Section 4.10). Seleno-methionine
(^{75}Se-methionine) is a γ emitter and so is very easy to detect, especially in whole-body systems.
It has the significant disadvantage that the radioactive moiety may be cleaved *in vivo* and so is
not always a reliable tracer for the original amino acid.

- Sufficient incorporation of labelled precursor may be achieved by incubation times of only
3–4 h. This may be necessary if the tissue culture conditions are not ideal for cell maintenance.

- Tissue culture media prepared for biosynthetic labelling by the omission of an amino acid
should not be used for the determination of the rate of protein synthesis by incorporation of
isotopically labelled amino acids, as the rate of uptake and incorporation is often crucially
dependent on the external concentration of amino acids.

- Biosynthetic labelling *in vivo* may be achieved by injecting mice intraperitoneally with
1.85 × 10^7 Bq of a ^{3}H-labelled amino acid mixture: inject once daily on days 7–10 after the

initial inoculation of hybridoma cells. Collect the ascitic fluid by drainage and dialyse against phosphate-buffered saline until no ^{3}H is detectable in the dialysis fluid. For an IgG monoclonal antibody, all of the radioactivity should be TCA precipitable, approximately 30% should be retained by a protein A column and the specific activity of the protein A-purified material should be approximately 3.7 GBq/mmol. *Remember that the mice will excrete ^{3}H after day 7, so appropriate precautions to contain the radioactivity and prevent personal contamination must be taken.*

4.9.5 Conjugation labelling

Most proteins can be labelled easily by one of the direct methods, but some antibodies, particularly those with many tyrosines within the combining site, can be damaged by these methods.

Bolton and Hunter designed a compound, *N*-succinimidyl-3-(4-hydroxyphenyl) propionate, which can be labelled easily by the chloramine T method (see Bolton & Hunter 1973). The labelled ester is isolated by gel filtration and then mixed with the protein so that conjugation occurs via an amide linkage to lysine residues on the protein. The ester (Bolton and Hunter reagent) is also available commercially ready labelled with ^{125}I.

4.10 Autoradiography and fluorography

The utility and sensitivity of SDS-PAGE gels can be greatly increased by the use of radioactively labelled molecules, particularly in combination with immunoprecipitation. It is also possible to convert this essentially qualitative technique into a quantitative one, as explained in the Technical notes below.

4.10.1 Direct autoradiography

MATERIALS AND EQUIPMENT
SDS-PAGE gel, containing radioactively labelled proteins (see Appendix B.2.1)
X-ray film
Polyacrylamide gel drier
3 MM paper
Cling film or Saran wrap
Intensifying screen
Metal X-ray cassette

METHOD

1 Remove the polyacrylamide gel from the electrophoresis apparatus and cut away the stacking gel with a scalpel blade.
2 Fix the gel for 4 h in an aqueous solution of 40% v/v methanol and 10% v/v acetic acid and then soak for 15 min in a 5% solution of acetic acid containing 0.1% glycerol.

Continued

3 Lay the gel on a sheet of water-saturated 3 MM paper just larger than the gel and cover with a sheet of cling film. Take care to remove all excess water and air bubbles before trimming away the excess cling film with a scalpel blade.

4 Seal the gel into a commercial drier, preferably connected to a high-efficiency oil vacuum pump via two solid CO_2/acetone water traps. A water vacuum pump will do, provided the water pressure is high enough.

5 Turn on the vacuum and heating and dry the gel completely. This may be determined by the change in profile of the gel or when the gel no longer feels cool to the touch, in each case as judged through the rubber sheet of the drier. Do not release the vacuum until the gel is hot.

6 In the dark room, load a metal X-ray cassette with an intensifying screen (if required; see Technical notes), film and the gel (face down on the film).

7 If an intensifying screen has been used put the cassette at $-70°C$, otherwise leave it at room temperature away from direct sunlight, volatile chemicals and any external source of penetrating radiation.

8 Develop the X-ray film according to the manufacturer's instructions. The length of exposure will vary according to the type and amount of radioactivity and should be determined empirically. In some gels, it might be necessary to have both a long and short exposure to gain maximum information; for example, see Fig. 3.15.

9 Blackening of the film in areas corresponding to the protein tracks may be used to infer the presence of radioactive material in the original gel.

TECHNICAL NOTES

- Direct autoradiography is only possible with the penetrating radiations emanating from ^{131}I, ^{125}I, ^{32}P, etc., Weaker emitters ^{14}C, ^{35}S, ^{3}H, etc., require fluorography: see below.
- The sensitivity of detection may be increased by the use of:
  (a) *Intensifying screens.* These are plastic sheets impregnated with heavy metal ion phosphor crystals and are used to trap radiations which pass through the X-ray film. As a consequence, they emit photons and so blacken the X-ray film on the side away from the polyacrylamide gel. In principle, it is possible to use two intensifying screens, one on either side of the film. In practice, however, this can blur the final image because of the greater distance travelled by the radioactive and photon radiations.
  (b) *Preflashed film.* X-ray film is relatively insensitive and therefore single silver atoms may be induced in the silver halide crystals by transient exposure to an electronic flash. The duration of the flash and its intensity (varied by changing the distance between film and electronic flash-gun) is critical and should be determined empirically. Set the shortest duration on the flash-gun and position the gun at varying distances (increasing in steps of 1 m) from film test strips. Develop the film (and a piece of unflashed original) and use the conditions which just give barely visible fogging.
  Exposure of the gel with intensifying screens and preflashed film at $-70°C$ gives maximal stability of both the nascent image and the sensitized preflashed areas.
- It is convenient to use a mixture of purified radioactive proteins as molecular weight markers in these gels. Suitable mixtures for different fractionation ranges may either be bought commercially as a ^{14}C-methylated protein mixture or prepared from an 'in-house' mix of purified

proteins treated with ^{14}C-formaldehyde. Intensely coloured 'rainbow markers', which are also radioactive, are available commercially and offer the dual convenience of visibility during electrophoretic separation and fogging of the X-ray film.

- Much has been written about the artefacts associated with autoradiography. The two most commonly seen are:

  (a) A homogeneous fogging of the film, often in areas away from contact with the gel. This is due to chemical fogging and probably means that the acetic acid failed to volatilize during drying. Dry the gel with a hot air drier and re-expose to X-ray film.

  (b) Lightning strikes. This is caused by an electrostatic discharge from either your fingers or dampness causing the surfaces of the gel, screen or film to adhere. When you peel the surfaces apart an electrostatic charge is generated. Earth your fingers by touching the bench and make sure the interior of the cassette is warm and dry—especially if it has been exposed at –70°C—before you open it.

- If your cassettes are used communally, it is a wise precaution to line them with plastic benchcote or candy paper. If one becomes contaminated then the liner rather than the cassette can be replaced. Similarly, it is good practice to clean the intensifying screens regularly with an anti-static screen cleaner.

- As noted in Fig. 3.15, this technique is usually used qualitatively; however, it is relatively simple to quantify the radioactivity contained in the gel, although there is considerable loss of sensitivity. If you intend to measure the radioactivity, it is helpful to stain the gel, prior to drying the gel down. This will help you to locate the individual tracks. Remember that quantification can be carried out after the gel has been exposed to X-ray film, provided that sufficient radioactivity remains.

  (a) Lay the stained, dried gel on a glass plate and cut it up into its individual lanes using a scalpel blade and straight edge.

  (b) Cut strips of 1-mm tracing graph paper approximately the same size as the gel tracks.

  (c) Use spray adhesive to attach a strip of graph paper to each gel track, at right angles to the polypeptide bands.

  (d) Cut each track into 1-mm strips using a sharp pair of scissors, place each strip in a γ spectrometer and plot a graph of the amount of radioactivity.

  (e) Count in a γ spectrometer and plot a graph of the amount of radioactivity against the distance travelled down the gel.

  (f) Compare the result with that obtained from the X-ray film.

4.10.2 Fluorography

Weak α and β emitters would be detected very inefficiently by direct autoradiography because of the relatively short distances travelled by these radiations. Instead a scintillant is incorporated directly into the gel and the energy from the decay of the radioisotope is transferred to the X-ray film as photons of light.

In the original method for gel impregnation, the scintillant (usually 2,5-diphenyloxazole—PPO) was dissolved in dimethyl sulphoxide (DMSO), thus causing considerable shrinkage and distortion of the gel. Aqueous preparations are now commercially available (e.g. Amplify, APBiotech; see Appendix C. In both cases they are available as liquid or spray). The gel is fixed in an aqueous solution of methanol–acetic acid as above and then soaked in the scintillant solution.

After drying (without glycerol), the gel is loaded into a metal cassette with X-ray film and exposed at −70°C.

4.10.3 Ultrasmall gold probes

The advantage of labels such as enzymes is that they amplify the reaction and lead to an easily visible product. In so doing they can lead to some diffuseness with loss of structural detail. Gold provides a useful label where this fine structure is critical. Colloidal gold particles can be coupled to proteins and so used as the label coupled to antibodies or detection molecules, such as protein A. Best resolution is achieved using small particles (> 1 nm), and then enhancing the detection by deposition of silver on top of the gold. Gold-coupled reagents are available commercially together with silver enhancement systems. These may be visualized with a light microscope, an electron microscope and in protein blotting.

4.11 Western blotting

A sheet of nitrocellulose is placed against the surface of an SDS-PAGE protein fractionation gel (see Appendix B.2.1) and a current applied across the gel (at right angles to its face), thus causing the proteins to move out of the gel and onto the nitrocellulose where they bind firmly by covalent forces. Two variants of the basic apparatus are available to achieve the electrophoretic transfer, the so-called wet and semidry blotters:

wet blotters: the gel and transfer membrane are immersed in large volumes of buffer;

semi-dry blotters: use filter paper pads moistened with buffer.

4.11.1 Immuno- or Western blotting of SDS-PAGE

MATERIALS AND EQUIPMENT

Wet blotting apparatus (see Appendix C)

Polyacrylamide running buffer, 0.1 M tris(hydroxymethyl)-aminomethane (Tris)–glycine, pH 8.3, with 500 ml of methanol added to 2 l of blotting buffer (see Appendix A)

Nitrocellulose paper

Whatman no. 1 filter paper

Scotch-brite pads

METHOD

1 Equilibrate the SDS-PAGE gel (containing the fractionated protein) in blotting buffer for 30–60 min.

2 Assemble the blotting sandwich within the blotting cassette taking, in order, Scotch-brite pad, nitrocellulose sheet, polyacrylamide gel and Scotch-brite pad (anode → cathode) (Fig. 4.7). Take care to avoid any air bubbles between the gel and the nitrocellulose.

3 Insert the cassette into the blotting buffer and connect the power supply. The cathode should be on the gel side.

4 Blot for about 3 h at 60 V or overnight at 35 V.

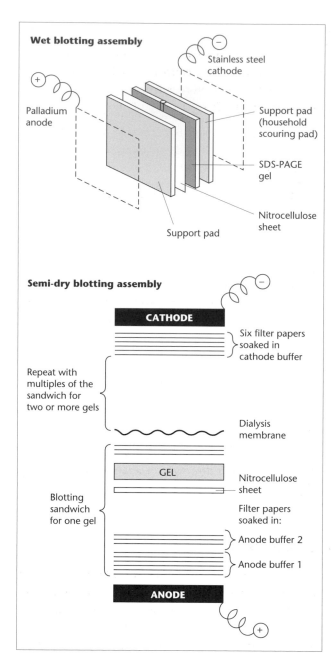

Fig. 4.7 Assembly sequence for sandwich for wet and semi-dry blotting. The precise details of the components will vary with the apparatus used; however, the order of assembly—anode, nitrocellulose sheet, SDS-PAGE gel, cathode—is vital. If it is reversed by mistake, the carefully separated proteins will be electrophoretically transferred to 5 l of tank buffer. The semi-dry blotter not only avoids the use of large volumes of buffer but also can be run as a sandwich of several gel–nitrocellulose sheets interspersed with low molecular weight cut-off dialysis membranes. The dialysis membrane permits the passage of ions but not of proteins.

TECHNICAL NOTES

- Methanol is used in the blotting buffer to prevent the gel swelling.
- Take great care to ensure that the blotting cassette is assembled in the correct order. Proteins transferred into the filter pads rather than the nitrocellulose will be lost.
- It is good practice to stain the gel for proteins after blotting over, to ensure that the transfer was complete. Some proteins, e.g. the relatively insoluble cytoskeletal components, tend to transfer inefficiently and non-quantitatively.
- Blots may be dried, sealed in a plastic bag and stored at –20°C for up to 6 months.

4.11.2 Staining Western blots

Blots may be stained with the usual protein stains. If it is intended to visualize the polypeptide bands by deposition of enzymically generated colours, 0.02% Ponceau S in 3% trichloroacetic acid can be used as a temporary stain, but may cause some protein denaturation. The blots are differentiated in running tap water. This stain is completely reversible and removed by washing in tap water.

4.11.3 Blocking protein-binding sites

Before visualization of protein bands with labelled antibodies it is necessary to block the remaining protein-binding sites on the nitrocellulose. Bovine serum albumin, haemoglobin or skimmed milk powder are frequently used for blocking, sometimes with the addition of 0.05% Tween 20. Tween 20 alone may be used and has the advantage that, after visualization with specific antibodies, the whole blot can be stained with protein stains. Moreover, the added advantage is that it reveals the markers for molecular weight determination, allowing the visualization of protein bands which have failed to bind antibody. A word of caution: Tween 20 alone is not an efficient blocking agent, so when concentrated protein solutions are used, such as serum or ascitic fluid, the background can be unacceptably high.

MATERIALS AND EQUIPMENT
Phosphate-buffered saline (PBS), containing 0.05% Tween 20 and 1% w/v bovine serum albumin (BSA)
Plastic box

> **METHOD**
>
> Place the nitrocellulose blot in the PBS–Tween–BSA and gently rotate on an orbital shaker for about 2 h at room temperature, or overnight in the cold.

4.11.4 Immunostaining nitrocellulose blots

Although proteins separated by SDS-PAGE and blotted onto nitrocellulose have been subjected to harsh denaturing conditions (detergent treatment, boiling, reducing agents and distortion due to adsorption to the highly charged surface of the nitrocellulose membrane) a large proportion of antigenic determinants remain intact and can be revealed by the addition of labelled antibodies. In the past, radiolabelled antibodies or antibodies detected by radiolabelled protein A have been extensively used. Although the technique offers high sensitivity, preparation for autoradiography can be complex and time consuming, and carries the risk of chronic exposure to low levels of radioactivity. The techniques for the use of enzyme-labelled antibodies have been improved greatly and a range of substrates developed which are not carcinogenic and can be used to deposit a variety of coloured, insoluble products on top of the protein band.

Biotinylated antibodies followed by streptavidin–peroxidase give well visualized bands with 4-chloro-1-naphthanol as substrate. Carbohydrate determinants maintain their immunogenic properties after SDS-PAGE fractionation and can be detected with biotinylated lectins or antibodies.

Nitrocellulose blot with immunoglobulin bands

Biotinylated antibody, e.g. biotinylated goat anti-human IgG streptavidin–peroxidase

Phosphate-buffered saline (PBS) containing 0.05% v/v Tween 20 with and without 1% w/v bovine serum albumin (BSA) (PBS–Tween–BSA)

4-chloro-1-naphthanol

0.05 M tris(hydroxymethyl)-aminomethane (Tris)–HCl buffer, pH 7.6

Hydrogen peroxide

METHOD

1 Prepare a dilution of biotinylated antibody in PBS–Tween–BSA; as a guide, high-titred antibodies can be used at a dilution of 1 : 1000. Prepare a sufficient volume of diluted antibody to cover the blot.

2 Immerse the blot in the antibody solution and agitate gently for 2 h on an orbital shaker.

3 Wash the blot thoroughly by immersing in excess PBS–Tween (0.05%); no BSA. Mix gently for 10 min on the orbital shaker.

4 Repeat the wash step three more times.

5 Add sufficient streptavidin–peroxidase conjugate (diluted 1 : 1000 in PBS–Tween–BSA) to cover the blot. Mix gently for 1 h on the orbital shaker.

6 Wash the blot by immersing in four changes of PBS–Tween as before.

7 During the final wash prepare the substrate solution by dissolving 6 mg 4-chloro-1-naphthanol in 20 ml methanol and adding it to 100 ml Tris–HCl buffer, pH 7.6, plus 12 μl hydrogen peroxide (30 volumes' strength).

8 Immerse the washed blot in the substrate solution. Mix gently on the orbital shaker. Bands should develop sufficient colour within a few minutes.

9 Remove the blot and wash with distilled water.

10 Dry the blot and analyse immediately. Although the coloured bands fade with time, the rate of colour loss can be retarded if the blots are kept in the dark.

TECHNICAL NOTES

- If the antibody is expensive, or the supply limited, a smaller volume of diluted antibody may be applied to the nitrocellulose sheet by means of saturated filter paper. It is essential to achieve good contact between the paper and the nitrocellulose. This may be achieved by sealing the nitrocellulose–filter paper sandwich into a plastic bag or by clamping it between two glass slides.

- Some of the substrates still in use are known carcinogens, e.g. bisdiazotized benzidine. *These should only be handled in a fume cupboard.*

- The colour reaction can be quantified by scanning densitometry and a permanent record made by photography, e.g. the Biogene Documentation System.

4.11.5 Western blotting with radiolabelled probes

1 Proceed as method above but at step 5 add ^{125}I-streptavidin instead of the enzyme-labelled material. Use about 1×10^6 c.p.m. per track.

2 After washing, dry the blot for 10–20 min between filter papers.

3   Wrap in cling film and insert into an X-ray cassette with autoradiographic film.

4   Leave the autoradiograph to expose at −70°C for between 12 h and 1 week depending upon the amount of radioactivity bound. Develop the film according to the manufacturer's instructions.

TECHNICAL NOTES

- The sensitivity of the detection system may be increased using:
  - (a) *Preflashed film.* The duration of the flash and its intensity (varied by changing the distance between film and electronic flash-gun) is critical and should be determined empirically. Set the shortest duration on the flash-gun and position the gun at varying distances (increasing in steps of 1 m) from film test strips. Develop the film and use the conditions that just give barely visible fogging. Exposure of preflashed film at −70°C gives maximal stability of both the nascent image and the sensitized preflashed areas.
  - (b) *Intensifying screens.* Screens should be placed on either side of the blot–film sandwich. The screens are impregnated with heavy metal ions coupled to a scintillation system. The efficiency of capture of the emitted radiations is therefore increased and more of them are recorded on the X-ray film because of the photon emissions from the screens. Screens are important for the efficient capture of [131]I.
- The system described above may also be adapted for analysis using ^{125}I-labelled antibodies or unlabelled antibodies detected by ^{125}I-labelled protein A.

4.11.6 Chemiluminescence as a non-radioactive method for detecting antigens by Western blot analysis

This non-radioactive method is available for detecting antigens by Western blot analysis. This utilizes a chemiluminescent reagent which reacts with enzyme-labelled antibodies, e.g. horseradish peroxidase. Here is an outline of the basic technique.

- Horseradish peroxidase oxidizes a peracid salt which then leads to a raised oxidation state of the haem group within the horseradish peroxidase itself.
- As this raised state decays, luminol radicals are formed, which on decaying emit light.
- In an enhanced assay, enhancer phenolic molecules are placed between the haem group and the luminol which results in increased (1000-fold) and prolonged emission of light with a half-life of around 60 min.

The above technique has been further developed by Lumigen Inc. with the enzymatic generation of an acridinium ester which produces an intense light emission this is the more sensitive alternative ECL Plus (Code RPN 213, available from AP Biotech) where the light emission is of longer duration than the original ECL system. Both the ECL and ECL Plus system can be used on either nitrocellulose (Hybond C) or polyvinylidene difluoride (PVDF) (Hybond P) blotting membranes.

MATERIALS

Non-fat dried milk powder
Phosphate-buffered saline (PBS) containing 0.1% (v/v) Tween 20
Tris(hydroxymethyl)-aminomethane (Tris)-buffered saline, pH 7.6
PBS, pH 7.5
Nitrocellulose membrane
Primary antibody (raised against antigen of interest)

Horseradish peroxidase (HRP)-conjugated second antibody (to react with the primary antibody)
Streptavidin biotinylated HRP conjugate
ECL reagents 1 and 2
X-ray film

METHOD

1 Prepare and electrophorese antigens on the SDS-PAGE gel, then blot by the usual protocol.
2 Block the nitrocellulose membrane with PBS, pH 7.5, containing 0.1% (v/v) Tween 20 and 5% (w/v) non-fat dried milk powder.
3 Leave the membrane in the blocking solution overnight at 4°C.
4 Wash the membrane with 3 × 2-min washes of PBS–Tween 20.
5 Dilute the primary antibody to the appropriate dilution in PBS–Tween 20.
6 Incubate the washed membrane with the first antibody solution at 20°C with continuous shaking for 60 min.
7 Wash the membrane with 2 × 2-min washes of PBS–Tween 20.
8 Dilute the second antibody (biotinylated or HRP-labelled) in PBS–Tween 20.
9 Incubate the membrane with the HRP-labelled second antibody solution at 20°C with continuous shaking for 60 min.
10 Serially wash the membrane in PBS–Tween 20 at 20°C for:
   2 × 1 min
   1 × 15 min
   3 × 5 min.
   Note: If using HRP-labelled antibody, go to step 13.
11 Make the working dilution of the biotinylated streptavidin–HRP complex in PBS–Tween 20, then incubate with the membrane at 20°C with continuous shaking for 60 min.
12 Serially wash the membrane in PBS–Tween 20 at 20°C for:
   2 × 1 min
   1 × 15 min
   3 × 5 min.
13 Substrate preparation. The peracid salt is kept separate from the luminol/enhancer mixture and mixed just prior to use. Mix equal volumes of reagent 1 and 2 (ECL working solution).
14 Lay blot flat on cling film (Saran wrap) with the protein side uppermost.
15 Pipette ECL working solution on to the blot and leave for 1 min.
16 Drain and wrap in cling film.
17 In a dark room, place the wrapped blot against the X-ray film and expose for 15 s (longer or shorter times may be necessary).
18 Develop using standard X-ray developing chemicals.

TECHNICAL NOTES

- The pH will need to be adjusted to pH 7.5 with concentrated sodium hydroxide when the milk powder has been added.
- BSA may not be used as a blocking agent with the ECL Plus detection reagents.
- The incubation with the dried milk powder is for blocking any non-specific binding sites.
- Obviously the dilution of the antibody (first and second) will vary, depending on the antigen–antibody system being used. A 'typical' polyclonal antibody may work at around 1 : 10 000.

Therefore it is advisable to perform the first assay with a reasonably low dilution of antibody and then make further dilutions up or down, depending on the results obtained. If using the ECL HRP-conjugated antibodies, the recommended dilution range is 1 : 3000–1 : 12 000.

• Following ECL detection, it is possible to reprobe the membrane several times.

4.12 Anti-idiotype antibodies

Many anti-idiotype antibodies will bind to determinants around the outside of the combining site, but a proportion will bind within the paratope (see Fig. 4.8). In so doing they will bear some resemblance to the antigen that would normally fit within the site. This subset of anti-idiotypes can be substituted for the antigen, and have been used to immunize animals instead of using the antigen itself.

Anti-idiotype antibodies provide ideal reagents for probing receptor sites where the ligand is available but the receptor is unknown or difficult to obtain. Using the ligand to produce the anti-ligand antibody, this in turn can be used as the 'antigen' to produce an anti-idiotype that will bind to the receptor (see Fig. 4.8).

4.12.1 Production of anti-idiotypes

Production of anti-idiotype antibodies does not differ in principle from the production of any other type of antibody. The following protocol works well for the production of monoclonal anti-idiotype antibodies.

METHOD

1 Concentrate and purify the monoclonal antibody. In the case of tissue culture supernatants, purification by ammonium sulphate precipitation will probably be sufficient, whereas separation from polyclonal immunoglobulin will be necessary with ascitic fluid.

Continued on p. 156

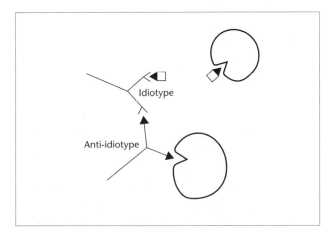

Fig. 4.8 Polyclonal antibody to the ligand is used to produce monoclonal anti-idiotype. Labelled anti-idiotype will then detect the receptor for the ligand on the cell, and may be used to isolate the receptor by immunoprecipitation.

2 Give a total of three subcutaneous injections of 50 μg purified monoclonal antibody to BALB/c mice, with an interval of 2 weeks between each injection. For the first injection the antibody should be combined with Freund's complete adjuvant, for the second use incomplete Freund's adjuvant, and in the third the antibody should be adsorbed onto alum.

3 Give each mouse a final intravenous boost with 20–50 μg antibody 3 days prior to removing the spleens for fusion.

4 Fuse the spleen-cell suspensions with the hybridoma parent by conventional hybridoma technology.

5 Screen each hybridoma supernatant against idiotype and normal immunoglobulin of the same subclass, using radio- or enzyme immunoassay.

4.13 Antibodies in molecular biology

The majority of techniques in molecular biology are beyond the scope of this book, but some of the contributions of immunology to this important discipline deserve mention.

If monoclonal antibodies had not already existed, then they would certainly have had to be invented for molecular biology. Similarly, the ability of polyclonal sera to 'view' a polypeptide as a series of discrete epitopes has been crucially important for the detection of incompletely expressed protein sequences fused in the middle of completely unrelated proteins.

Antibodies provide a means for defining and testing the function of previously unknown protein molecules. They are an essential tool for the characterization of the protein via recombinant DNA technology.

4.13.1 Analysis of *in vitro* translation products

Routes from the first definition of an antigen, for example a novel, functionally important cell-surface glycoprotein, to a full determination of its amino acid sequence, are now well established. Often the first step in characterization is to determine its apparent molecular weight by immuno-precipitation (see Section 3.13) and SDS-PAGE analysis (see Appendix B).

Some of the questions to be resolved before attempting the full cycle of cloning, expression and sequencing are:

(a) Does the cell really make the antigen or has it been acquired exogenously?

(b) Is the antigenic determinant protein- or carbohydrate-based?

(c) Is the epitope sequence- or conformation-based? If the latter is the case then it is unlikely that the antibody would react with the unglycosylated, incomplete segment of the original molecule expressed in the middle of a bacterial protein.

Immunoprecipitation of *in vitro* translation products from cell-derived mRNA not only definitively resolves these questions but also provides confirmation that the mRNA is acceptable for the preparation of cDNA.

A typical result is shown in Fig. 4.9. The mRNA was extracted from the cell expressing the antigen of interest and mixed with ^{35}S-methionine and micrococcal nuclease-treated rabbit reticulocyte lysate (the latter is a rich source of all the molecules to make protein, but devoid of the

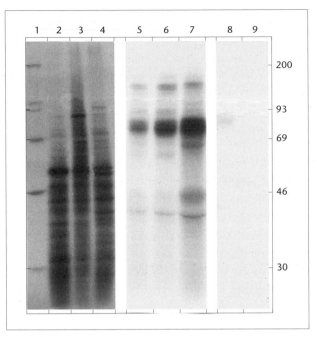

Fig. 4.9 Immunoprecipitation of *in vitro* translation products. Messenger RNA, extracted from three different stages of the life-cycle of a protozoan parasite, was translated *in vitro* in the presence of ^{35}S-methionine. The resulting polypeptides were fractionated on an SDS-PAGE gel, either immediately (tracks 2–4), or after immunoprecipitation with either a monoclonal antibody (tracks 5–9) which reacted with a polypeptide in a single life-cycle stage (track 4), or an irrelevant antibody (results not shown). Track 1 contains radiolabelled molecular weight standards, molecular weight is in thousands and migration position is indicated by arrowheads. Tracks 2–4 show polypeptides in the starting material with a molecular weight of up to 100 000, indicating good translation. Tracks 5–7 show the effect of increasing the amount of monoclonal antibody added as ascitic fluid. Although the 85-kDa band increases in intensity, so does the non-specific binding. Tracks 8 and 9 show the lack of binding of the antibody to other life-cycle stages (represented in tracks 2 and 3).

'message'). The polypeptides synthesized *in vitro* have been visualized by fluorography after immunoprecipitation and SDS-PAGE analysis. Significantly, the photograph shows discrete polypeptides some of which are in excess of 90 kDa apparent molecular weight, indicating that the mRNA is in good condition. The single, large polypeptide band precipitated by the monoclonal antibody, which is slightly smaller than that synthesized by intact cells (not shown), confirms that the epitope is not carbohydrate dependent, either directly or for its conformation. (The techniques for *in vitro* translation are explained in full in Hames & Higgins 1999.)

4.13.2 Screening of expression libraries

Antibody can provide a powerful tool by which a mature molecule, for example a cell-surface glycoprotein expressed by a eukaryotic cell, can be related to a set of partial sequences expressed in bacterial fusion proteins.

The method described was used to screen a cDNA library from a protozoan parasite expressed in the bacteriophage λgt11. The methods in recombinant DNA technology referred to below are fully described in Glover (1996) or Sambrook and Russel (2000).

Preparation in advance

1   Calculate the titre of the recombinant phage stock and dilute to produce about 300 discrete plaques per plate (adjust the total number per plate according to the size of the plaques).

2   Grow up a stock of the *Escherichia coli* (Y1090) plating cells and mix an aliquot with the appropriate dilution of phage and plate out.

3   Incubate the culture plates at 42°C until plaques appear (between 3 and 4 h, but longer if the *E. coli* has been cooled for storage).

4   Transfer the cultures to a 37°C incubator, overlay each plate with a sterile, isopropyl-β,D-thiogalactopyranoside (IPTG)-impregnated nitrocellulose filter (previously soaked in 10 mM IPTG and dried before use) and incubate overnight to induce fusion protein expression.

5   Before removing the filters, use a syringe loaded with dye and fitted with a large gauge needle to pierce each filter at three places round its periphery to provide orientation marks in the filter and agar. (By this means it will ultimately be possible to match up the black spots on the autoradiograph or coloured spots on the filter with phage plaques on the original culture plate.)

6   Unless you are using a monoclonal antibody produced *in vitro*, it will be necessary to exhaustively absorb all antisera or ascitic fluids to remove the naturally occurring anti-*E. coli* and antibacteriophage antibodies. Commercial preparations are now available which will allow this to be accomplished conveniently, according to the manufacturer's instructions.

MATERIALS AND EQUIPMENT

Nitrocellulose filters bearing replicates of recombinant phage plaques

Antibody, poly- or monoclonal, specifying antigen of interest

10 mM tris(hydroxymethyl)-aminomethane (Tris), pH 9.6, containing 150 mM sodium chloride and 0.05% v/v Tween 20 (wash buffer)

Bovine serum albumin (BSA), RIA grade

3 MM paper

Clear acetate sheets

Pen with water-insoluble ink

Radioactive ink

Orbital shaker

Bag sealer

Role of continuous plastic tube

In addition:

Materials for autoradiography or enzyme labels

METHOD

1   Remove the nitrocellulose filters from each plate and immerse them in a large volume of 10 mM Tris, pH 9.6, containing 150 mM sodium chloride and 0.05% v/v Tween 20 (wash buffer). Store the agar plates face down at 4°C until immunoscreening is complete.

2   Leave the filters in the wash buffer on the orbital shaker for 10 min at room temperature. Use sufficient buffer to ensure that the filters are moving freely.

3   Transfer the filters to wash buffer containing 3% w/v BSA (RIA grade) and leave rocking for 30 min at room temperature. (The BSA will block the unoccupied protein-binding sites on the filters and so prevent non-specific uptake of antibody protein.)

Continued

4 Seal the filters into a plastic sac, excluding as much air as possible.

5 Dilute the pre-absorbed antibody (see step 6, Preparation in advance) in wash buffer containing 3% w/v BSA, allowing 5 ml of solution for every 20 filters, and load it into the sac using a syringe and needle. As a guide, dilute the antibody 1 : 100 or use neat tissue culture supernatant from hybridoma cells.

6 Reseal the plastic sac and leave it rocking for 1 h at room temperature.

7 Cut open one edge of the sac and recover the antibody solution. So little is consumed during this procedure that it may be stored at –20°C for further use.

8 Transfer the filters to a tank of wash buffer and rock gently for 10 min at room temperature. For efficient washing, use sufficient buffer to allow the filters to move freely.

9 Wash twice more under the same conditions.

10 Remove the filters from the final wash, gently blot each one dry on 3 MM paper and seal all together into a plastic sac, excluding as much air as possible.

11 Dilute the anti-immunoglobulin antibody or protein A in wash buffer containing 3% BSA. See Technical notes for selection of label.

12 Add the labelled second reagent to the plastic sac, using a syringe and needle, and reseal the sac.

13 After incubating on the rocking platform for 1 h at room temperature, open the sac, recover and store the labelled reagent, and wash the filters three times in wash buffer as in step 8 above.

A *For immunoscreening with enzyme labels*

14 After the final wash, blot each filter dry on 3 MM paper, and process with chromogenic substrate to reveal the binding sites of the enzyme-conjugated second reagent, as described in Section 4.11.4.

B *For immunoscreening with radioactive labels*

14 Remove each filter from the final wash solution, blot dry on 3 MM paper and mount onto a sheet of card covered with Saran wrap. (Saran wrap is best but cling film may be used if necessary.) Finally, cover the filter and card tightly with Saran wrap.

15 Cover each orientation hole on the filters with a small sticky label and mark the position of the hole with radioactive ink (this aids orientation of the autoradiograph when preparing the template for isolation of the phage plaques).

16 Expose to X-ray film using tungsten intensifying screens and process photographically.

17 Prepare a duplicate of the coloured dots on the filter (enzyme labels) or the black dots on the autoradiograph (radioactive labels) using a clear acetate sheet and a fine pen. Remember to transfer the orientation marks.

18 Mark the regions of the positive plaques on the acetate sheet and use this to guide a Pasteur pipette to remove a plug of agar from the corresponding region in the original plate.

The plugs of agar are each dispersed in individual tubes containing a storage buffer. If the original phage plaques were discrete and optimally spaced, each plug should contain one, or a limited number, of types of recombinant phage. It is necessary to repeat the 'screening and picking' process until the phage plaques are uniformly positive on immunoscreening (Fig. 4.10).

You should now have a series of recombinant phages containing segments of the DNA coding for the protein defined by the original antibody.

(a)   (b)

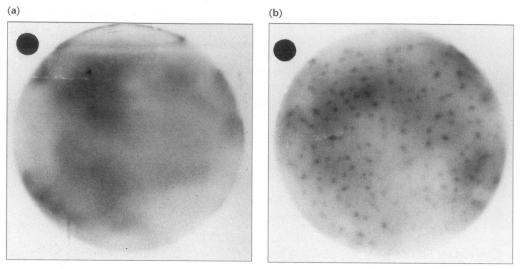

Fig. 4.10 Screening of a λgt11 expression library with antibodies. A λgt11 genomic library of the protozoan parasite *Trypanosoma cruzi* was screened with a mixture of antisera from infected patients. (a) The first round of screening identified a single-phage colony in this plate (corresponding to the black dot on the photograph of the nitrocellulose filter) producing a fusion protein which contained one or more parasite-derived epitopes. Once the agar plug containing the recombinant phage had been replated onto a fresh culture of *Escherichia coli* (b) the proportion of positive colonies increased dramatically.

TECHNICAL NOTES
- It is necessary to remember that polyclonal sera or ascitic fluids are biological materials and not chemical reagents. The pre-absorption step, to remove the anti-*E. coli* and antiphage antibodies, must be carried out to completion.
- Binding of the first antibody can be visualized with an anti-immunoglobulin antibody or protein A, labelled with either a radioactive or enzyme label.
- It is good practice to keep the filters moist during autoradiographic exposure as it is possible to continue the washing procedure if the radioactive background is unacceptably high, or to repeat the immunoscreening if no signal is detected after 7 days' exposure. This is not possible with enzyme labels.
- All materials and equipment should be sterile and aseptic technique should be used throughout. The screening can take between 7 and 9 days; therefore, even at 4°C, microbial contaminants can overgrow and make plaque identification difficult.
- Monoclonal antibodies raised against short peptides, especially C-terminal, are likely to be better reagents than antibodies which recognize conformational determinants.

4.13.3 From partial sequence to mature protein

The rapid progress seen in the characterization of important proteins in infectious organisms has been made possible by the application of the techniques of molecular biology, rather than those of protein chemistry. Consequently, there is a frequent need to relate an incomplete, and often unknown, sequence of DNA expressed in a prokaryote to the mature molecule expressed in the eukaryotic cell. The multiperspective specificity of polyclonal antibodies combined with the discriminatory power of immunoblotting allow this link to be established with relative ease.

Once an unknown sequence has been expressed, e.g. as a plasmid-derived fusion protein in β-galactosidase, then the whole bacterial lysate may be used to immunize a mouse and so produce an antiserum suitable for immunoblotting.

An important note: adequate specificity controls are needed when using the antiserum for immunoblotting. It is essential to blot against not only the organism or cell of interest but also the E. coli host strain (not infected with the recombinant plasmid). Only then is it possible to be reasonably confident that the mature polypeptide identified on the blot of the SDS-PAGE-fractionated organism really does relate to the fusion protein.

It is possible to adsorb the fusion protein onto nitrocellulose and use it for affinity purification of antibodies from polyclonal sera. This has been particularly useful in clinical situations, where immunization with fusion protein is not possible.

The technique

- A small square of nitrocellulose filter is placed in contact with a single clone of recombinant phage growing in E. coli. After induction of the fusion protein, the filter is 'blocked' with BSA and pre-eluted with 0.1 M glycine–HCl buffer, pH 2.5, containing 150 mM sodium chloride.
- Antibody is absorbed from the patient's serum onto the filter, which is then extensively washed and eluted by immersion in a small volume of glycine–HCl buffer.
- After neutralization with a few crystals of solid Tris, the affinity-purified antibody can be used for a miniature immunoblot (Section 4.11 and Miniblotter apparatus).

This technique both relates the fusion protein to the mature protein (identified by size in the blot) and establishes its importance to the patient's response to infection.

It has been possible to relate a DNA sequence of unknown function to a gene product using an antiserum raised against the synthetic oligopeptide inferred from the triplet code. Oligopeptides of < 10 amino acids are relatively poor immunogens; however, once their chain length exceeds 10–15 the chance of obtaining an antiserum is high. This approach tends to favour detection of epitopes in accessible regions of high hydrophilicity and N- or C-terminal regions, even when the resulting antisera are used in immunoblotting.

4.14 **Further reading**

Allan, V.J. (2000) *Protein Localization by Fluorescence Microscopy: A Practical Approach*. Oxford University Press, Oxford.

Basham, L.E., Pavliak V., Li, X. *et al.* (1996) A simple, quantitative, reproducible avidin-biotin ELISA for the evaluation of group B streptococcus type-specific antibodies in humans. *Vaccine* **14**(5), 439–445.

Bolton, A.E. & Hunter, W.M. (1973) The labelling of proteins to high specific radioactivities by conjugation to a ^{125}I-containing acylating agent. *Biochem J* **133**, 529–539.

Borrebaeck, C.A.K. (2000) Antibodies in diagnostics—from immunoassays to protein chips [Review]. *Immunol Today* **21**(8), 379–382.

Caponi, L. & Migliorini, P. (1999) *Antibody Usage in the Lab*. Springer Verlag, New York.

Casey, J.L., Coley, A.m., Tilley, L.M. & Foley, M. (2000) Green fluorescent antibodies: novel *in vitro* tools. *Protein Eng* **13**, 445–452.

Dunbar, B.S. (ed) (1994) *Protein Blotting: A Practical Approach*. Oxford University Press, Oxford.

Durrant, I. (1990) Light-based detection of biomolecules. *Nature* **346**, 297–8.

Glover, D.M. (ed) (1996) *DNA Cloning*, Vols I, II, III and IV. IRL Press, Oxford.

Hainfield, J.F. & Powell, R.D. (2000) New frontiers in gold labelling. *J Histochem Cytochem* **48**, 471–480.

Hames, B.D. (1999) *Protein Expression: A Practical Approach*. Oxford University Press, Oxford.

Hames, B.D. & Glover, D.M. (1996) *Molecular Immunology: Frontiers in Molecular Biology*. IRL Press, Oxford.

Hames, B.D. & Higgins, J. (1999) *Post-translational processing: A Practical Approach*, 2nd edn. Oxford University Press, Oxford.

Harlow, E. & Lane, D. (1998) *Using Antibodies: A Laboratory Manual*. Cold Spring Harbor Laboratory Press, Cold Spring Harbor.

Homburger, H.A., Cahen, Y.D., Griffiths, J. & Jacob, G.L. (1998) Detection of antinuclear antibodies: comparative evaluation of enzyme immunoassay and indirect immunofluorescence methods. *Arch Pathol Lab Med* **122**(11), 993–999.

Kerr, M.A & Thorpe, R. (eds) (1994) *Immunochemistry labfax. bios*, Blackwell Science Ltd, Oxford.

Lan, H.Y., Hutchinson, P., Tesch, G.H., Mu, W. & Atkins, R.C. (1996) A novel method of microwave treatment for detection of cytoplasmic and nuclear antigens by flow cytometry. *J Immunol Meth* **190**(1), 1–10.

McMahon, M.J. & O'Kennedy, R. (2000) Polyreactivity as an acquired artefact, rather than a physiologic property of antibodies: evidence that monoreactive antibodies may gain the ability to bind to multiple antigens after exposure to low pH. *J Immunol Meth* **241**(1–2), 1–10.

Nejsum, L.N., Elkjaer, M., Hager, H,. Frokiaer, J., Kwon, T.H. & Nielsen, S. (2000) Localization of aquaporin-7 in rat and mouse kidney using RT-PCR, immunoblotting, and immunocytochemistry. *Biochem Biophys Res Commun* **277**(1), 164–170.

Phillips, T.M. & Dickens, B.F. (2000) *Affinity and Immunoaffinity Purification Techniques*. Eaton Pub Co, BioTechniques Press, Westborough MA.

Sambrook, J. & Russel, D. (2000) *Molecular Cloning*. Cold Spring Harbor Laboratory Press, Cold Spring Harbor.

Shata, M.T., Stevceva, L., Agwale, S., Lewis, G.K. & Hone, D.M. (2000) Recent advances with recombinant bacterial vaccine vectors [Review]. *Mol Med Today* **6**(2), 66–71.

Skerra, A. (2000) Engineered protein scaffolds for molecular recognition. *J Mol Recognit* **13**(4), 167–187

Stahl, D., Lacroix-Desmazes, S., Mouthon, L., Kaveri, S.V. & Kazatchkine, M.D. (2000) Analysis of human self-reactive antibody repertoires by quantitative immunoblotting [Review]. *J Immunol Meth* **240**, 1–14.

Stumpf, W. & Solomon, H. (1994) *Autoradiography and Correlative Imaging*. Academic Press Inc., USA.

Van de Plas, P. & Leunissen, J.L.M. (1993) Ultrasmall gold probes: Characteristics and use in immuno(cyto)chemical studies. In: *Antibodies in Cell Biology* (ed. DJ Assai). Academic Press, London.

Van Gijlswijk, R.P., van Gijlswijk-Janssen, D.J., Raap, A.K., Daha, M.R. & Tanke, H.J. (1996) Enzyme-labelled antibody–avidin conjugates: new flexible and sensitive immunochemical reagents. *J Immunol Meth* **189**(1), 117–127.

Vincent, P. & Samuel, D. (1993) A comparison of the binding of biotin and biotinylated macromolecular ligands to an antibiotin monoclonal antibody and to streptavidin. *J Immunol Meth* **165**, 177–182.

Webster, D. (2000) *Protein Structure Prediction: Methods and Protocols Methods in Molecular Biology*. Blackwell Science Ltd, Oxford.

Weeks, I., Beheshti, I., McCapra, F., Campbell, A.K. & Woodhead, J.S. (1983) Acridinium esters as high-specific activity labels in immunoassay. *Clin Chem* **29**(8), 1474–1479.

Wilchek, M. & Bayer, E.A. (eds) (1990) *Methods in Enzymology* [Volume 184 is dedicated to Avidin-Biotin techniques.] Academic Press, London.

Williams, M.A. (1990) *Autoradiography and Immunocytochemistry*. North-Holland, Amsterdam.

5 Immunoassay

5.1 What is the basis of an immunoassay?

An immunoassay is the mixing of an antigen with an antibody with the formation of a complex, followed by the discrimination between the amount of bound versus free reactants. To aid this, either the antigen or antibody is labelled, most often with an enzyme or radioisotope. There is no fundamental difference between assays using antibodies as the analytical reagent and assays involving other reagents. Thus it can be helpful to think in the assayists' terms of the analytical reagent and the analyte (the substance to be analysed), particularly in immunology where frequently it is the antibody which is being assayed and so the antigen becomes, in effect, the analytical reagent. The basis of all immunoassays is the formation of a complex between analyte and analytical reagent, followed by estimation of bound versus free components. At virtually every step in the general assay procedure it is possible to choose from a wide variety of different techniques, i.e. enormous methodological flexibility is possible to achieve an optimized system. For example, there are solid versus soluble phase assays, radioisotope versus enzyme, competitive versus non-competitive assays.

The original immunoassays involved a saturation analysis in which a limiting amount of antibody was reacted with excess labelled antigen. If a known amount of unlabelled antigen is added to an assay of this type they will inhibit the binding of labelled antigen to the antibody (Fig. 5.1). Thus a set of standards may be used to construct an inhibition curve from which the amount of an unknown analyte may be determined by the degree of inhibition induced.

For optimal sensitivity

The concentration of antibody should be as low as possible but, as the concentrations of reactants decrease, other factors such as the speed of reaction and accuracy become limiting (see Box). Sensitivity is also dependent on a combination of the antibody affinity and the error in determining the bound fraction.

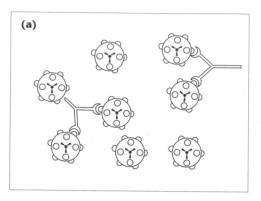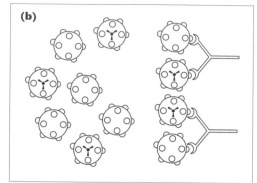

Fig. 5.1 Saturation immunoassay. (a) An excess of antigen competes for a limiting amount of antibody. (b) Unlabelled antigen inhibits the binding of labelled antigen.

ANTIBODY AFFINITY AND IMMUNOASSAY

- Once assay procedures have been optimized, the limiting factor becomes the ability to raise antisera containing high-affinity antibodies.
- Affinity is unlikely to exceed 1×10^{12} l/mol and as it is impractical to lower the experimental error to less than 1%, this imposes a theoretical limit on sensitivity of 1×10^{-14} mol/l.
- Using the Avogadro constant this gives just under 10^7 molecules/ml as the theoretical lower limit of detection (Ekins 1981, 1985; for a fuller discussion of these points see Further reading).

Labelled antibody (immunometric) assay: use of excess antibody rather than an excess of antigen

Standard amounts of antigen are reacted with excess labelled antibody then, following separation of bound and free reactants, the bound antibody is estimated. An important feature: no matter how low the antigen concentration, if sufficient antibody is added, some of the antibody will combine to form a complex within a given time; the rate of complex formation being equal to $K1[Ag][Ab]$ (see Section 3.1.1). In principle, therefore, a single molecule of antigen may be detected.

Sensitivity and specificity are important considerations in immunometric assays, as the antibody is in excess, and any cross-reactivity in the antiserum could allow side reactions with inappropriate antigens. Weak and possibly spurious cross-reactions have probably been under-estimated in some studies.

The need for pure and highly specific antibodies was a considerable hindrance to the widespread application of immunometric assays based on polyclonal antisera. However, the development of highly efficient affinity chromatographic techniques and, more especially, the introduction of techniques for the routine preparation of monoclonal antibodies has reduced this problem to trivial proportions.

Advantage of immunometric assays

Two analytical reagents can be used to characterize the analyte as long as it has two distinct epitopes. Most frequently, the assay is performed in 'sandwich' form, as shown in Fig. 5.2.

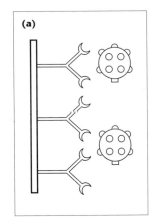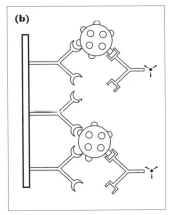

Fig. 5.2 Immunometric assay. (a) An excess of antibody, usually on a solid phase, binds to one epitope on the antigen while (**b**) a second labelled antibody binds to an unrelated epitope and detects the bound antigen.

This may be exploited using a combination of an antibody and another analytical reagent to secure specificity, as was done when we estimated circulating IgG-containing immune complexes, using both C1q and rabbit anti-human IgG antibody.

5.1.1 Classification of immunoassays

Immunoassays may be classified in various ways, such as whether:

- one of the components is labelled or unlabelled;
- the label is a radioactive isotope or non-isotopic, e.g. fluorochrome, an enzyme;
- it is competitive or non-competitive, e.g. immunometric;
- the assay involves separation of bound from free components—heterogeneous assay—or the degree of antibody–antigen reaction is estimated without separation, such as with fluorescence polarization or surface plasmon resonance.

5.2 Choice of label

When choosing a 'label' for use as means of detection within an immunoassay, the following should be considered:

- the nature of the label;
- the characteristics of signal generation; and
- the detection system used to measure it.

Radioisotopes and enzymes have so far found wide application in immunoassay. The type of label can have a marked effect on the maximum sensitivity of the assay system.

Please refer to the following websites for comprehensive details on radioisotope health and safety procedures as well as useful information regarding detection and half-life:

http://www.practicingsafescience.org

http://www.hse.gov.uk

5.2.1 Radiolabels

Two main factors contribute to the accuracy and sensitivity of signal detection:

(i) the level of background; and

(ii) the number of measurable units of activity generated per unit time for each labelled molecule. Sensitivity will be at its greatest when the background is near zero and each molecule of bound antibody emits an observable signal.

The radioisotope ^{125}I has been frequently used as it has the advantages of:

(i) a low natural background in the environment and in biological fluids; and

(ii) a radioactive disintegration that is independent of the chemical or physical nature of the assay.

The main problem with this seemingly useful isotope is a handicap of about six orders of magnitude on assay sensitivity; e.g. under normal conditions, the background count in a radioassay is unlikely to be less than 30 c.p.m. Assuming a detection efficiency of 50% of radioactive disintegrations, if each reagent molecule is labelled with a single ^{125}I molecule, we will need about 250 000 molecules of antibody to obtain a count rate of 1 c.p.m. To get a statistically significant result compared to background, many millions of antibody molecules need to be bound, rather than the theoretical threshold for immunometric assays of a single molecule. The half-life of the chosen isotope must be considered since an isotope with a short half-life will have a limited shelf life.

5.2.2 Enzyme labels

Enzymes offer a distinct advantage over radioisotopes in that each enzyme-labelled antibody can contribute to the signal during the time of the assay, as each enzyme molecule can convert many molecules of substrate to detectable product. Most enzyme assays are limited by the sensitivity of the detection apparatus (photometer, spectrophotometer) and the poor optical and chemical reproducibility of the cuvettes, microtitre trays, etc., used for the assays. The strategy adopted by Harris *et al.* (1979) was to use an enzyme label (alkaline phosphatase) to convert a radioisotopically labelled substrate (^{3}H-adenosine monophosphate), rather than a chromogenic substrate, into a labelled product (^{3}H-adenosine). This procedure permits the sensitivity of radioactive detection to be combined with enzyme amplification, thus giving a detection sensitivity of 10^{-21} moles (about 600 molecules), much closer to the theoretical threshold.

In competition immunoassay, as the threshold of detection is high and depends upon antibody affinity rather than on the ability to detect single molecules of reagent, increases in specific activity only contribute to increased assay speed. Thus conventional radioisotopic methods are still the method of choice in many of these assays.

For details of biotinylation and its use in assays, see Section 4.7.

5.2.3 Methods for detection of label

The method depends on the label; e.g. ^{125}I is easily detected in a γ spectrometer scintillation counter and many systems are now available for counting multiple samples at the same time.

Detection by liquid scintillation, e.g. for ^{3}H, can be a very sensitive method, but there is the problem of quenching in that some biological molecules within the reagents may quench the scintillant (see also Stokke *et al.* 1990).

Enzymes are generally used to produce coloured products from colourless substrates that can be determined easily in a spectrophotometer or colorimeter. Automated plate readers are commercially available which make reading large numbers of samples relatively easy.

5.3 Separation procedures

All heterogeneous immunoassays require the separation of bound from free components. There is always some lack of efficiency in whatever separation technique is used, such as:
- trapping of free ligand in the bound fraction; or
- physical adsorption of free ligand to assay plastics, e.g. plates, test tubes, etc.

Assays try to minimize this but care must be taken to preserve the binding of antigen to antibody while reducing non-specific binding as far as possible.

A wide range of techniques have been used to ensure good separation:
- Adsorption via:

  activated charcoal, e.g. vitamin B_{12} assay; or

  ammonium sulphate (50% saturated solution), e.g. assay involving a precipitation of the antibody component.
- Precipitation via:

  polyethylene glycol;

  anti-antibody, e.g. mouse anti-human IgG; or

  antibody on particles, tubes, plates.
- Solid phase using:

  antigen on particles, tubes, plates.

Activated charcoal has now been largely superseded and although less often used than solid-phase systems, precipitation assays can still provide useful information and are easy to set up.

Solid-phase assays have a delightful simplicity but it is easy to assume greater reliability than the system can provide. Care must be taken to check for batch variability and to control for temperature and time of reagent delivery.

5.4 Immunoassay procedures

To illustrate these different separation procedures a range of techniques is included below. The use of ammonium sulphate to separate bound from free antigen has already been discussed in Chapter 3.

5.4.1 Competition radioimmunoassay

The basic common feature of these assays is the separation of bound from free reactants. There are a number of systems available, such as:
- molecular sieving;
- solvent and salt precipitation;

- second antibodies; and
- solid-phase systems.

In the radioimmunoassay for IgG, precipitation with polyethylene glycol (PEG) is used to separate bound from free antigen. One of the problems is that the antigen (human IgG) and the antibody (rabbit IgG) are of the same molecular weight and precipitability by PEG. This can be overcome by the use of human ^{125}I-Fab as the labelled antigen since it is soluble in PEG. Ideally, the labelled antigen and the 'cold' antigen to be assayed should be as alike as possible.

Radioimmunoassay of human IgG

Preparation of ^{125}I-Fab

MATERIALS AND EQUIPMENT
Human IgG
Sodium ^{125}I iodide, carrier free
Bovine serum albumin (BSA), RIA grade
0.1 M tris(hydroxymethyl)-aminomethane (Tris)-buffered saline (TBS), pH 8.0
Chicken serum
Whatman GF/B glass-fibre filter

METHOD

1 Obtain human IgG and prepare the Fab fragment.
2 Label 10 µg protein with 18.5×10^6 Bq ^{125}I and store in 5 ml TBS.
3 Immediately before use, dilute with TBS containing 10% chicken serum and filter under gentle pressure through a Whatman GF/B glass-fibre filter.

Determination of binding curve

MATERIALS AND EQUIPMENT
Anti-human IgG
^{125}I-Fab (prepared as above)
Bovine serum albumin (BSA), RIA grade
0.1 M Tris-buffered saline (TBS), pH 8.0
Polyethylene glycol (PEG) 6000 (15% w/v in TBS)
Microtitre plates
Cell-harvesting machine
Whatman GF/B glass-fibre filter strips, for harvester
Gamma spectrometer

METHOD

1 Dilute the anti-IgG serum 1 : 100 and then prepare a range of two- to three-fold dilutions in TBS containing 0.1% BSA.
2 Add 100 µl of ^{125}I-Fab (dilute to yield 10^5 c.p.m. in TCA precipitable material per well, as in step 3 above) to each well of the microtitre tray. (Use sufficient wells for triplicates of each antibody dilution.)
3 Add 50 µl aliquots of the diluted anti-IgG serum to appropriate wells, mix thoroughly and incubate at room temperature for 16 h.

Continued

4 Add 200 µl of 23% w/v PEG solution to each well and incubate at room temperature for 2 h.

5 Collect the contents of each well onto Whatman GF/B glass-fibre filter strips using a cell-harvesting machine.

6 Wash each precipitate with 1.5 ml of PEG, 15% w/v in TBS.

7 Determine number of c.p.m. per sample using a γ spectrometer and plot a curve of c.p.m. against antiserum dilution, i.e. an antibody-binding curve to determine the dilution of antibody that binds 50% of the antigen.

In all future assays with the same reagents use the dilution of antiserum binding 50% of the added radioactivity.

Construction of inhibition curve

MATERIALS AND EQUIPMENT

Human IgG

Anti-human IgG serum (standardized as above)

^{125}I-Fab (diluted in chicken serum to half dilution used above)

0.1 M Tris-buffered saline (TBS) pH 8.0

Bovine serum albumin (BSA), RIA grade

Polyethylene glycol (PEG) 6000, 23% w/v in TBS

Cell-harvesting machine

Whatman GF/B glass-fibre filter strips, for harvester

METHOD

1 Prepare a stock solution of IgG, final concentration 0.3 mg/ml in TBS containing 1% w/v BSA (aliquot and store at –20°C for use).

2 To perform the assay, prepare standard IgG solutions in the range 2 ng to 2 µg/ml in TBS containing 0.1% w/v BSA.

3 Add 50 µl aliquots of standard IgG to 50 µl of an appropriate dilution (determined as in section above) of anti-IgG serum (in triplicate).

4 Mix samples and incubate for 16 h at room temperature.

5 Add 50 µl of ^{125}I-Fab (diluted in 20% chicken serum to half dilution used above) and incubate for 4 h at room temperature.

6 Precipitate complex by the addition of 200 µl of PEG solution (23% w/v in TBS). Incubate and harvest precipitates as in steps 4–7 of the section above.

7 Plot the inhibition of binding of ^{125}I-labelled Fab on a linear scale (i.e. c.p.m. in precipitate) against the concentration of unlabelled IgG added on a log scale.

Use this standard curve to determine the concentration of IgG in unknown solutions.

TECHNICAL NOTE

If an anti-immunoglobulin antibody is used to enhance complex formation, only a 2% solution of PEG is required in this method. This offers the significant advantage that whole IgG may then be used as a labelled antigen.

5.4.2 Immunometric assays

Immunometric assays almost invariably require solid-phase systems. They can be performed in many different ways, for example: (a) with antibody on the solid phase to capture antigen, which is then detected by a second labelled antibody directed against another epitope on the antigen; or (b) for the detection of antibody by adsorption of antigen on the solid phase, followed by binding of the antibody to be determined, which, in turn, is detected by the addition of a labelled second antibody directed against the Fc region. We describe a method based on the latter type of assay.

5.4.3 Enzyme-linked immunosorbent assay (ELISA)

General method for ELISA

MATERIALS AND EQUIPMENT

Antigen; for example, human serum albumin (HSA)

0.05 M carbonate–bicarbonate buffer, pH 9.6

Phosphate-buffered saline (PBS) containing 0.05% Tween 20 (PBS–Tween)

Hydrogen peroxide (30%)

0.18 M citrate–phosphate buffer, pH 4.0

2,2'-azinobis (3' ethylbenzthiazoline sulphonic acid, ABTS)

Casein

Bovine serum albumin (BSA)

Normal sheep serum

Sodium fluoride (80 mg in 25 ml distilled water)

Horseradish peroxidase–anti-immunoglobulin conjugate; for example, sheep anti-mouse Ig conjugate

Test sera; for example, sera from mice immunized with HSA

Enzyme immunoassay microtitre plates

ELISA reader

Preparation in advance

PREPARATION OF ENZYME SUBSTRATE

Prepare this just before adding to the plates.

1 Add 50 mg ABTS to 100 ml 0.18 M citrate–phosphate buffer, pH 4.0.

2 Add 30 µl of 30% hydrogen peroxide.

Hydrogen peroxide is gradually lost from the stock solution with storage. Therefore it is advisable to calculate the exact amount needed to be added each week.

3 Make a 1 : 1000 dilution of hydrogen peroxide by adding 50 µl H_2O_2 to 50 ml distilled water.

4 Determine the absorbance at 240 nm in a 1-cm cell against a distilled water blank.

5 The percentage concentration of original H_2O_2 = absorbance 240 × 77.98.

6 Volume of original H_2O_2 solution needed per 100 ml substrate solution:

$$= \frac{1}{\% \text{ concentration}} \text{ml}$$

For example, absorbance of 1 : 1000 dilution of H_2O_2 = 0.37, therefore percentage concentration = 0.37 × 77.98 = 28.9% therefore volume of H_2O_2 needed per 100 ml = 1/28.9 = 0.035 ml.

METHOD

1 Dissolve the antigen in carbonate–bicarbonate buffer. The optimum concentration should be determined for each antigen but a concentration of 1–10 μg/ml should give acceptable results for most antigens.

2 Add 200 μl to each well of a micro-ELISA plate cover and incubate overnight at 4°C in a humid chamber.

3 Wash to remove unbound antigen and fill the wells with 250 μl 1% w/v casein to block any remaining protein-binding sites (gelatin, BSA or skimmed milk powder are often used instead of casein).

4 Incubate at room temperature for 1 h.

5 Wash the plates twice with PBS–Tween by filling, then inverting and shaking the plates.

6 Dilute the test sera in PBS–Tween containing 1% BSA. (The optimum dilution must be determined in advance; it will generally be about 1 : 1000.)

7 Add 200 μl diluted test serum and incubate for 2 h at room temperature in a humid chamber.

8 Wash the plates three times with PBS–Tween.

9 Prepare the peroxidase–antibody conjugate by mixing 100 mg casein, 1 ml sheep serum, 100 μl Tween 20 with 50 μl peroxidase–antibody and adjust to a final volume of 100 ml with PBS. Allow to dissolve with gentle stirring. (The exact dilution of conjugate will vary and must be determined by experiment. As a guide, this will generally be between 1 : 1000 and 1 : 10 000 for good antibody preparations.)

10 Add 200 μl diluted conjugate to each well.

11 Incubate at room temperature for 1 h.

12 Wash three times with PBS–Tween.

13 Prepare the substrate solution and add 200 μl substrate to each well. Leave in the dark at room temperature for the colour to develop, usually 10–30 min.

14 Stop the reaction by adding 50 μl sodium fluoride solution to each well.

15 Quantify the colour reaction in an ELISA reader set at 650 nm.

TECHNICAL NOTES

- Strictly, each assay should include dilutions of a standard reference serum for the calibration of unknown samples. In practice, however, the test is reasonably reproducible and some workers record their results directly in absorbance units.

- The same assay could be performed with radiolabelled antibody. In this case flexible polystyrene plates should be used so that each well may be punched out and the bound radioactivity measured in a γ spectrometer after step 12, instead of processing for enzyme activity.

- An alternative substrate for the peroxidase enzyme is 34 mg O-phenylene diamine and 50 μl hydrogen peroxide (20 volumes) to 100 ml 0.1 M citrate–phosphate buffer, pH 5.0. The reaction is stopped by the addition of 50 μl 12.5% sulphuric acid and the absorbance measured at 492 nm.

- If an alkaline phosphatase-labelled enzyme is used, the substrate should be made up as follows: 50 mg 4-nitrophenyl phosphate in 50 ml diethanolamine buffer, pH 9.8. The reaction is stopped by the addition of 50 μl 3 M NaOH and the absorbance is measured at 405 nm.

- Material from detergent-solubilized cells binds very poorly to ELISA plates because of the surfactant effect: for example, protein dissolved in < 0.1% Triton X-100 shows little and variable binding; > 0.1% detergent inhibits binding completely. The problem of poor adherence may be overcome (for many antigens) by denaturation with Bouin's fixative: add 50 µl antigen solution to each well (approximately 40 µg/ml initial protein concentration) and 200 µl Bouin's fluid. Centrifuge at 500 g for 10 min, remove the fixative, wash once with 50% v/v ethanol and twice with PBS. Block plates with PBS containing 3% w/v BSA and 0.01% w/v thiomersal for 1 h. Such plates can be stored at 4°C for 1 week. This does not work for all cell-derived antigens and needs to be determined empirically.

Marked increases in sensitivity can be obtained by substituting a bioilluminescent detection system for the enzyme in solid-phase assays. Jackson *et al.* (1996), using identical assay systems, have shown a > 10^4-fold increase in sensitivity with luminometry, using a covalent conjugate of streptavidin and aequorin. Aequorin is a bioluminescent molecule that releases a blue light upon the addition of Ca^{2+}.

Matrices for solid-phase assays

Plastic surfaces

The majority of assays are now performed with the antigen or antibody passively adsorbed onto a plastic solid phase. Improved manufacturing processes have resulted in plastic supports with reproducible binding characteristics, although there is batch-to-batch variation, so researchers must optimize each system. Various proteins adsorb to differing degrees to the same plastic so trials must be carried out to determine the best support for a particular protein. Plates may now be obtained which have been irradiated to allow covalent interactions following the generation of free radicals. Some proteins (especially smaller molecules), bind very differently to the various makes of plate, whereas others seem to be 'plate-indifferent'.

For radioassays, use flexible polystyrene plates which can be easily cut into separate wells for counting.

For enzyme assays, use flat-bottomed plates with good optical as well as binding properties.

Particles

Cellulose, Sephadex, Sepharose, Sephacryl and many other particles are available as supports that have the advantage of a large surface area for derivatization.

For assay quantification, the particles must be recovered from suspension by centrifugation or, alternatively, the use of particles containing iron oxide, that can be rapidly sedimented with a magnet prior to decantation of the supernatant.

Papers and membranes

Cellulose comes in a convenient form as everyday paper, small discs of which can be coupled with antigen.

Nitrocellulose membranes have a strong surface charge and bind proteins tightly, a property taken advantage of in Western blotting. They are suitable for the dot blotting of samples; the paper is blocked with non-specific protein such as albumin, then assayed with specific antibodies.

For use in radioisotopes, the paper may be cut for counting. In enzyme assays, an insoluble coloured product is deposited on the membrane, which can be quantified in a densitometer.

ELISA optimization

ELISA systems are so robust that there is a strong temptation to select an 'average' set of conditions, find the assay that works, and stick with it. Marked increases in sensitivity and reproducibility can be obtained by optimizing each of the steps. Sittampalam *et al.* (1996) have applied experimental design techniques to optimize an ELISA to reproducibly measure in the 10–1000 pg/ml range.

5.5 Solid-phase radioimmunoassay for cell-surface antigens

Cells may be used in solid-phase assays; centrifugation and fixation are necessary to firmly attach the cells to the plastic surface. Enzyme detection systems can be used but care must be taken that cellular enzymes do not interfere with the assay. To avoid these problems, complete radiolabelled antibodies may be used as shown below.

5.5.1 Preparation of cell-coated assay plates

MATERIALS AND EQUIPMENT
Cells carrying antigen of interest
Glutaraldehyde
Phosphate-buffered saline (PBS)
PBS containing 5% w/v bovine haemoglobin and 0.2% w/v sodium azide
Microtitre plate with U-shaped wells, flexible polyvinyl chloride

Note: Azide is a dangerous chemical—do not discard down the sink.

METHOD

1 Harvest the cells by centrifugation and wash three times in PBS by centrifugation (150 *g* for 10 min at 4°C).
2 Count and adjust the cell numbers to 2×10^7/ml.
3 Dispense 50 μl aliquots of fresh 0.25% glutaraldehyde in PBS into each well of the microtitre plate.
4 Add 50 μl of cell suspension to each of 95 wells of the plate and centrifuge at 100 *g* for 5–10 min at 4°C. The 96th well is used as a control for non-specific binding in the final assay.
5 Remove the glutaraldehyde solution by tapping the inverted plate over a sink.
6 Flood the plate with PBS and roll a glass rod over the surface to remove air bubbles. Washing may also be performed by immersing the plate in a beaker of PBS.
7 Flood the plate with PBS containing bovine haemoglobin (5% w/v) and sodium azide (0.2% w/v). Again, roll a glass rod over the surface to remove air bubbles.

Continued on p. 174

> **8** Incubate the plate for 1 h at room temperature. This will saturate the protein-binding sites on the plastic.
>
> **9** The plates may be used immediately or stored for up to 10 weeks without removing the haemoglobin buffer.

TECHNICAL NOTES

- Soluble proteins will adsorb directly to these polyvinyl plates. Add 50 µl of protein solution (at 50–200 fmol/ml) in PBS to each well and incubate for at least 1 h at room temperature. Remove the supernatant (keep for re-use) and wash the plate three times with PBS containing bovine haemoglobin (5% w/v) and sodium azide (0.2% w/v). The protein solution must be free of detergent as this will inhibit binding.
- Antibody may also be linked to the plate and used to adsorb viable cells which are then fixed with glutaraldehyde.
- The relatively low concentration of glutaraldehyde used to fix the cells does not seem to alter surface antigens.

5.5.2 Radioiodinated anti-mouse immunoglobulin antibody (see Section 4.9)

Either: Prepare antibody to mouse immunoglobulin by affinity chromatography and then label with ^{125}I using Iodogen.

Or alternatively: Label anti-mouse immunoglobulin antibody while it is still attached to the affinity column using the chloramine T technique. Elute the ^{125}I-labelled antibodies with 0.2 M glycine–HCl buffer, pH 2.5, containing carrier protein.

5.5.3 Binding assay

MATERIALS AND EQUIPMENT

Cultures of fused cells

Assay plates coated with cells

Phosphate-buffered saline (PBS)

PBS containing 5% w/v bovine haemoglobin, and 0.2% w/v sodium azide

^{125}I-labelled anti-mouse immunoglobulin antibody

Plate sealers

Vacuum trap for radioactive washings

Nichrome wire, electrically heated, for cutting up plates

Gamma spectrometer

> **METHOD**
>
> **1** Remove the haemoglobin buffer by tapping the inverted test plate.
>
> **2** Remove 50 µl of supernatant from each hybrid well to be tested and transfer to the assay plate according to the following.
>
> *Continued*

Protocol.

Well number	Test antigen	Antibody	^{125}I-anti-mouse immunoglobulin
1	+	Hybrid supernatant	+
↓		↓	
93	+	Hybrid supernatant	+
94	+	Positive control*	+
95	+	Negative control*	+
96	−	Positive control*	+

* See Technical notes, item 3.

3 Incubate for 1 h at room temperature.

4 Wash the plate three times by immersing it in PBS and emptying it into a sink.

5 Add 25 μl of haemoglobin buffer containing 5×10^4 c.p.m. ^{125}I labelled anti-mouse immunoglobulin antibody to each well and incubate for 1 h at room temperature.

6 Remove the unbound radioactive antibody using a Pasteur pipette attached to a suction trap.

7 Wash five times by adding 3 drops of PBS to each well and then suck the solution into a vacuum trap.

8 Leave the plates to dry in a fume cupboard.

9 Cut up the tray with an electrically heated Nichrome wire to release the wells. For convenience, a plate sealer can be stuck to the bottom of the tray during cutting.

10 Load the wells directly into γ-counter tubes with forceps and determine their radioactive content.

TECHNICAL NOTES

- The baseline counts in wells 95 and 96 should be less than 200 c.p.m.
- Provided the baseline counts are reproducible, a count of more than 500 c.p.m. usually indicates antibody activity in the test supernatant.
- Because hybridoma supernatants have low total protein concentrations they give much 'cleaner' results in these assays than conventional antisera. Accordingly, the best controls are positive and negative supernatants from already established hybrids. Although it is often possible to beg hybrid supernatants with unrelated antibody activity to serve as controls in initial experiments, it is usually necessary to use diluted conventional antisera as positive controls.
- When working with parasites we have found that monoclonal antibody-defined antigens are sometimes not expressed uniformly by all members of a population. Under these conditions it is necessary to use a binding assay that gives information on the population distribution of binding; for example, indirect immunofluorescence using either a UV microscope or a fluorescence-activated cell sorter (see Chapter 8).
- As soon as positive cultures have been identified the cells should be cloned and, if possible, some of each uncloned positive well should be expanded and stored in liquid nitrogen as an insurance against a failure during cloning.

5.6 **Homogeneous immunoassays**

The degree of antigen–antibody interaction is determined with separation of bound and free components and has the advantage that equilibrium established in the assay is not disturbed. Many techniques have been used, including fluorescence polarization and fluorescence quenching, but the technique is now becoming more common with the availability of sophisticated surface plasmon resonance equipment that can very sensitively detect the interaction of antibody with antigen.

5.6.1 **Plasmon resonance**

This technique utilizes a surface sensitive detector which consists of:

(a) a ligand immobilized to the detector; and

(b) the detector which can measure the absorption of an analyte on the same spot and at the time when it occurs.

Biosensors allow real-time biomolecular interactions to be monitored without having to use a label. They can analyse interactions between proteins, nucleic acids, carbohydrates, lipids and low molecular weight molecules, such as signalling substances and drugs. The main advantage is that molecules do not need to be purified, but can be studied in crude extracts, lipid vesicles, viruses and bacteria as well as eukaryotic cells.

The first system to be commercially available was the BIAcore® (Pharmacia Biosensor, Uppsala, Sweden). This system combines a detector, a gold sensor chip, and integrated liquid-handling fluidic components for transport of samples and reagents to the site of interaction. The ligand is immobilized to a surface, such as dextran coated on the gold sensor chip. When the analyte is injected into the instrument, it passes over the immobilized ligand by means of the fluidic system. Adsorption of the analyte from the continuous flow of sample is measured as a function of time. After the pulse has passed the chip surface, the analyte dissociates and this can be monitored. The surface optical detection technique of BIAcore® uses surface plasmon resonance (Jonsson *et al.* 1991). Polarized light illuminates the sensor and is reflected into the detector array. Through surface plasmon resonance, light is displaced at one angle of incidence, and this is measured as a dark spot on the detector. This angle for extinction of light is changed when analyte associates or dissociates from the ligand.

An alternative to the BIAcore® is the IAsys® (Affinity Sensors, Cambridge, UK) which has a different optical detection system using a resonance mirror, and uses a stirred cuvette instead of a fluidic system.

Bisensors are used to monitor biomolecular interactions, such as molecular recognition, affinity, kinetics and multimolecular interactions. Kinetics and affinity measurements are determined from the curves generated in response to the association or dissociation of analyte from ligand (Altschuh *et al.* 1992). The association phase is a function of the kinetic properties of the reaction as long as the mass transport of analyte to the immobilized ligand is not a limiting factor in the reaction. The association constant (k_a) is obtained from a series of analyte concentrations and the detection range extended from 10^3 to 10^6/M/s. The dissociation rate constant (k_d) is ascertained by measuring the dissociation of bound analyte in buffer flow after the sample has passed the chip surface. The association equilibrium constant (K_a), or affinity constant, is calculated from the ratio of k_a to k_d. Analyte concentration ($\geq$ ng/ml) can be measured in crude extracts after calibrating the biosensor with known concentrations of analyte.

5.7 Further reading

Altschuh, D., Dubs, M.C., Weiss, E., Zeder-Lutz, G. & Van Regenmortel, M.H. (1992) Determination of kinetic constants for the interaction between a monoclonal antibody and peptides using surface plasmon resonance. *Biochemistry* **31** (27): 6298–304.

Arason, G.J., D'Ambrogio, M.S., Vikingsdottir, T., Sigfusson, A. & Valdimarsson, H. (1999) Enzyme immunoassays for measuring complement-dependent prevention of immune precipitation (PIP) and solubilization of preformed antigen–antibody complexes (SOL). *J Immunol Meth* **223**(1), 37–46.

Bicamumpaka, C. & Page, M. (1998) Development of a fluorescence polarization immunoassay (FPIA) for the quantitative determination of paclitaxel. *J Immunol Meth* **212**(1), 1–7.

Bolton, A.E. & Hunter, W.M. (1997) Radioimmunoassays and related methods. In: *Weir's Handbook of Experimental Immunology* (eds L.A. Herzenberg, D.M. Weir & C. Blackwell), 5th edn. Blackwell Science, Oxford.

Boraker, D.K., Bugbee, S.J. & Reed, BA. (1992) Acoustic probe-based ELISA. *J Immunol Meth* **155**(1), 91–4.

Borrebaeck, C.A.K. (2000) Antibodies in diagnostics—from immunoassays to protein chips [Review]. *Immunol Today* **21**(8), 379–382.

Brickelmaier, M., Hochman, P.S., Baciu, R., Chao, B., Cuervo, J.H. & Whitty, A. (1999) ELISA methods for the analysis of antibody responses induced in multiple sclerosis patients treated with recombinant interferon-beta. *J Immunol Meth* **227**, 121–135.

Bright, S.W., Tinsley, F.C., Dominianni, S.J., Schmiegel, K.K., Fitch, L.L. & Gold, G. (1997) Competitive particle concentration fluorescence immunoassays for measuring anti-diabetic drug levels in mouse plasma. *J Immunol Meth* **207**(1), 23–31.

Butler, J.E. (ed.) (1991) *Immunochemistry of Solid-Phase Immunoassay*, 2nd edn. Iowa State University Press, Iowa.

Chard, T. (1986) *An Introduction to Radioimmunoassay and Related Techniques: Laboratory Techniques in Biochemistry and Molecular Biology*, 3rd edn. Elsevier, Amsterdam.

Choi, J., Kim, C. & Choi, M.J. (1998) Comparison of capillary electrophoresis-based immunoassay with fluorescence polarization immunoassay for the immunodetermination of methamphetamine using various methamphetamine antibodies. *Electrophoresis* **19**, 2950–5.

Crowther, J.R. (ed.) (2000) *The ELISA Guidebook*. Humana Press, New Jersey.

Datta, P. & Dasgupta, A. (1998) Bidirectional (postive/negative) interference in a digoxin immunoassay: importance of antibody specificity. *Ther Drug Monit* **20**, 3352–7.

Diamandis, E.P. & Christopoulos, T.K. (1996) *Immunoassay*. Academic Press, London.

Ekins, R.P. (1981) Merits and disadvantages of different labels and methods of immunoassay. In *Immunoassays for the 80s* (eds A. Voller, A. Bartlett & D. Bidwell). MTP Press, Lancaster. [Many types of immunoassay and their applications are dealt with in this book.]

Ekins, R.P. (1985) Current concepts and future developments. In *Alternative Immunoassays* (ed. W.P. Collins). John Wiley and Sons, London. [There are many other useful chapters in this book.]

Findlay, J.W., Smith, W.C., Lee, J.W. *et al.* (2000) Validation of immunoassays for bioanalysis: a pharmaceutical industry perspective. *J Pharm Biomed Anal* **6**, 1249–73.

Giraudi, G., Anfossi, L., Rosso, I., Baggiani, C., Giovannoli, C. & Tozzi, C. (1999) A general method to perform a noncompetitive immunoassay for small molecules. *Anal Chem* **71**(20), 4697–4700.

Gosling, J. (2000) *Immunoasssay—A Practical Approach*. Oxford University Press, Oxford.

Gregorius, K., Mouritsen, S. & Elsner, H.I. (1995) Hydrocoating: a new method for coupling biomolecules to solid phases. *J Immunol Meth* **181**(1), 65–73.

Gudmundsson, B.M., Young, N.M. & Oomen, R.P. (1993) Characterization of residues in antibody binding sites by chemical modification of surface-adsorbed protein combined with enzyme immunoassay. *J Immunol Meth* **158**(2), 215–227.

Harris, C.C., Yolken, R.H., Krokan, H. & Chang Hsu, I. (1979) Ultrasensitive enzymatic radioimmuno-assay; application to detection of cholera toxin and rotavirus. *Proc Natl Acad Sci USA* **76**, 5336–5339.

Herzenberg, L.A., Weir, D.M., Herzenberg, L.A. & Blackwell, C. (eds) (1997) *Weir's Handbook of Experimental Immunology*, 5th edn. Blackwell Science. Oxford.

Ishikawa, S., Hashida, S., Hashinaka, K. & Ishikawa, E. (1998) Rapid and ultrasensitive enzyme immuno-assay (thin aqueous layer immune complex transfer enzyme immunoassay) for HIV-1 p24 antigen. *J Clin Lab Anal* **12**(4), 205–12.

Jackson, R.J., Fujhashi, K., Kiyono, H. & McGhee, J.R. (1996) Luminometry: a novel bioluminescent immunoassay enhances the quantification of mucosal and systemic antibody responses. *J Immunol Meth* **190**, 189–197.

Jonsson, U., Fagerstam, L., Ivarsson, B. *et al.* (1991) Real time biospecific interaction analysis using surface plasmon resonance and a sensor chip technology. *Biotechniques* **11**, 620–627.

Koskinen, S., Hirvonen, M. & Tolo, H. (1995) An enzyme immunoassay for the determination of anti-IgA antibodies using polyclonal human IgA. *J Immunol Meth* **179**(1), 51–58.

McCloskey, N., Turner, M.W. & Goldblatt, D. (1997) Correlation between the avidity of mouse-human chimeric IgG subclass monoclonal antibodies measured by solid-phase elution ELISA and biospecific interaction analysis. *J Immunol Meth* **205**, 67–72.

Miles, L.E.M. & Hales, C.M. (1968) Labelled antibodies and immunological assay systems. *Nature* **219**, 186–189.

Noel, D., Bernardi, T., Navarro-Teulon, I. *et al.* (1996) Analysis of the individual contributions of immunoglobulin heavy and light chains to the binding of antigen using cell transfection and plasmon resonance analysis. *J Immunol Meth* **193**(2), 177–187.

Pellequer, J.L. & Van Regenmortel, M.H.V. (1993) Measurement of kinetic binding constants of viral anti-bodies using a new biosensor technology. *J Immunol Meth* **166**, 133–143.

Perrin, A., Theretz, A., Lanet, V., Vialle, S. & Mandrand, B. (1999) Immunomagnetic concentration of anti-gens and detection based on a scanning force microscopic immunoassay. *J Immunol Meth* **224**, 77–87.

Pokric, B. (2000) Precipitation at equivalence and equilibrium: a method for the determination of equilibrium constants of reaction between multideterminant antigen and specific polyclonal antibodies. *J Chem Inf Comput Sci* **40**(3), 524–529.

Price, C.P. (1998) Progress in immunoassay technology. *Clin Chem Lab Med* **36**, 6341–347.

Raju, T.S., Nayak, N., Briggs, J., O'Connor, J.V. & Lerner, L. (1999) A convenient microscale colourimetric method for terminal galactose on immunoglobulins. *Biochem Biophys Res Commun* **261**(1), 196–201.

Shan, G., Huang, W., Gee, S.J., Buchholz, B.A., Vogel, J.S. & Hammock, B.D. (2000) Isotope-labelled immunoassays without radiation waste. *Proc Natl Acad Sci USA* **97**(6), 2445–9.

Sittampalam, G.S., Smith, W.C., Miyakawa, T.W., Smith, D.R. & McMorris, C. (1996) Application of experimental design techniques to optimize a competitive ELISA. *J Immunol Meth* **190**, 151–161.

Sonezaki, S., Yagi, S., Ogawa, E. & Kondo, A. (2000) Analysis of the interaction between monoclonal anti-bodies and human haemoglobin (native and cross-linked) using a surface plasmon resonance (SPR) biosensor. *J Immunol Meth* **238**(1–2), 99–106.

Stokke, T., Holte, H., Davies, C.D., Steen, H.B. & Lie, S.O. (1990) Quenching of Hoechst 33258 fluorescence in erythroid precursors. *Cytometry* **11**(6), 686–690.

Tani, A., Noda, M. & Ichimori, Y. (2000) Development of EIA systems for active-form MAP kinase. *J Immunol Meth* **238**(1–2), 87–97.

Tijssen, P. (1985) *Practice and Theory of Enzyme Immunoassays. Laboratory Techniques in Biochemistry and Molecular Biology*. Elsevier, Amsterdam.

Venkatesh, N. & Murthy, G.S. (1996) Dissociation of monoclonal antibody–antigen complexes: implications for ELISA procedures. *J Immunol Meth* **199**(2), 167–174.

Volland, H., Pradelles, P., Ronco, P. *et al.* (1999) A solid-phase immobilized epitope immunoassay (SPIE-IA) permitting very sensitive and specific measurement of angiotensin II in plasma. *J Immunol Meth* **228**(1–2), 37–47.

Wild, D. (ed.) (2001) *The Immunoassay Handbook*, 2nd edn. Grove's Dictionaries, Nature, MacMillan Press.

Yu, H. (1998) Comparative studies of magnetic particle-based solid-phase fluorogenic and electrochemilu-minescent immunoassay. *J Immunol Meth* **218**(1–2), 1–8.

6 Isolation of cells

6.1 Peritoneal cells

Peritoneal-derived immune cells are essentially made up of macrophages and lymphocytes (predominantly CD5 -B1 lymphocytes) and may be prepared by washing the peritoneal cavity of normal mice or guinea-pigs. For many purposes it is possible to elicit larger numbers of macrophages by producing a local inflammatory response, e.g. with starch, sodium trioleat, paraffin oil, etc. However it is important to remember that macrophages elicited in this wash will contain engulfed particles and will not be normal.

6.1.1 Isolation of normal peritoneal macrophages

MATERIALS

Mice or guinea-pigs

Tissue culture medium containing 10% fetal bovine serum

1% w/v neutral red in saline

METHOD

1 Kill the mouse or guinea-pig by cervical dislocation.

2 Inject 8.0 ml of tissue culture medium into the mouse's peritoneal cavity (80 ml for guinea-pigs).

3 Knead the abdomen gently to bring the cells into suspension.

4 Open the abdominal skin to expose the peritoneum.

5 Using a syringe with a 21-gauge needle, push the needle into the peritoneum, roll the mouse on its side and aspirate the medium. Alternatively, insert the needle into the peritoneal cavity towards the xiphisternum with the needle bevel directed downwards. The ventral peritoneal wall can be raised slightly with the syringe needle and the internal organs tend to settle, this reduces the possibility of fat bodies blocking the needle during withdrawal of the fluid.

Continued on p. 180

---

6 Collect the peritoneal cells by centrifugation (150 *g* for 10 min at room temperature) using siliconized glassware or plastic.

7 Estimate the number of phagocytes using a haemocytometer by the uptake of a 1% neutral red solution.

TECHNICAL NOTES

- A normal mouse will yield 5×10^6 peritoneal exudate cells, up to 50% of which will be lymphocytes.
- Although more of the peritoneal infusion can be collected by using a pipette after opening the peritoneum, care is needed if the cells are intended for sterile use.
- Most of the phagocytic cells will be macrophages, but there is likely to be a small amount of contamination with neutrophils.

6.1.2 Eliciting peritoneal exudate cells

MATERIALS

Mice or guinea-pigs

1% starch in 0.14 M saline

Tissue culture medium

1% w/v neutral red in saline

METHOD

1 Inject 2 ml of starch suspension into the peritoneal cavity of the mouse (25 ml for guinea-pigs).

2 Kill the animals after 3 days.

3 Inject 2–5 ml of tissue culture medium into the peritoneal cavity and gently press the abdomen to bring the cells into suspension (80 ml for guinea-pigs).

4 Open the abdominal skin of the animal and hold up the centre of the peritoneum with forceps.

5 Make a small hole in the peritoneum and remove the medium with a pipette.

6 Finally, open the animal fully and suck out all the medium. To handle these peritoneal exudate cells you must use either siliconized glassware or plastic.

7 Estimate the number of phagocytes by the uptake of a 1% neutral red solution (haemocytometer count).

The exudate should contain approximately 75% phagocytes and 25% other cells; this may be confirmed by non-specific esterase staining. Although more cells are obtained after starch treatment, remember that some of them will be activated as the starch induces a mild inflammatory response.

6.1.3 Non-specific esterase staining of macrophages

Peritoneal macrophages stain more strongly for non-specific esterase activity (particularly if they have been elicited by an inflammatory stimulus) than macrophages and monocytes elsewhere in the body. The latter types of cells are still easily distinguished by this staining reaction.

MATERIALS AND EQUIPMENT

Source of macrophages or monocytes

1 g pararosaniline

10 M HCl

Phosphate buffers

Acetone

Formaldehyde solution

Sodium nitrite, 4% w/v in water, freshly prepared

0.1 M sodium hydroxide

α naphthyl acetate

Methyl green dye, 0.4% w/v in water

DePeX artificial mountant

Equipment for smear preparation

Preparation in advance

1 Prepare a stock solution of the stain by mixing 1 g pararosaniline with 5 ml concentrated HCl (10 M) and 20 ml distilled water.

2 Heat to 70°C, allow to cool to room temperature, filter and store at 4°C in the dark.

METHOD

1 Prepare a smear of the cells on a microscope slide, either manually, or using a cytocentrifuge (see Section 11.6).

2 Fix the cells for 30 s at 4°C in 30 ml of 0.1 M phosphate buffer, pH 6.6, mixed with 45 ml acetone and 25 ml formaldehyde solution.

3 Wash three times with distilled water and air dry.

4 Immediately prior to use, prepare the active diazonium salt, hexazotized pararosaniline by mixing 6 ml of 4% w/v sodium nitrite (freshly prepared) with an equal volume of the pararosaniline stock solution and dilute to 200 ml with 0.067 M phosphate buffer, pH 5.0.

5 Adjust the activated dye solution to pH 5.8 with 0.1 M sodium hydroxide; this is the optimum pH for esterase activity.

6 Dissolve 50 mg α-naphthyl acetate in 2 ml acetone and add to the staining solution in step 5.

7 Incubate the smears in the stain for 4 h at room temperature or 45 min at 37°C, rinse in distilled water and counterstain for 1–2 min in a 0.4% aqueous solution of methyl green dye.

8 Wash the smears in distilled water, air dry and mount with DePeX.

6.2 Preparation of lymphocytes from blood

Differential centrifugation on a density gradient gives high-purity lymphocyte preparations. All equipment and solutions for these techniques must be sterile.

6.2.1 Mouse lymphocytes

Blood is layered onto a density gradient formulated such that only the erythrocytes form a pellet.

MATERIALS

Triosil 75 (available commercially, and is sterile)
Ficoll
Mouse blood sample
Tissue culture medium (see Appendix B.6)
Centrifuge tubes to prepare gradient
Pasteur pipettes

METHOD

1 Prepare a 9.2% w/v Ficoll solution in distilled water and autoclave.
2 Mix 43.4 ml of Ficoll solution and 6.6 ml of Triosil 75 under sterile conditions.
3 Dilute the blood 1 : 1 with sterile tissue culture medium without serum.
4 Layer 5 ml of diluted blood onto 2 ml of the gradient mixture and centrifuge at 300 *g* for 15 min at 4°C. The lymphocytes should not enter the gradient, but remain at the plasma–density gradient interface as a band.
5 Remove and discard the medium above the lymphocyte band.
6 Recover the lymphocyte band and wash three times by centrifugation (150 *g* for 10 min at 4°C).

TECHNICAL NOTES

- This technique works with heparinized blood.
- Discarding the supernatant above the lymphocyte band removes much of the platelet contamination. Washing in tissue culture medium will reduce the numbers of remaining platelets. The supernatant of the first wash will appear turbid because of unsedimented platelets; consequently, it is good practice to check by eye that a well-defined pellet has formed before discarding the wash supernatant.
- Do not collect too much of the density gradient; this contains neutrophils.
- Lymphocyte yield is $1-2 \times 10^6$/ml of venous blood.
- Commercial preparations of the density gradient are prepared gravimetrically and give more reproducible results. There are many suppliers, e.g. Lymphoprep™.

6.2.2 Human lymphocytes

Preparation of human peripheral blood mononuclear cells from whole blood

In this technique peripheral blood mononuclear cells (PBMC) are isolated from defibrinated or anticoagulated human blood using a density-interface centrifugation technique. It is adapted from Mutch and Westwood (2001).

MATERIALS AND EQUIPMENT

Human blood
Tissue culture medium, e.g. RPMI 1640 medium supplemented with 2.0 g/l sodium bicarbonate, 2 mM L-glutamine, 5 mM 4-(2-hydroxyethyl)piperazine-1-ethane sulphonic acid (HEPES)

buffer, 50 μg/ml gentamicin antibiotic solution (from a 50 mg/ml stock solution freshly prepared just before use)

Centrifuge tubes (50 ml with screw caps)

Ficoll–Paque (Ficoll–sodium diatrizoate, $\rho = 1.077$; Amersham Pharmacia Biotech)

Disposable syringes

Flexible 30-cm plastic cannula

Pasteur pipette

Note: *All equipment and solutions for this technique must be sterile.*

METHOD

1 Dilute 20 ml of human defibrinated blood with 10 ml of tissue culture medium, then add to a 50-ml centrifuge tube.

2 Carefully underlay 13–15 ml Ficoll–Paque using a sterile flexible cannula and disposable syringe, then centrifuge at 450 g for 25 min at 20°C.

3 Remove all but 3 ml of the serum above the layer of PBMC; this can be done carefully using a sterile pipette.

4 Heat inactivate the serum removed in step 3 by heating for 30 min at 56°C and keep serum for use in step 8.

5 Carefully remove the PBMC layer with minimal underlying Ficoll–Paque and add to a sterile 50-ml centrifuge tube. Samples from a single donor may be pooled (up to 25 ml per 50-ml centrifuge tube).

6 Wash the PBMC by adding an equal volume of tissue culture medium, then gently mix by resuspending the cells.

7 Centrifuge the cells at 150 g for 15 min at 20°C, remove the supernatant and then resuspend the cells in culture medium.
(Note that the PBMC layers contain enough serum within the suspension so serum need not be added at this stage.)

8 Resuspend the final pellet in complete medium containing 10% (v/v) heat-inactivated autologous serum (as prepared in step 4).

TECHNICAL NOTE

Use autologous serum rather than human AB serum as a supplement for the tissue culture medium for cells to be isolated for proliferative assays, as it avoids the need to pretest the serum. Do *not* use fetal bovine serum as it is likely to totally destroy the assay!

Human lymphocytes and peripheral blood mononuclear cells

MATERIALS

Human blood

Endotoxin-free heparin

Hank's balanced salt solution (Sigma)

Lymphoprep™ (Nycomed Amersham)

Pasteur pipettes

20-ml centrifuge tubes

RPMI 1640 containing 2 mM L-glutamine, 1 mM sodium pyruvate, 100 U/ml penicillin, 100 µg/ml streptomycin, 0.5 µg/ml fungizone and 10% heat-inactivated pooled human serum (e.g. human AB serum or autologous serum—see Appendix B.6)

METHOD

1 Collect human peripheral blood into tube containing endotoxin-free heparin (10 U/ml blood).
2 Add an equal volume of Hank's balanced salt solution and mix gently by inversion.
3 Overlay 10 ml aliquots of the diluted heparinized blood onto 5 ml of Lymphoprep™. Then centrifuge at 800 g for 20 min at 20°C.
4 The middle interface contains the lymphocytes (see Fig. 6.1). Remove cells using a sterile Pasteur pipette, taking care not to disturb the upper layer.
6 Wash the cells with 10 ml of Hank's balanced salt solution. Pellet the cells by centrifugation at 250 g for 15 min at 20°C.
7 Resuspend the cells for culturing in RPMI 1640 containing 2 mM L-glutamine, 1 mM sodium pyruvate, 100 U/ml penicillin, 100 µg/ml streptomycin, 0.5 µg/ml fungizone and 10% heat-inactivated serum.

6.2.3 Chicken lymphocytes

Although dextran sedimentation techniques are available to prepare chicken leucocytes, they give poor cell yields. Chicken erythrocytes are much larger than the white cells and so separation by differential centrifugation is possible without a density gradient. Chicken PBMC tend to clump readily under normal conditions and so these are also removed from the plasma.

MATERIAL
Chicken blood containing heparin

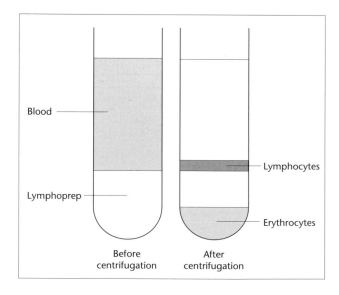

Fig. 6.1 Lymphoprep: before and after centrifugation. Lymphocytes are found at the interface.

METHOD

1 Cool the blood to 4°C.
2 Centrifuge at 150 *g* for 3 min at 4°C.
3 Reduce the centrifugal force to 35 *g*, and continue spinning for a further 10 min at 4°C.

The supernatant plasma will contain lymphocytes virtually free of all other cells; lymphocyte yield 3–5 × 10^6/ml whole blood. It is essential to use blood containing heparin, as citrated saline reduces the viscosity of the plasma and reduces cell yield and purity. As cockerel blood has a lower viscosity than hen blood due to its lower lipid content, a loose buffy coat often forms during centrifugation. This should be resuspended by gentle stirring.

6.3 Preparation of lymphocytes from solid lymphoid organs

Lymphocyte suspensions may be prepared from solid lymphoid organs, for example spleen, lymph nodes, bursa, thymus.

METHOD

1 Tease the organs apart using forceps or needles over fine nylon gauze to retain the connective tissue capsule of the organ.
2 Wet the gauze with a few ml of tissue culture medium. Lymphocyte viability tends to vary with the amount of fibrous tissue in the organ and the 'deftness of touch' of the operator.

Approximate cell yields from each of the organs are given in Fig. 6.2. Cell viability should be as follows: thymus 95%, spleen 80–90% and lymph node 70–80%. The lymphocyte subpopulations of each organ are summarized in Table 6.1. If uniformly viable cell suspensions are required, e.g. for antibody-mediated cytotoxicity assays, dead cells may be removed as described in Section 6.4.

Table 6.1 Percentage lymphocyte subpopulations of murine lymphoid organs

Organ	% T lymphocytes	% B lymphocytes	% 'null' cells
Thymus	97	1	2
Lymph node	77	18	5
Spleen	35	38	27
Blood	70	24	6
Thoracic duct lymph	80	19	1

T lymphocyte: thymus-derived small lymphocyte, with Thy-1-positive, surface immunoglobulin-negative phenotype.
B lymphocyte: in chickens B lymphocytes are bursa-derived (i.e. from the bursa of Fabricius); in mammals, B lymphocytes may be defined serologically by their expression of surface immunoglobulin but not Thy-1 antigens.
'Null' cells: resemble small lymphocytes morphologically, but do not have Thy-1 or surface immunoglobulin surface markers. This is a mixed cell lineage, some members of which are undoubtedly of the lymphoid series and, having IgG Fc receptors, are capable of antibody-dependent cytotoxic activities. These cells have some of the characteristics of monocytes and express some T-lymphocyte markers. Typically, these have the morphology of large granular lymphocytes (Fig. 7.2c). Natural killer (NK) cells also belong to this population.

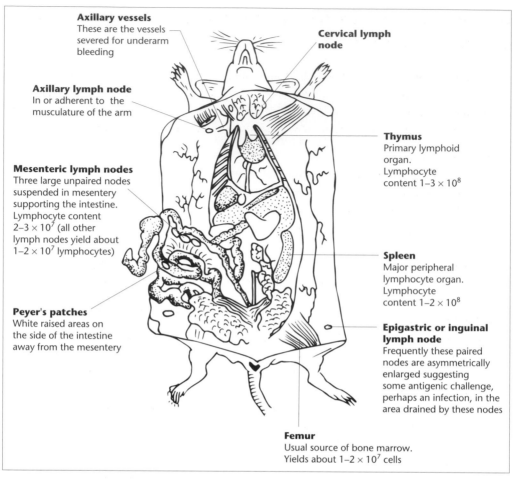

Axillary vessels
These are the vessels severed for underarm bleeding

Cervical lymph node

Axillary lymph node
In or adherent to the musculature of the arm

Thymus
Primary lymphoid organ.
Lymphocyte content 1–3×10^8

Mesenteric lymph nodes
Three large unpaired nodes suspended in mesentery supporting the intestine. Lymphocyte content 2–3×10^7 (all other lymph nodes yield about 1–2×10^7 lymphocytes)

Spleen
Major peripheral lymphocyte organ.
Lymphocyte content 1–2×10^8

Peyer's patches
White raised areas on the side of the intestine away from the mesentery

Epigastric or inguinal lymph node
Frequently these paired nodes are asymmetrically enlarged suggesting some antigenic challenge, perhaps an infection, in the area drained by these nodes

Femur
Usual source of bone marrow.
Yields about 1–2×10^7 cells

Fig. 6.2 The major lymphoid organs of the mouse. One of the major lymphoid organs not obvious in the drawing is the blood; it contains about 3–10×10^6 lymphocytes/ml in a total leucocyte count of 4–12×10^6/ml. As a guide, the differential leucocyte count of mice is approximately neutrophils 25%, eosinophils 2%, basophils < 0.1%, lymphocytes 65% and monocytes 8%. The data for lymphocyte content of the various organs were derived from a specific pathogen-free (SPF) stock of CBA mice aged about 4–8 weeks old. At this age the total blood volume is about 6.3 ml/100 g body weight. The change in blood volume with weight (age) shows a curvilinear relationship probably due to an enhanced fat deposition after 20 g. It follows the general form

$y = 0.097x - 0.002x^2$

where y is blood volume (ml) and x is body weight (g).
Other strains of mice, particularly if they are outbred, show a linear relationship between body weight and blood volume. For example, the relationship for Swiss mice is:

$y = 0.072x$

where unknowns are as above.
The cell content of each lymphoid organ is known to vary with age (especially the thymus), strain, sex, health and immune status of the individual.

Sterile cell suspensions may be prepared from solid lymphoid organs by pressing the organ through autoclaved nylon gauze in tissue culture medium (see Appendix B.6) using the piston from a 5- or 10-ml disposable syringe. The debris adheres to the nylon gauze and the cell suspension may be dispersed by aspiration with a Pasteur pipette.

6.4 Removal of dead cells

The surface charge difference between dead and viable cells is very great when they are suspended in media with a low ionic strength (isotonicity is maintained by the addition of glucose). Filtration of such cell suspensions through a column of hydrophilic cotton wool results in the retention of dead cells; cells in the effluent volume will then be uniformly viable.

MATERIALS AND EQUIPMENT
Phosphate-buffered saline (PBS)
0.308 M glucose in water
Siliconized Pasteur pipettes (see Technical notes)
10-ml conical centrifuge tubes, siliconized
Absorbent cotton wool
Fetal bovine serum (FBS)
All steps in this procedure should be carried out with solutions equilibrated on ice or at 4°C.

METHOD

1 Mix 1 volume of PBS with 19 volumes of the glucose solution (low ionic strength buffer).
2 Spin down lymphocytes and resuspend to $2-4 \times 10^7$/ml in low ionic strength buffer.
3 Cut end from a siliconized Pasteur pipette just below the drawn-out shoulder, and pack with cotton wool (to about 5 mm in height).
4 Add up to 4 ml of cell suspension to each pipette, allow the suspension to flow through under 1 g and collect the effluent in a siliconized tube.
5 Wash through with 0.5 ml of low ionic strength buffer, underlay the cell suspension with 1 ml FBS and centrifuge at 220 g for 15 min at 4°C.
6 Resuspend the cells in tissue culture medium and perform a viability count.

TECHNICAL NOTES
- This method of dead-cell removal is often of crucial importance in microscale assays, where the sensitivity of the assay depends on high initial cell viability.
- If a sterile cell suspension is required, autoclave PBS, glucose and prepacked columns. Using solutions precooled on ice, the columns may be run in a laminar flow hood at room temperature.
- Siliconizing of plastic and glassware (see Appendix B). Large containers may be coated with a thin film of silicon by rinsing them with one of the proprietary siliconizing solutions in heptane. Small items, such as pipettes, etc., may be treated in bulk with dichlorodimethylsilane vapour (this chemical is highly volatile and extremely toxic: handle it only inside a fume hood).

6.5 Removal of phagocytic cells

Macrophages can be removed from a cell suspension using either their adherence or phagocytic properties.

6.5.1 Adherence to Sephadex

MATERIALS AND EQUIPMENT

Cells for depletion

Sephadex G-10

Tissue culture medium containing 10% (v/v) fetal bovine serum

Syringe barrel, 20 ml

Phosphate-buffered saline (PBS)

METHOD

1 Hydrate the Sephadex in PBS and settle for 10 min to remove 'fines'.
2 Autoclave in glass bottles at 138 kPa for 15 min.
3 Pack 10 ml of sterile Sephadex into a 20-ml syringe barrel fitted with a sintered plastic disc, and wash with 10 ml of warm tissue culture medium.
4 Add a maximum of 3×10^8 cells in 1 ml and allow them to become included into the column bed.
5 Wash out the non-adherent cells with 20 ml of warm tissue culture medium, collect the effluent and concentrate the cells by centrifugation (150 g for 10 min at 4°C).

TECHNICAL NOTES

- Sephadex G-10 filtration is known to remove rat dendritic cells, even though they are not adherent to glass or plastic surfaces. Human and mouse suppressor T cells are also adherent to Sephadex.
- Although adherent cells may also be removed by filtration through glass beads or fibres, the resulting cell suspensions show a greater depletion of B lymphocytes compared with the technique described above.

6.5.2 Phagocytosis of iron powder (for removal of actively phagocytic cells)

MATERIALS AND EQUIPMENT

Iron powder

Samarium cobalt magnet

Cell suspension in medium containing 5% fetal bovine serum

10-ml conical plastic tubes

METHOD

1 Wash the iron powder in ethanol and then in distilled water; autoclave at 138 kPa for 15 min if required for sterile cell separation.
2 Adjust the cell suspension to $2–3 \times 10^7$ lymphocytes/ml.
3 Add 4 mg of iron powder and mix thoroughly.
4 Incubate at 37°C for 30 min, mixing occasionally.
5 Stand the plastic tube on one of the poles of the magnet and leave at 4°C for 10 min.

Continued

6 Remove the cells in suspension (with the tube still standing on the magnet) and transfer to a second plastic tube.

7 Resettle the cells on the magnet for a further 10 min at 4°C.

These are not preparative techniques. Phagocytic cells attached to Sephadex or containing iron powder are *not* functional.

6.6 B-cell depletion for T-cell enrichment

6.6.1 Anti-immunoglobulin columns

MATERIALS AND EQUIPMENT

Degalan V26 plastic beads

0.1 M phosphate buffer, pH 6.4

Phosphate-buffered saline (PBS)

10 mg purified rabbit anti-mouse immunoglobulin antibodies

METHOD

1 Wash 5 g of Degalan beads with distilled water, and then equilibrate with 30 ml phosphate buffer. Remove all liquid with a pipette.

2 Add 10 mg purified antibody (initial concentration 5 mg/ml).

3 Incubate at 15°C for 2 h, then at 4°C overnight.

4 Recover unbound antibody and calculate amount adsorbed to beads.

Control column

Many cells passing down a column of protein coated onto plastic beads will stick non-specifically because of the strong non-covalent intermolecular forces at the surface of the bead. Hence retention of the cells will not only be related to the antiserum on the column. As a control for non-specific retention of cells a column of an irrelevant antibody, e.g. anti-keyhole limpet haemocyanin, must be prepared and used in an identical manner to that described for the anti-immunoglobulin column.

Cell fractionation

MATERIALS AND EQUIPMENT

Mouse spleen or lymph-node cells

Two 20-ml plastic syringe barrels

Sintered plastic discs for columns

Tissue culture medium containing 5% fetal bovine serum and ethylene diamine tetra-acetic acid (EDTA), 5 mM

Degalan beads coated with (a) anti-Ig and (b) an unrelated antibody

1 Pour the coated plastic beads into separate syringe barrels fitted with sintered plastic discs and equilibrate each with 30 ml of medium.

2 Seal off the column with a needle and rubber bung.

3 Incubate the column at 37°C for 30 min.

4 Cool to 4°C for 30 min before use.

5 Prepare a single-cell suspension of mouse spleen or lymph-node cells and deplete of phagocytic cells. Wash in medium and adjust to 10^7 lymphocytes/ml.

6 Pipette 1 ml of lymphocytes onto each column.

7 Allow the cells to enter the column bed and reseal column.

8 Add 1 ml of medium to the column; allow it to enter the column.

Under the conditions described the anti-Ig column will be able to deplete 10 aliquots of lymphocytes. The depleted population may be collected either as individual aliquots or as a pool.

9 After the last aliquot of cells, wash the column through with 15 ml of medium. Collect effluent.

10 Concentrate the effluent cells by centrifugation and count in a haemocytometer.

TECHNICAL NOTES

- The high non-specific retention by these columns can be minimized by a high flow rate. At a flow rate of 2–3 ml/min about 20–30% non-specific loss may be expected.
- All cell fractionation procedures must be carried out at 4°C.
- T lymphocytes prepared by this technique may be contaminated by a variable proportion of null cells (see Table 6.1).

Biomagnetic separation of cells

Rapid separation of subsets of cells from a heterogeneous population has been very much simplified by the development of Dynabeads. In the direct technique, magnetic beads are coupled to antibodies which target a specific cell-surface antigen. Once added to the heterogeneous mixture of cells, the beads bind to the target ligand. Cell-bound beads can be separated from rest of the suspension using a Dynal magnet particle concentrator. The indirect technique may be used to isolate the cell subset of interest indirectly by the removing other cell types from the heterogeneous suspension of cells, i.e. depleting the cell suspension of unwanted subsets of cells.

6.6.2 General protocol for the isolation of cells using Dynabeads

MATERIALS

Dynabeads M-450 coated with primary antibody (see Table 6.2)
Dynal magnetic particle concentrator (Dynal MPC)
Phosphate-buffered saline (PBS), pH 7.4

Table 6.2 Dynabeads available for the isolation of human immune cell subsets from whole blood, buffy coat or peripheral blood mononuclear cells

	Dynabeads M-450 coated with
Leucocytes	anti-CD45
B lymphocytes	anti-CD19
T lymphocytes	anti-CD3, anti-CD2
	anti-CD4, anti-CD8
Granulocytes	anti-CD16, anti-CD15
Haemopoietic progenitor cells	anti-CD34
Antigen-presenting cells	anti-HLA class II
Monocytes/ macrophages	anti-CD14
Natural killer cells	anti-CD56, anti-CD16

Dynabeads are also available for the isolation of murine immune cell types.

METHOD

1 Use 1×10^7 Dynabeads M-450 per ml of cell suspension. Gently vortex the Dynabeads, then allow to separate using the Dynal MPC.

2 Remove the liquid and wash three times with an equal volume of PBS.

Direct isolation of cells

3 Add the washed Dynabeads M-450 to the heterogeneous cell suspension which contains the cells to be isolated.

4 Incubate with gentle mixing at 4°C for 30 min.

5 Insert the tube containing the cells and Dynabeads M-450 into the Dynal MPC, and allow to stand for 5 min. Cells possessing the target cell's surface ligand are rosetted on the side of the test tube.

6 Discard the supernatant and wash the rosetted cells in PBS (or cell culture media).

7 Insert the tube containing the cells and Dynabeads M-450 into the Dynal MPC, and allow to stand for 3 min.

8 Repeat steps 6 and 7 three times.

Indirect isolation of cells

9 Add the washed Dynabeads M-450 to the heterogeneous cell suspension which contains the cells to be isolated.

10 Incubate with gentle mixing at 4°C for 30 min.

11 Insert the tube containing the cells and Dynabeads M-450 into the Dynal MPC, and allow to stand for 5 min. Cells possessing the target cell's surface ligand are within the supernatant.

12 Transfer the supernatant to another test tube.

6.6.3 Nylon wool columns

Spleen-cell suspensions may be fractionated on the basis of their differential adherence to nylon fibres. At 37°C and in the presence of serum, B lymphocytes will bind avidly to nylon wool columns, giving an effluent population of virtually pure T lymphocytes and 'null' cells. This technique has the obvious advantages of speed, convenience and low cost.

MATERIALS AND EQUIPMENT

Nylon wool, sterile

Tissue culture medium containing 5% fetal bovine serum (FBS)

Syringe, 20 ml, plastic, sterile

METHOD

1. Pack 600 mg of sterile nylon wool (approximately 6 ml) into a 20-ml syringe barrel and wash with tissue culture medium containing 5% FBS.
2. Seal the column and incubate at 37°C for 1 h.
3. Prepare cells, depleted of phagocytic cells, and adjust to 5×10^7 lymphocytes/ml.
4. Flush column with 5 ml of warm tissue culture medium. (This will correct any change in pH during incubation.)
5. Add 2 ml of cell suspension dropwise to the top of the column. After it has all entered, add 1 ml of warm tissue culture medium.
6. Seal the column and incubate at 37°C for 45 min.
7. Wash the column with 25 ml of warm tissue culture medium and collect the unbound cells in the effluent.
8. Concentrate the cells by centrifugation (150 g for 10 min at 4°C) and determine the number of viable lymphocytes.

The effluent population should be depleted of B lymphocytes, as evidenced by anti-immunoglobulin immunofluorescence, and will consist of T lymphocytes and 'null' cells. A proportion of the bound cells may be recovered by mechanical elution as follows.

1. Wash the column with 100 ml of warm tissue culture medium and discard the effluent.
2. Seal the column with a needle and rubber bung.
3. Add 2 ml of warm tissue culture medium and squeeze the nylon wool with blunt stainless steel forceps.
4. Unseal the column and wash with 10 ml of warm tissue culture medium. Finally, replace the syringe piston and expel all the tissue culture medium.
5. Collect the effluent cells and concentrate by centrifugation (150 g for 10 min at 4°C).
6. Count number of viable lymphocytes/ml.

The cells recovered by mechanical elution will consist of B lymphocytes, as evidenced by anti-immunoglobulin immunofluorescence, contaminated with a variable number of T lymphocytes and 'null' cells.

6.7 Propagation of antigen-responsive normal T-lymphocyte lines

Under the conditions described below, normal T lymphocytes may be expanded into lines capable of extensive *in vitro* proliferation and yet still retain their effector capacity and antigen selectivity.

Immunogens used range from allogeneic cells to processed antigen expressed by MHC-compatible antigen-presenting cells or viral antigens expressed on infected autologous host cells.

There are many different methods for isolating antigen-specific T-cell clones *in vitro*. We will describe here methods that we have used for the isolation of murine and, in Section 6.8, human antigen-reactive T-cell lines and clones.

6.7.1 Dose–response curve for antigen

MATERIALS AND EQUIPMENT

Inbred mice for immunization (it is important to use inbred mice of known haplotype as
   Ia-identical animals have to be used as a source of feeder cells)

Antigen

Freund's complete adjuvant

Tissue culture medium

Fetal bovine serum (FBS)

2-mercaptoethanol

Antibiotics   streptomycin and penicillin

96-well culture plates

^{3}H-thymidine

Automated cell harvester

Beta spectrometer

METHOD

1 Immunize mice by a subcutaneous injection at the base of the tail with antigen emulsified in Freund's complete adjuvant (100 µl total volume per injection site).

2 Anaesthetize the mice 3–4 days after the last injection and bleed for serum.

3 Kill the mice by cervical dislocation and remove the para-aortic and inguinal lymph nodes (draining the base of the tail) using aseptic technique.

4 Prepare a sterile single-cell suspension as described in Section 6.3.

5 Wash the cell suspension twice by centrifugation and resuspend the cells in complete medium (containing 10% FBS, 2×10^{-5} M 2-mercaptoethanol, 100 U/ml penicillin and 100 µg/ml streptomycin) and resuspend at 2×10^6 cells/ml.
   A control population should be prepared in an identical manner using cells from mice immunized with Freund's complete adjuvant alone.

6 Dispense 100 µl aliquots of cells into the wells of a 96-well microtitre tray (U-shaped wells) and add a range of antigen concentrations in triplicate, each in 100 µl of medium.

7 Incubate for 4–6 days, depending on the peak of the mitogenic response, and during the last 18 h of incubation add 37×10^3 Bq per well of ^{3}H-thymidine.

Continued on p. 194

8 Harvest with an automated cell harvester and measure radioactive incorporation using a β scintillation counter.

9 Calculate the proliferation index according to the equation:

$$\text{Stimulation index} = \frac{\text{c.p.m. cells with antigen} - \text{c.p.m. cells without antigen}}{\text{c.p.m. cells without antigen}}$$

Repeat the calculations for cells from animals immunized with Freund's adjuvant alone to check that the antigen being used reacts specifically with the cells primed with antigen *in vivo*.

10 Plot a dose–response curve for the antigen to determine the optimum concentration for *in vitro* stimulation.

TECHNICAL NOTE

The immunization protocol must be varied to take account of the antigen being used. A single injection of a highly immunogenic antigen is often sufficient. However, for some antigens a booster injection 7 days after the first (or an even more extensive boosting) may be advantageous. In any case harvest the lymph nodes 3–4 days after the last injection.

6.7.2 **Murine T-lymphocyte line production**

METHOD

1 Immunize four to six mice as described above and prepare a single-cell suspension of lymph-node cells (see Section 6.3).

2 Resuspend the cells in tissue culture medium containing 10% FBS and aliquot at $2–5 \times 10^6$ cells per well in 24-well culture plates.

3 Add antigen at the optimum concentration (determined above) to achieve a total culture volume of 1.5 ml and incubate for 4–6 days at 37°C in a humidified incubator gassed with 5% CO_2 in air.

4 Harvest the cells by centrifugation (150 *g* for 10 min at room temperature) and isolate the blast cells by density gradient centrifugation (Section 6.2).

5 Wash the cells twice by centrifugation, resuspend in tissue culture medium containing 5% FBS and count in a haemocytometer.

6 Prepare a single-cell suspension from the spleens of syngeneic mice (see Section 6.3) for use as feeder cells.

7 Irradiate the normal spleen cells with 25 Gy irradiation, wash and resuspend in tissue culture medium containing 5% FBS.

8 Plate $1–2 \times 10^6$ irradiated feeder cells with 1×10^5 T-cell blasts per well in a total volume of 2 ml.

9 Incubate for 7–14 days.

10 Repeat steps 3–6 and plate $1–2 \times 10^6$ irradiated feeder cells with $1–2 \times 10^5$ T cells plus antigen at the optimum concentration.

11 Incubate for 4 days.

12 Repeat steps 3–7.

T-cell lines can be maintained long-term by this regime of regular stimulation and 'rest'. When larger numbers of cells are required for assays, the cells can be expanded in tissue culture flasks (start with 25 cm^2 growth area flasks). To maintain maximum cell density at the beginning of an expansion phase, incubate the flasks upright or at a slight angle to vertical. It is possible to maintain antigen-reactive T-cell lines in culture for up to about 14 days without antigen stimulation by adding exogenous interleukin 2 (IL-2) to the medium. Activated (antigen-stimulated) T-cell lines which express IL-2 receptors will respond by vigorous growth and proliferation. However, growth declines rapidly within a few days because of a decrease in the expression of the IL-2 receptor. Restimulation with the appropriately presented antigen or a mitogen is then required to induce re-expression of high levels of the Il-2 receptor.

Laboratories vary in their techniques for production of T-cell lines and many factors can influence the outcome; persistence is obligatory and 'green fingers' are helpful.

6.7.3 T-lymphocyte cloning

MATERIALS AND EQUIPMENT
Antigen-reactive T-cell line
Syngeneic irradiated feeder cells
Antigen
Tissue culture medium containing 5% fetal bovine serum
96-well microculture plates (flat wells)
Interleukin 2 (IL-2) (see Technical note)

METHOD

1 Prepare T-cell blasts as described in previous section.
2 Dispense 5×10^5 irradiated feeder cells in tissue culture medium containing IL-2 and the optimum concentration of antigen into the wells of the microtitre trays.
3 Prepare suspensions of the T-cell blasts at: (a) 100 cells/ml; (b) 33 cells/ml; (c) 10 cells/ml; and (d) 3.3 cells/ml.
4 Dispense aliquots of 100 µl of each suspension, preparing one plate each for (a) and (b), and three plates each for (c) and (d). The higher concentrations are used to check that the cells will grow.
5 Examine the plates under an inverted microscope with phase-contrast optics after 7 days.
6 Wells in which T lymphocytes have grown can easily be identified, as the phase-bright T cells grow as a clump amongst the dying, phase-dark feeder cells.
7 Positive wells should be transferred into 24-well culture plates containing fresh, irradiated syngeneic feeder cells (2×10^6 per well), the optimum concentration of antigen and IL-2.
8 To ensure that monoclonality is obtained the selected 'cloned lines' should be recloned by plating at 1 cell/ml.

Once cloned populations have been selected and expanded, aliquots should be cryopreserved against accidental loss or clonal exhaustion. By this stage the T lymphocytes will have adapted (probably been intensively selected) to the *in vitro* conditions and so can be maintained relatively easily by repeated cycles of antigen stimulation and 'rest'. Some T-cell clones can be maintained in IL-2-supplemented medium alone for several days but will need stimulation with antigen plus feeder cells to sustain proliferation and their differentiated function.

TECHNICAL NOTE

It is preferable to use recombinant IL-2 for technical convenience: titrate the units of activity to determine the optimum concentration in your system. This is likely to be around 2000 U/ml. Alternatively, IL-2-containing supernatants can be prepared from T-lymphocyte lines (MLA-144 (gibbon line) for use with human cells or EL4 for use with murine cells) or from normal lymphocytes (e.g. rat spleen) stimulated in bulk with concanavalin A (mitogenic stimulation as for phytohaemagglutinin—PHA). IL-2 is constitutively produced by the cell lines; however, its production may be maximized by growing the cells to their plateau density, washing them into serum-free medium and incubating overnight at 37°C in a humidified atmosphere containing 5% CO_2 in air.

Interleukin-2 from any of these sources will maintain murine T-lymphocytes, but human T-lymphocytes need primate IL-2.

6.8 Production of human T-lymphocyte lines

6.8.1 Human T-lymphocyte lines

Procedures for deriving human T-lymphocyte lines are essentially similar to those described for the mouse (see Section 6.7), but with some important differences and limitations. Human lines are usually derived using either ethical (vaccination) or fortuitous (usually an infection) immunization. They invariably need repeated donations from the same individual to provide both T lymphocytes (a minor requirement) and feeder cells (a massive requirement). Although it is possible to select a panel of HLA-D-matched individuals to supply feeder cells or to transfect the required major histocompatibility complex (MHC) molecules into antigen-presenting cells, this requires sophisticated laboratory back up. Attempts have been made to establish lines of Epstein–Barr virus-transformed autologous B cells from the T-lymphocyte donor and use these as antigen-presenting cells, but without uniform success.

MATERIALS AND EQUIPMENT

Peripheral blood drawn from an antigen-sensitized individual (see Technical notes)
Antigen
Tissue culture medium
Pooled normal human serum (NHS)
^{3}H-thymidine
96-well microculture plates, U-shaped wells
24-well culture plates
Tissue culture flasks, 25 cm^2
Automated cell harvester
Beta spectrometer

As with the murine T cells, it is important to establish a dose–response curve for the antigen to be used.

1 Fractionate peripheral blood mononuclear cells (PBMC) from heparinized blood by density gradient centrifugation (Section 6.2.2).
2 Wash the cells twice by centrifugation and resuspend in tissue culture medium containing 10% pooled NHS.
3 Dispense 100 μl aliquots of cells (2×10^6/ml) into the wells of U-shaped well microtitre plates. Add 100 μl aliquots of antigen in doubling dilutions in 100 μl medium.
4 Incubate at 37°C in a humidified atmosphere of 5% CO_2 in air for 5 days.
5 Add 37×10^3 Bq of ^{3}H-thymidine to each well and incubate for a further 6 h.
6 Harvest the wells using an automated cell harvester and measure isotope incorporation using a β counter.
7 The results are expressed as an index of stimulation, as defined for murine lymphocytes above.
8 Plot a dose–response curve to determine the optimum antigen concentration required to give maximum T-lymphocyte proliferation.

TECHNICAL NOTES

- Although many of the antigenic constituents of human vaccines or common infectious organisms have been used to produce T-lymphocyte lines, those of the influenza virus have been particularly useful because parallel developments in molecular biology have made a wide range of defined 'flu peptides readily available.
- Please refer to the following websites for comprehensive details on radioisotope health and safety procedures as well as useful information regarding detection and half-life:
  http://www.practicingsafescience.org
  http://www.hse.gov.uk

Human T-lymphocyte line production

MATERIALS AND EQUIPMENT
Heparinized human peripheral blood
Tissue culture medium
Pooled normal human serum (NHS)
Source of IL-2, either supernatant from the cell line MLA-144, or recombinant human material
Antigen
96-well microculture plates, flat wells
Tissue culture flasks, 25 cm² growth area
24-well culture plates

1 Prepare human peripheral blood lymphocytes from heparinized blood by density gradient centrifugation (Section 6.2.2) and resuspend in tissue culture medium containing 10% pooled NHS.

Continued on p. 198

2 Adjust the cell concentration to $1–2 \times 10^6$/ml and dispense in 10 ml aliquots into 25-cm^2 tissue culture flasks or in 2 ml aliquots in 24-well cluster plates. Add the required antigen at its optimum concentration.

3 To maintain high cell density incubate the flasks upright at 37°C in a humidified atmosphere of 5% CO_2 in air for 6–7 days.

4 Harvest the cells and separate the blasts by density gradient centrifugation (Section 6.2.2) and wash the cells in tissue culture medium by centrifugation.

The T-cell lines can be maintained in IL-2-containing medium with repeated rounds of stimulation with antigen and feeder cells. They are much easier to grow than their murine equivalents, to the extent that they can be cloned at or soon after primary plating.

6.8.2 **Human T-lymphocyte cloning**

MATERIALS AND EQUIPMENT

As previous section, but including phytohaemagglutinin (PHA)

METHOD

1 To prepare autologous irradiated feeder cells, separate leucocytes from heparinized blood, wash and irradiate with 40 Gy from a high-energy source.

2 Adjust the cell concentration to 1×10^6/ml in medium containing 10% pooled NHS, IL-2, antigen at the optimum concentration and a submitogenic concentration of PHA (e.g. 0.01–0.1 µg/ml—it is necessary to titrate the concentration with each new batch of PHA).

3 Resuspend fractionated T-cell blasts after *in vitro* stimulation as described in the previous section. Prepare suspensions at 100, 33, 10, 3.3 and 1 cell/ml in tissue culture medium containing 10% human serum. Prepare sufficient for 48 microcultures of each of the three higher concentrations and 96 cultures for each of the two lower concentrations.

4 Plate out 100 µl aliquots of the T-lymphocyte suspensions and incubate at 37°C in a humidified atmosphere of 5% CO_2 in air for 7 days.

5 Examine the plates under a phase-contrast inverted microscope for growth. The clones tend to grow in clumps and so are very easy to identify.

6 Positive wells can be expanded into 24-well cluster plates containing 1×10^6 irradiated autologous feeder cells per well in medium supplemented with serum, IL-2, antigen and PHA.

7 After a further 7 days' incubation the T-cell blasts can be further expanded on an irradiated feeder layer grown in 25-cm^2 culture flasks with antigen stimulation.

To ensure monoclonality, repeat steps 1–6. T-cell clones can be maintained for short periods in IL-2-containing medium but will need stimulation with antigen and feeder cells every 6–14 days.

6.9 T-lymphocyte hybridomas

T-cell hybridomas have been used for studies on the T-cell receptor and as a source of T-cell-derived cytokines and other regulatory effector molecules, particularly suppressor factors. They are also used for evaluating cell recognition reactions. The methods used to prepare T-cell hybridomas are essentially the same as for B-cell hybrids: an activated population of T cells primed to respond to a particular antigen, or activated with mitogen (phytohaemagglutinin–PHA, or concanavalin A–Con A) is fused with a tumour-cell line of T-cell origin, usually the murine AKR thymoma BW-5147. Fusion products are assessed for phenotype and karyotype (to determine that they are true T-lymphocyte–tumour-cell hybrids) and finally cloned and functionally selected depending upon the activity (or activities) desired.

MATERIALS AND EQUIPMENT

Activated murine lymphocytes (see Technical notes)

8-azaguanine-resistant variant of the murine AKR thymoma BW-5147 (but see also
    Technical notes)

Tissue culture medium (Appendix B.6), alone or with 10% fetal bovine serum (FBS)

Polyethylene glycol solution PEG-1500 (prepared as in Section 2.5)

Concentrated HAT medium (see Section 2.5.4)

96-well microtitre plates

24- and 48-well tissue culture plates

Irradiated (25 Gy) spleen cells and thymocytes, syngeneic with the lymph-node donor

---

METHOD

1 Mix 2×10^7 washed BW-5147 cells in serum-free medium with 1×10^8 washed stimulated murine lymphocytes in a 50-ml conical tube and centrifuge (150 g for 15 min at room temperature).

2 Carefully remove the supernatant by aspiration and tap the tube to resuspend the cells.

3 Place the tube in a water bath at 37°C and add 1 ml of a 1 : 1 mix of PEG-1500 in serum-free medium; add dropwise over 45 s.

4 Allow the tube to stand for 45 s and then over 5 min add 50 ml of serum-free medium prewarmed to 37°C with gentle mixing.

5 Leave the cell suspension at 37°C for 5 min and then centrifuge to pellet the cells (150 g for 15 min at room temperature).

6 Remove and discard the supernatant before resuspending the cells in serum-free medium. Centrifuge and resuspend in tissue culture medium containing 10% FBS.

7 Dispense in 100 µl aliquots into 96-well microtitre plates.

8 Incubate at 37°C for 24 h, and then add 50 µl of threefold concentrated HAT medium to each well.

9 Every 5 days, remove half of the supernatant and replace with fresh single-strength HAT medium, for at least 3 weeks.

First hybrids will begin to appear after about 10 days and new ones will continue to appear for the next 3 weeks. Growing hybrids should be karyotyped, phenotyped and screened for antigen reactivity as soon as possible. T-cell hybrids tend to be unstable in the expression of their selected function and so positive lines should be cloned by limiting dilution once their hybrid status has been confirmed. Cloning may be facilitated by the addition of 1×10^5 per well irradiated syngeneic spleen cells. Feeder cells also act as antigen-presenting cells if required by an antigen-specific response. The cells should be freshly prepared and irradiated immediately before they are required. Samples of each clone of interest should be cryopreserved after screening, in case of *not only* accidental loss, but also population drift resulting in loss of function.

TECHNICAL NOTES
- Activate T-lymphocytes by:
    (a) priming *in vivo* by injection of antigen in adjuvant subcutaneously at the base of the tail, restimulation *in vitro* and expansion in IL-2-containing medium to achieve the required cell numbers; or
    (b) stimulation with mitogen (PHA or Con A); stimulation *in vitro* followed by expansion in IL-2-containing medium.

    Hybridomas derived from these cell populations would not be expected to show antigen specificity.
- The BW-5417 line should be cultured every 2–3 months in 2×10^5 M 6-thioguanine to maintain sensitivity to aminopterin in HAT.
- Other murine tumour-cell lines such as FS6-14.13 can also be used for fusion to murine T-cells to produce T-cell hybridomas. Human T-lymphocyte hybridomas can be produced using appropriate human T-cell tumour lines, e.g. MOLT-4.
- The activated lymphocyte population may be enriched for T cells by nylon wool column fractionation (Section 6.6.3) under sterile conditions prior to fusion.
- To facilitate phenotypic analysis (Section 6.9.3), it is convenient to use a T-lymphocyte donor that expresses the Thy-1.2 gene product such as C3HeB/Fe and many other strains, in contrast to the Thy-1.1 expressed by the AKR-derived BW-5147 line.

6.9.1 Screening for functional T hybrids

The techniques used to analyse the T hybridomas will depend upon the effector function rescued and whether the cells are antigen-specific. In general, the techniques cited in Section 9.4 may be adapted for use with T-hybrid lines. T-cell hybrids tend to be unstable, often exhibiting very high ploidy numbers immediately after fusion, but rapidly losing chromosomes thereafter. Clones of interest should be cryopreserved and growing clones checked and recloned to maintain their antigen-specific effector function.

6.9.2 Karyotype analysis

MATERIALS AND EQUIPMENT
Actively growing T hybrids
Colchicine (usually supplied as Colcemid) 0.1% w/v solution
Trypsin, 1.0% w/v solution
Potassium chloride, 0.5% solution
Buffered Giemsa stain, freshly made prior to use (see Section 11.7)

1 Transfer about 10^7 actively growing and dividing T-hybridoma cells into a tissue culture grade conical centrifuge tube. Add 0.1 ml of 0.1% colchicine and incubate at 37°C for 2 h. This arrests the cells in mitosis.

2 Centrifuge to pellet the cells and remove the supernatant.

3 Resuspend the cells vigorously, using a vortex mixer, add 10 ml of 0.5% potassium chloride and incubate for 10 min to allow the lymphocytes to swell and burst.

4 Centrifuge to pellet the contents of the tube, remove the supernatant and slowly resuspend the pellet in 1 : 3 solution of glacial acetic acid and methanol to fix the nuclei.

5 Repeat the centrifugation and fixing twice and finally resuspend the pellet in about 10 drops of fixative.

6 Wash a clean microscope slide with a few drops of fixative and wipe dry with a clean tissue to completely degrease.

7 Breathe onto the slide to warm and moisten it. Using a Pasteur pipette deposit a single drop of the cell suspension onto the slide from a height of 15–30 cm. Tilt the slide to drain the fixative away and allow the slide to dry.

This procedure ruptures the nuclei and allows the chromosomes to spread. It requires a certain amount of practice to achieve good separation of the chromosomes.

8 Dip the slide in the trypsin for 20 s and wash with tap water.

9 Stain with buffered Giemsa (Section 11.7).

10 Wash with tap water.

11 Observe under a transmitted light microscope: at × 40 magnification to select a suitable nuclear spread, and then to × 100 magnification for counting.

6.9.3 Phenotypic analysis

Karyotypic analysis (Section 6.9.2) provides the definitive demonstration of hybrid status, but in the initial stages it is convenient to select on the basis of a hybrid cell-surface phenotype. Most strains of mice express the Thy-1.2 gene product, whereas AKR mice, from which the tumour-cell line BW-5147 was derived, express Thy-1.1. Thus hybrids are HAT resistant, express the Thy-1.2 antigen and sometimes coexpress Thy-1.1. Lines selected after HAT treatment which express only Thy-1.1 should be discarded as they are probably HAT-resistant revertants of the tumour-cell line.

MATERIALS AND EQUIPMENT

Anti-Thy-1.1 and anti-Thy-1.2 monoclonal antibodies (for direct or indirect immunofluorescent staining; Section 4.2.5)

Phosphate-buffered saline (PBS) containing 2% fetal bovine serum (FBS)

UV microscope or continuous-flow cytofluorimeter

METHOD

1 Wash 6×10^6 of the hybrids by centrifugation and divide into 3 aliquots.

2 Process for direct or indirect immunofluorescence using anti-Thy-1.1, anti-Thy-1.2 and irrelevant (control) antibodies (Section 8.2.1).

3 Examine by fluorescence microscopy or by flow cytometry (Section 8.5).

6.10 **Further reading**

Davis, J.M. (1995) *Basic Cell Culture Techniques: A Practical Approach.* Oxford University Press, Oxford.

Fisher, D., Francis, G.E. & Rickwood, D. (eds) (1998) *Cell Separation: A Practical Approach.* Oxford University Press, Oxford.

Fitch, F.W. & Gajewski, T.F. (1997) Production of T cell clones. *Current Protocols in Immunology,* Supp. 24: 3.13. John Wiley & Sons, New York.

Gajewski, T.F., Schell, S.R., Nau, G. & Fitch, F.W. (1989) Regulation of T cell activation: Differentiation amongst T cell subsets. *Immunol Rev* **111**, 79–110.

Graziani-Bowering, G.M., Graham, J.M. & Filion, L. (1997) A quick, easy and inexpensive method for the isolation of human peripheral blood monocytes. *J Immunol Meth* **207**(2), 157–168.

Herzenberg, L.A., Weir, D.M., Herzenberg, L.A. & Blackwell, C. (eds) (1997) *Weir's Handbook of Experimental Immunology,* 5th edn. Blackwell Science, Oxford.

Kjeldsen, L., Sengelov, H. & Borregaard, N. (1999) Subcellular fractionation of human neutrophils on Percoll density gradients. *J Immunol Meth* **232**(1–2), 131–143.

Kompala, D.S. & Todd, P. (eds) (1999) *Cell Separation Science and Technology.* Oxford University Press, Oxford.

Mutch, D. & Westwood, O.M.R. (2001) In: *Epitope Mapping—A Practical Approach* (eds O.M.R. Westwood & F.C. Hay). Oxford University Press, Oxford.

Partington, K.M., Jenkinson, E.J. & Anderson, G. (1999) A novel method of cell separation based on dual parameter immunomagnetic cell selection. *J Immunol Meth* **223**(2), 195–205.

Pelegri, C., Rodriguez-Palmero, M., Morante, M.P., Comas, J., Castell, M. & Franch, A. (1995) Comparison of four lymphocyte isolation methods applied to rodent T cell subpopulations and B cells. *J Immunol Meth* **187**(2), 265–271.

Robinson, J.P., Darzynkiewicz, Z, Tanke, P. *et al.* (eds) (1997) *Current Protocols in Cytometry.* John Wiley & Sons, New York.

Rubbi, C.P., Patel, D. & Rickwood, D. (1993) Evidence of surface antigen detachment during incubation of cells with immunomagnetic beads. *J Immunol Meth* **166**, 233–241.

Todd, D., Singh, A.J., Greiner, D.L., Mordes, J.P., Rossini, A.A. & Bortell, R. (1999) A new isolation method for rat intraepithelial lymphocytes. *J Immunol Meth* **224**(1–2), 111–127.

Westwood, O. & Hay, F. (eds) (2001) *Epitope Mapping—A Practical Approach.* Oxford University Press, Oxford.

7 Phagocytosis, complement and antibody-dependent cytotoxicity

7.1 **Phagocytosis**

This process of binding and ingesting particles is a key part of the immune response. In the 19th century Metchnikoff originally demonstrated the phenomenon, at the macro level, by introducing a splinter into the body of a starfish larva.

7.1.1 *In vivo* phagocytosis

Microorganisms, or their experimental equivalent of carbon, iron or latex particles, are readily engulfed by circulating and tissue-fixed phagocytes. The cells of the reticuloendothelial system are capable of ingesting and degrading foreign material by means of intracellular enzymes in phagosomes, i.e. neutrophils (polymorphonuclear leucocytes), monocytes, histiocytes or tissue macrophages (microglia—brain, Kupffer cells—liver, glomerular mesangial cells—kidney, synovial macrophages—joints, etc.) and vascular endothelial cells.

Reticuloendothelial cell clearance can be monitored *in vivo* using colloidal carbon particles or microorganisms. Following the intravenous injection of colloidal carbon the clearance is determined by the light transmission through lysed blood samples. Similarly the clearance of microorganisms can be estimated by culturing blood samples taken at time intervals following intravenous injection.

7.1.2 *In vitro* phagocytosis

Phagocytosis is a two-stage process in which particles are first bound to the cell surface and then ingested. *In vitro* it is important to distinguish these two processes.

7.1.3 Microscopical determination of phagocytosis of yeasts

Yeasts bind to lectin-like receptors on the surface of phagocytic cells principally through the mannose receptor, this binding being blockable with α-mannans. Moreover yeasts are also potent activators of the alternative complement pathway and, following exposure to fresh serum, bind to CR1 and CR3 receptors for C3b and C3bi deposited on the yeast surface, this binding not being blockable with α-mannans.

However, some of the problem with using yeasts to measure phagocytosis is determining whether the organisms have been internalized or are simply binding to the surface. With fresh yeast this is difficult but autoclaved yeasts exhibit staining properties which allow the differentiation of ingested particles (Giamis *et al.* 1992). Autoclaved yeasts stain light pink with May–Grünwald/Giemsa unless pretreated with tannic acid, when they stain deep violet. Tannic acid is unable to reach cell-ingested yeasts, therefore they stain light pink, whereas surface-bound particles stain violet.

Preparation of phagocytic cells

Mouse macrophages can be obtained simply by washing out the peritoneal cavity but they will be contaminated with about 50% lymphocytes. This is not usually a problem as most methods for studying phagocytosis involve allowing the cells to adhere to glass or plastic surfaces and this considerably enriches the preparation. Larger numbers of macrophages may be elicited by producing a local inflammatory response, e.g. with starch, sodium trioleat, paraffin oil, but these cells (see Section 6.1) will be stimulated and may contain engulfed particles.

Human monocytes and neutrophils

Neutrophils and monocytes may be prepared from anticoagulant-treated whole blood by dextran sedimentation followed by density gradient sedimentation on Percoll A.

Dextran sedimentation

MATERIALS
Blood—heparin treated
3.5% w/v T-250 dextran in 0.14 M saline
Centrifuge tube

METHOD

1　Layer 5 ml blood on 10 ml dextran and incubate for 1 h at 37°C.
2　Remove and retain leucocyte-rich supernatant and wash by centrifugation.

Percoll A density gradient centrifugation

MATERIALS
Leucocytes (from dextran sedimentation, above)
Centrifuge tube
Percoll A, 60% and 80% solutions in tissue culture medium

1   Add 5 ml of 80% Percoll to centrifuge tube.
2   Layer on 5 ml 60% Percoll.
3   Place 5 ml cell suspension on top of gradient.
4   Centrifuge at 240 g for 30 min at 4°C.
5   Collect monocytes from the medium–60% Percoll interface.
6   Collect neutrophils from the 60–80% Percoll interface.

TECHNICAL NOTE

The monocytes will be contaminated with lymphocytes but can be enriched by adherence to a glass or plastic surface for 30 min at 37°C. The non-adherent lymphocytes (about 50% of the total population) may then be washed away.

Phagocytic assay

MATERIALS AND EQUIPMENT

Macrophages—prepared as above in RPMI 1640 medium

Yeast—*Saccharomyces cerevisiae*

YPD (yeast culture medium available from Sigma, UK)

Water bath sonicator

Autoclave

Calcium- and magnesium-free phosphate-buffered saline (PBS)

RPMI 1640 medium (no fetal bovine serum (FBS) or antibiotics)

Glass coverslips 14 mm diameter

24-well multiwell plates

May–Grünwald and Giemsa stains

Giemsa buffer

Light microscope

1% w/v tannic acid

Heat-inactivated FBS

A Preparation of yeast

1   Culture yeast in YPD for 48 h at 30°C.
2   Autoclave at 120°C for 45 min in culture medium.
3   Wash three times in calcium- and magnesium-free PBS.
4   Aliquot and store at 4°C.
5   Just before use, sonicate gently in a water bath to disrupt clumps and dilute to 10^8/ml in RPMI 1640 medium without FBS and antibiotics.

B Assay

1   Place a sterile glass coverslip in each well of a multiwell plate.
2   Add 1 ml of macrophage/monocyte suspension, at 10^5/ml, to each well.

Continued on p. 206

3 Incubate at 37°C for 2 h.

4 Remove culture medium and wash with medium.

5 Add 1 ml medium to each well and incubate for 2 h at 37°C.

6 Add 100 μl yeast suspension (10^8 particles/ml).

7 Incubate for 1 h at 37°C in a 5% CO_2 humidified incubator.

8 Wash twice gently with culture medium.

9 Add 1 ml 1% w/v tannic acid solution.

10 Leave 1 min.

11 Wash with medium.

12 Cover coverslip with a drop of heat-inactivated FBS.

13 Dry coverslips in air.

14 Stain with May–Grünwald freshly diluted 1 : 2 with buffer, for 5 min.

15 Rinse coverslips in buffer.

16 Stain in Giemsa solution, freshly diluted with buffer, for 15 min.

17 Rinse in buffer.

18 Invert coverslips on microscope slides and observe at × 1000 magnification.

TECHNICAL NOTES

- Surface-bound yeasts stain deep violet while intracellular particles are light pink.
- Phagocytosis may be stimulated or inhibited by adding reagents 15 min prior to adding the yeast particles, e.g. a 10 mg/ml solution of α-mannans will almost completely inhibit binding to the macrophages.

7.1.4 Flow cytometric and plate fluorometric phagocytic techniques

Counting ingested particles is a reliable way of measuring phagocytosis but laborious for large numbers of samples. Alternatively, fluorescein-labelled *Escherichia coli* and *Saccharomyces cerevisiae* are available commercially and monitor uptake of these particles in the flow cytometer or in 96-well microplates using a microplate fluorescence reader. Please note: It is necessary to distinguish ingested from cell-bound particles but this may be accomplished by quenching the fluorescence of the external particles with the addition of Trypan blue (Buschmann & Winter 1989; Wan *et al.* 1993).

7.2 Neutrophil function tests

In vitro assays are available for many of the key neutrophil activities, e.g. chemotaxis, phagocytosis and microbicidal activity. However the precise relationship between the parameter being measured and its *in vivo* expression is not always clear. The nitroblue tetrazolium reduction assay described below can be used to measure both phagocytosis (this is the only way in which the dye enters the cell) and one of the metabolic pathways responsible for microbial killing (hexose monophosphate shunt activation).

7.2.1 Nitroblue tetrazolium (NBT) test

Addition of the yellow NBT dye to plasma results in the formation of a NBT–heparin or NBT–fibrinogen complex, which may be phagocytosed by neutrophils. Normal neutrophils show little incorporation of the complex unless they are 'stimulated' to phagocytic activity, e.g. by the addition of endotoxin.

This technique may be used to measure the degree of 'stimulation' of untreated cells or their capacity for phagocytosis after stimulation.

Stimulated neutrophils incorporate the dye complex into phagosomes and, after lysosomal fusion, intracellular reduction results in the formation of blue insoluble crystals of formazan. The percentage of phagocytic cells may be determined using a light microscope or, as described below, the total dye reduction may be quantified spectrophotometrically after dioxan extraction.

MATERIALS AND EQUIPMENT

Sample of fresh venous blood in heparin (20 IU/ml)

Distilled water

Phosphate-buffered saline (PBS)

Escherichia coli endotoxin (1 mg/ml in PBS)

4 mM nitroblue tetrazolium (NBT) dye in PBS containing 340 mM sucrose

Dioxan

0.1 M HCl

Nylon wool, 100 mg in siliconized Pasteur pipette

Water bath at 70°C

Spectrophotometer

METHOD

1 Obtain blood sample in heparin (20 IU/ml) by venepuncture. Use a sample for total and differential leucocyte counts (see Figs 7.1 & 7.2). The NBT reduction activity of the sample must be determined within 60 min of venesection.

2 Add 15 μl of endotoxin solution (1 mg/ml in PBS, initial concentration) to 1.5 ml of blood and incubate at 37°C for 10 min.

3 Add 0.1 ml of freshly prepared NBT dye solution and mix gently.

4 After 20 min at 37°C, add blood dropwise to a nylon wool column.

5 Once the sample has entered the column wash twice with 2 ml of PBS and then 2 ml of distilled water. The distilled water will lyse any residual erythrocytes.

6 Add 2 drops of HCl to the column, to stop further reduction of the intracellular dye, and wash with 2 ml of distilled water.

7 Remove the nylon wool with forceps and place in 5 ml dioxan (in a glass container).

8 Incubate at 70°C with occasional vigorous shaking until the nylon wool returns to its original white colour (about 20 min).

9 Centrifuge the dioxan extract to remove any precipitate or nylon fibres (1000 *g* for 10 min at room temperature).

10 Measure the extinction at 520 nm using a spectrophotometer (use a dioxan standard).

The unstimulated control value is obtained by a parallel incubation of untreated blood, i.e. add 15 μl PBS alone at step 2, then assay as steps 3–10.

(a) (b)

(c) (d)

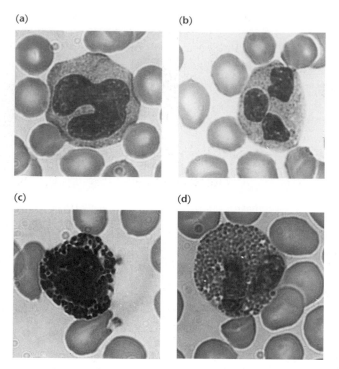

Fig. 7.1 **Light microscopy of non-lymphoid blood leucocytes.** Monocytes are the largest of the blood leucocytes and, in viable cell preparations, are not easily distinguished from cells of the lymphoid lineage. Granulocytes are classified according to the staining reaction of their granules in response to histological dyes, e.g. May–Grünwald/Giemsa staining. (**a**) Monocytes have a C-shaped nucleus and grey cytoplasm with a few azurophilic granules on May–Grünwald/Giemsa staining. They are the largest of the blood leucocytes and, on entering the tissues, differentiate into macrophages. (**b**) Neutrophils are polymorphonuclear cells with neutrophilic cytoplasm. Older cells have a more segmented nucleus and, in general, it is difficult to discern their cytoplasmic granules (except during infection—so-called toxic granulation). These cells account for about 90% of circulating granulocytes; they are about 15 μm in diameter and highly phagocytic. (**c**) There are very small numbers of basophils in circulation (< 1.0% of blood granulocytes). The characteristic deep blue granules obscure the nucleus and contain histamine—very important in type I anaphylactic-type hypersensitivity reactions. (**d**) The bilobed nucleus shown in the photograph is typical of a human eosinophil; the bright red granules make identification easy. These cells make up about 2–5% of blood leucocytes, but their frequency increases greatly in parasitic infections and allergic reactions. Typically these cells kill invading organisms by secretion of toxic cationic granules (exocytosis) rather than phagocytosis. Lymphocytes circulate for months, or even years; granulocytes circulate in the blood for about 7 h and thereafter are around in the tissues for only a few days.

TECHNICAL NOTES

- All glassware must be siliconized to prevent adherence of phagocytes.
- Both neutrophils and monocytes ingest NBT by phagocytosis.
- The conversion factor for the calculation of moles of formazan from extinction coefficient must be calculated for a sample of each batch of dye, after chemical reduction, as below.

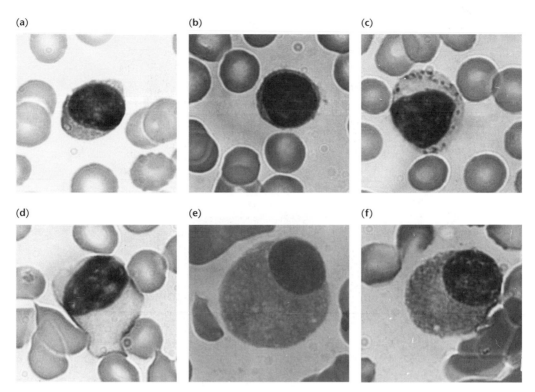

(a)

(b)

(c)

(d)

(e)

(f)

Fig. 7.2 **Morphology of lymphoid cells under the light microscope.** (a) and (b) show the morphology of typical small lymphocytes. The cells have a diameter of about 10 μm and are characterized by a large nucleus : cytoplasm ratio—typical of G0 or 'resting' cells. In May–Grünwald/Giemsa staining, the cells have a deeply staining nucleus, condensed chromatin and a thin rim of blue cytoplasm. (c) Large granular lymphocyte. Cells with this morphology have been associated with the majority of natural killer, lymphokine-activated killer and antibody-dependent cell-mediated cytotoxicity activity due to peripheral blood mononuclear cells. Their azurophilic granules contain perforins, which become integrated into the membrane of target cells during cytotoxic killing. These cells have a characteristic density which facilitates their purification from other lymphoid cells by density gradient centrifugation. (d) Reactive lymphocyte from a patient with infectious mononucleosis or glandular fever. Viable cell phenotyping of this cell would have shown it to be a T lymphocyte, in this case reacting to Epstein–Barr virus infection of B lymphocytes. The cell has extensive blue cytoplasm and an 'open' chromatin structure, as evidenced by the apparent holes in the nucleus shown in the photograph. T lymphocytes stimulated *in vitro* with an antigen or phytomitogen have a similar morphology and the same close 'wrapping' around the exterior of adjacent erythrocytes. (e) and (f) Plasma cells showing the typical characteristics of: large cytoplasm containing an eccentric nucleus with a 'cartwheel' chromatin structure; deep blue cytoplasm rich in RNA; and a lucid zone near the nucleus, corresponding to the Golgi apparatus. The cytoplasm is frequently vacuolated, presumably due to intracellular antibodies about to be secreted.

7.2.2 Determination of conversion factor

MATERIALS AND EQUIPMENT

Ascorbic acid

4 mM nitroblue tetrazolium (NBT) in distilled water containing 340 mM sucrose

0.1 M sodium hydroxide containing 24 mM sodium bicarbonate

Distilled water

Dioxan

Waterbath at 70°C

Spectrophotometer

METHOD

1 Add 150 µmol ascorbic acid to 0.2 ml of NBT solution and mix.

2 Add 2 ml of 0.1 M sodium hydroxide containing 24 mM sodium bicarbonate.

3 Incubate for 10 min at room temperature and add 5 ml distilled water.

4 Centrifuge at 1000 g for 15 min at room temperature.

5 Wash once in water by centrifugation (1000 g for 15 min at room temperature). Remove the supernatant and resuspend the blue insoluble formazan precipitate in 10 ml dioxan.

6 Dilute 1 ml of the suspension with 9 ml dioxan and incubate at 70°C for 20 min.

7 Cool to room temperature, and measure the extinction at 520 nm using a spectrophotometer (use a dioxan blank).

8 Calculate the conversion factor from the extinction value. As a rough guide, the conversion factor should be approximately 1 extinction unit ($E_{520\ nm}$) = 40 nmol of formazan.

7.2.3 Calculation of NBT uptake by phagocytes

1 Using the conversion factor determined above, determine the number of moles of formazan extracted from the untreated and endotoxin-stimulated blood.

2 Calculate the number of potential phagocytes used per assay (the percentage of the absolute count due to neutrophils and monocytes).

3 Express results as moles of formazan per phagocyte. Normal range: untreated blood, 0.92–3.62 fmol/phagocyte; endotoxin-stimulated blood, 2.52–4.90 fmol/phagocyte.

7.2.4 Neutrophil chemotaxis

The assay for neutrophil chemotaxis is a good guide to neutrophil function and is discussed in Section 10.9.

7.2.5 Continuous-flow cytometry for phagocytosis

A fluorescent dye is used which allows the use of the flow cytometer to carry out the measurements. 2′7′-dichlorofluorescein diacetate was the first dye to be used for this purpose (Bass *et al.* 1983; Vuorte *et al.* 1996) and gives a green fluorescent product on oxidation following the oxidative burst within the neutrophils.

2'7'-dichlorofluorescein diacetate (DCF-DA) 20 mM in ethanol; store below 0°C in the dark

Heparinized whole blood

Dulbecco's phosphate-buffered saline (PBS) (calcium- and magnesium-free), containing 5 mM glucose, 1% gelatin, 5 mM sodium azide and DCF-DA at 250 mM final concentration

EDTA

350 ng/ml phorbol myristic acetate (PMA) in ethanol

METHOD

1. Dilute 100 μl heparinized whole blood or cell suspension with Dulbecco's PBS containing DCF-DA.
2. Mix for 20 min at 37°C in a shaking water bath.
3. Add 0.5 ml EDTA and 350 ng/ml phorbol myristate acetate (PMA) in ethanol.
4. Treat with ice-cold distilled water for 20 s.
5. Centrifuge and resuspend in PBS–gelatin–glucose without DCF-DA.
6. Examine by flow cytometry.

TECHNICAL NOTES

- Azide inhibits enzymatic decomposition of H_2O_2 by cellular catalase and myeloperoxidase and does not impair H_2O_2 production.
- Ethanol depresses DCF fluorescence and so should be kept to a minimum concentration.
- Neutrophils produce between 50 and 70 nmol of superoxide/min 10^7 neutrophils in response to PMA.
- Other fluorescent indicators such as dihydrorhodamine 123 and hydroethidine have also proved useful.

7.3 Antibody-dependent cell-mediated cytotoxicity

In antibody-dependent cell-mediated cytotoxicity (ADCC) target cells coated with very small amounts of antibody are killed by non-immune effector cells. The effector cells (K cells) have receptors for the Fc regions of the antibody and appear to recognize immune complexes specifically. The exact killing mechanisms are unknown, but involve cell to cell contact and, in some of the effector cell types, may result from the release of lysosomal enzymes. With erythrocyte targets the effector cells tend to be of the granulocyte–macrophage lineage; but with tumour target cells, cells of the lymphocyte lineage predominate.

There is evidence to suggest a large overlap between the progenitors of ADCC effector cells and those of lymphokine-activated killer (LAK) cells. Some of these progenitors also show natural killer (NK) cell activity; the overlap is almost certainly confined to cells of lymphoid lineage in this case. It is possible to distinguish between the NK and LAK non-specific (non-antigen-specific) cytotoxic cells by the use of NK-resistant or -susceptible target cells. ADCC effector cells may be detected by their antibody dependence.

MATERIALS
Mouse

Chicken (has nucleated red blood cells)

Rabbit anti-chicken erythrocyte serum (diluted 1 : 6000 in tissue culture medium plus 10% fetal bovine serum)

Tissue culture medium

Fetal bovine serum (FBS)

Sodium ^{51}chromate ($^{51}CrO_4$)

Sheep erythrocytes (SRBC)

Eagle's minimum essential medium (MEM) containing 1% v/v FBS

5% CO_2 in air

7.3.1 Target cells

METHOD

1 Take 0.2 ml of blood from the chicken into a heparinized syringe. The main wing vein is a convenient site for venepuncture to obtain small volumes of blood.
2 Dilute 0.1 ml of blood with 1.9 ml of Eagle's MEM containing 10% FBS.
3 Use 0.1 ml of diluted blood and add 0.1 ml of sodium $^{51}CrO_4$.
4 Gas with 5% CO_2 in air.
5 Incubate at 37°C for 1 h.
6 Wash four times with medium containing 5% FBS. Centrifuge at 90 g for 7 min at 4°C.
7 Wash SRBC in tissue culture medium four times by centrifugation (450 g for 10 min).
8 Adjust SRBC concentration to 10^7/ml.
9 Add 10^5 labelled chicken red cells to each ml of sheep red cells.

TECHNICAL NOTE

The radioisotope ^{51}Cr has a half-life of around 28 days and is a γ emitter. The recommended safety guidelines for handling isotopes must be adhered to when using this Protocol. Refer to the following websites for comprehensive details on radioisotope health and safety procedures as well as useful information regarding detection and half-life:

http://www.practicingsafescience.org

http://www.hse.gov.uk

7.3.2 Effector cells

METHOD

1 Remove the spleen from the mouse and prepare a single-cell suspension.
2 Adjust to 2.5×10^6 leucocytes/ml.

7.3.3 Cytotoxic assay

1   Set up culture tubes according to the Protocol below.

Protocol.

Tube (in triplicate)	Spleen cells (µl)	Antibody (µl)	^{51}Cr-labelled chicken red cells (µl)
A	100	100	100
B	100	0	100
C	0	100	100
D	0	0	100
E	100 µl distilled water	100 µl distilled water	100

2   Cap the tubes and incubate, leaning at an angle of 30–45 degrees, in a gassed CO_2 incubator or a desiccator (5% in air) for 18 h.

3   Add 1 ml medium to each tube and then spin (90 g) for 10 min.

4   Remove 0.8 ml supernatant from each tube and assess this for ^{51}Cr release in a γ spectrometer.

TECHNICAL NOTES

- Tube A shows the ^{51}Cr release due to spleen cells plus antitarget antibody. The other cultures are controls. Tube B gives the amount of release due to spleen cells alone, while C measures the release due to antibody. Spontaneous release of the label by the erythrocytes is monitored by tube D.

- Refer to the following websites for comprehensive details on radioisotope health and safety procedures as well as useful information regarding detection and half-life:
  http://www.practicingsafescience.org
  http://www.hse.gov.uk/hsehome.htm

Calculation

Calculating the amount of cytotoxicity is complicated as there is some difficulty in choosing the correct control value against which to calculate the experimental ^{51}Cr release. The reason for this is that spleen cells, in the absence of antibody, exert a protective effect over the chicken erythrocytes. It will be seen that the ^{51}Cr release in tube B is usually less than the spontaneous release in tube D. Therefore, for the control culture, one may choose either effectors plus target cells (B) or target cells plus antibody (C).

The calculation of percentage cytotoxicity may then be as follows:

$$\% \, ^{51}\text{Cr release} = \frac{A - C}{E - C} \times 100$$

or

$$= \frac{A - B}{E - B} \times 100.$$

Letters in formulae correspond to culture tubes in the Protocol (see p. 213).

TECHNICAL NOTE
The assay for optimum conditions varies according to the ratio of effector to target cells.

7.4 Antibody-dependent cell-mediated cytotoxicity, lymphokine-activated and natural killer cells

In antibody-dependent cell-mediated cytotoxicity (ADCC), the apparent specificity of the killing reaction is superimposed on a non-specific effector cell by its acquisition of, or adsorption to, target cell-specific antibody. In the absence of antibody, a proportion of these non-specific killers can kill target cells directly and are referred to as natural killer (NK) cells. They are able to kill tumour cells without the need for previous immunization or passive antibody, and are greatly increased in numbers in mice carrying the *nu/nu* athymic mutation (where they presumably account for the resistance to spontaneous tumours shown by these T lymphocyte-deficient animals). They are virtually absent in the beige mutant of the C3H mouse.

Treatment of human or murine normal (non-immune) lymphocytes with IL-2 greatly enhances their non-specific killing capacity to many tumour targets. This led to the definition of a third functional class of non-specific cytolytic cells known as lymphokine-activated killer or LAK cells. These cells may have clinical use for antitumour therapy.

At present the lineage of cytolytic cells is confused but their functional classification is clear:

(a) There is a 'common pool' of antigen-specific and non-specific cytolytic effector cells, composed of several cell lineages.

(b) T lymphocytes are the only cytolytic effector cells known to date to have clonally distributed endogenous receptors for specific target-cell antigens.

(c) The so-called large granular lymphocytes, identified by virtue of their morphology (Fig. 7.2c), are able to mediate NK- and LAK-cell activity *in vitro*.

(d) Non-lymphoid cells are able to mediate NK and LAK activity.

(e) LAK and NK cells may be functionally distinguished by the judicious choice of tumour target cells; most tumour targets used to date have been LAK sensitive, but only a few are NK sensitive.

(f) Most primary cultures of freshly excised tumours are NK-resistant but LAK-sensitive, as are hapten-modified normal cells.

7.4.1 Assay of LAK- and NK-cell activity

MATERIALS AND EQUIPMENT
Heparinized, human venous blood
Density gradient, e.g. Lymphoprep™
Tissue culture medium containing 5% fetal bovine serum (FBA)
Recombinant IL-2

T-24 and K-562 cell lines

Sodium $^{51}CrO_4$

U-shaped microculture plates

Plastic tubes (circa 2ml), e.g. LP3

Microplate carrier for centrifugation

Gamma spectrometer

METHOD

1 Isolate peripheral blood mononuclear cells (PBMC) from heparinized venous blood by density gradient centrifugation and wash three times in tissue culture medium by centrifugation (150 g for 10 min at room temperature).

2 Adjust the PBMC to 5×10^6 cells/ml with tissue culture medium containing 5% FBA. For the assay of NK activity, no IL-2 or induction period is required: proceed to step 4.

3 For LAK-cell induction, supplement the PBMC suspension with recombinant IL-2 (500 U/ml) and dispense 100 µl aliquots into a U-shaped microculture tray as follows: allow for at least triplicate cultures at each dilution (see Protocol below), for each donor and each target (NK-resistant and -susceptible, see Technical notes), and leave five wells empty for each of the target cells for the determination of spontaneous isotope release. Culture in a humidified 37°C incubator gassed with 5% CO_2 in air.

   The time for optimum induction of LAK activity will vary with both donor and type of assay for which they are intended. Typically use cultures at 48–72 h after induction; however, LAK cells are still detectable at 7 days. It is conceivable that the early and late LAK activity might be due to varying proportions of the different cell types known to mediate this effector function.

4 Label the T-24 and K-562 target cells with $^{51}CrO_4$ by mixing 37×10^5 Bq of isotope with 10^6 T-24 or K-562 targets and incubate in a 37°C water bath for 1.5 h, mixing every 30 min.

5 Wash the target cells three times by centrifugation, resuspend and count cells using a haemocytometer. Retain an aliquot of labelled cells for freeze–thaw determination of maximum isotope release.

   For accurate determination of LAK activity it is necessary to determine isotope release over a range of different effector : target-cell ratios.

6 Prepare a series of target-cell suspensions according to the Protocol; add l00 µl of each to separate assay wells.

7 Add l00 µl of the highest target suspension to each of the five empty wells allowed for the determination of spontaneous release and supplement with l00 µl of tissue culture medium.

8 Centrifuge the plate at 50 g for 15 min at room temperature in a microplate carrier.

Protocol.

	Assay number			
	1	2	3	4
PBMC at 5×10^6/ml	100 µl ————————————————————→			
Target cells/ml (use 100 µl per culture)	3×10^7	6×10^7	12.5×10^7	25×10^7
Effector : target-cell ratio	6 : 1	12 : 1	25 : 1	50 : 1

Continued on p. 216

9 Incubate for 4 h at 37°C in a humidified incubator gassed with 5% CO_2 in air.

10 Remove 100 µl of supernatant into separate LP3 tubes, cap and count in a γ spectrometer.

11 Calculate specific lysis of each experimental well as follows:

$$\% \text{ specific lysis} = \frac{\text{experimental c.p.m.} - \text{spontaneous c.p.m.}}{\text{maximum c.p.m.} - \text{spontaneous c.p.m.}} \times 100$$

12 Determine the mean ± standard error of each set of replicates and display each donor's titration curve graphically for ease of comparison.

TECHNICAL NOTES

- LAK and NK effector functions are distinguished by differential killing of the two target cells used in the assay. T-24 cells are relatively NK-resistant, whereas K-562 cells are both NK- and LAK-susceptible. LAK activity varies widely between normal donors, between 30 and 100% specific lysis.
- As a guide, the maximum release from 10^4 target cells should be about 10 000 c.p.m. and the spontaneous release < 10% at 4 h. High spontaneous release is often due to the batch of FBS used as a tissue culture supplement; batches should be screened before purchase. FBA and autologous human serum give comparable results.
- It is also possible to generate LAK cells in bulk by culturing in flasks.
- The relatively high concentration of IL-2 used to generate these cells excludes the use of cell supernatants, e.g. from MLA 144, as an IL-2 source.
- Over a short induction period, < 48 h, LAK activity is resistant to hydroxyurea, cyclosporin and steroid treatment. However, when longer induction periods are used, up to 7 days, there is a decrease in the rate of LAK induction, suggesting that the cells participating in the early expression of LAK activity might be different to those involved at later time points.
- This assay may be adapted for using the non-radioisotope technique of time-resolved fluorescence as an alternative to using ^{51}Cr.

7.5 **Total haemolytic complement**

Lysis of antibody-coated erythrocytes has long been used as a means of estimating the complement activity of a serum. As complement is added to antibody-coated erythrocytes an increasing proportion of the cells are lysed as shown in Fig. 7.3. As the curve approaches 100% lysis asymptotically, it is difficult to determine the total lytic unit of complement (CH_{100}) and so one normally defines the 50% lysis point (CH_{50}). The von Krogh equation for the sigmoid dose–response curve of complement-mediated cytolysis was derived empirically and, in its basic form, may be written as:

$$x = k \left\{ \frac{y}{100 - y} \right\}^{1/n}$$

where x is amount of complement (ml of undiluted serum), y is proportion of cells lysed, k is 50% unit of complement and n is a constant.

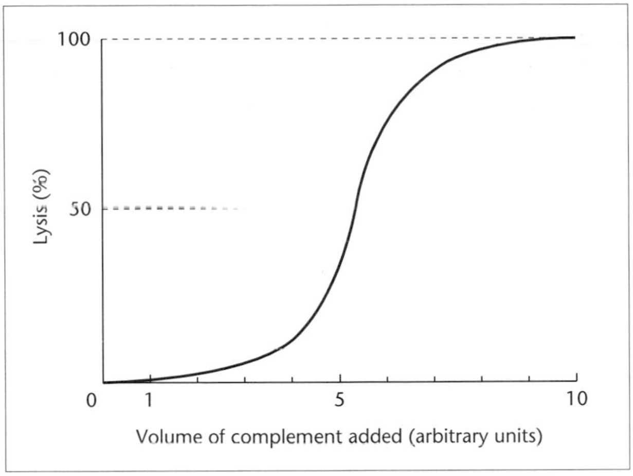

Fig. 7.3 Lysis of sheep erythrocytes (SRBC), sensitized by horse anti-SRBC, in the presence of human complement. The curve of complement-mediated lysis approaches the 100% lysis value asymptotically and so accurate determinations of serum complement levels are made on the 50% lysis point as shown in the graph.

The CH_{50} unit is determined under standardized conditions which depend upon:

(a) erythrocyte and antibody concentration;

(b) buffering conditions of the medium; and

(c) temperature.

Hence, the definition of the CH_{50} unit is arbitrary and depends on the conditions used. The assay may be performed in tubes without reference to a standard, or in agar with reference to a standard serum.

7.5.1 Standardization of erythrocytes

MATERIALS AND EQUIPMENT

Barbitone-buffered saline for complement tests (this contains essential calcium and magnesium ions)

Sheep erythrocytes (SRBC) in Alsever's solution

0.04% ammonia solution

Serum: this should be either fresh, or guinea-pig serum preserved specially for complement fixation assays

Horse haemolytic serum (source of anti-erythrocyte antibody)

Spectrophotometer

METHOD

1   Dilute the barbitone-buffered saline to working strength. Check for fungal or bacterial contamination, as these are anticomplementary.

2   Wash 4 ml of the erythrocyte suspension (supplied at ≈ 25% v/v in Alsever's solution) three times in barbitone-buffered saline (200 *g* for 3 min).

3   Resuspend the washed erythrocytes in 15 ml of barbitone-buffered saline (use a measuring cylinder).

4   Mix 1 ml of erythrocytes with 25 ml of ammonia solution to lyse the cells and read the absorbance at 541 nm. For a 6% SRBC suspension, in a 1-cm cuvette, the absorbance should be 0.48–0.50. Adjust the suspension as required.

Continued on p. 218

5 Mix 15 ml barbitone-buffered saline, 0.1 ml of horse haemolytic serum and 15 ml of 6% SRBC. Strictly, the anti-erythrocyte serum should be titred until the highest dilution still giving full complement fixation is reached; however, for most purposes it is sufficient to use a 1 : 150 dilution.

6 Incubate at 37°C for 15 min.

This method is for the preparation of 30 ml of 3% v/v sheep erythrocytes. Use the sensitized cells within 24 h.

7.5.2 Estimation of CH_{50} tube assay

METHOD

1 Set up the tubes as in the Protocol and remember to use fresh or specially preserved serum as the complement source.

2 Incubate at 37°C for 60 min.

3 Place the tubes on ice and add 2 ml of buffer to each tube.

4 Centrifuge at 200 g for 10 min at 4°C.

5 Remove a sample of each supernatant (tubes 1–7) and read their absorbance at 541 nm.

Protocol.

	Tube numbers						
	1	2	3	4	5	6	7
Buffer (ml)	1.10	1.05	1.00	0.90	0.80	1.20	1.20 ml ammonia solution
Guinea-pig serum (ml) initial dil. 1 : 30	0.10	0.15	0.20	0.30	0.40	0.00	
Sensitized erythrocytes (ml) suspension	0.3———————————————————→						

Calculation of results

1 Assuming that tube 7 represents total lysis, calculate the percentage lysis for each tube.

2 Plot the percentage lysis against the complement concentration (ml of undiluted serum). This will yield a sigmoid curve as in Fig. 7.3.

This dose–response curve follows the von Krogh equation given earlier. However, this equation may be logarithmically transformed so that the data fall on a straight line:

$$\log x = \log k + 1/n \log \frac{y}{100y}$$

where terms are defined as previously.

3 Plot log x against $\log[y/(100 - y)]$ for each dilution of complement used. The straight line has a slope of 1/n (the exact value depends on experimental conditions, but it should be within 20% of 0.2). The abscissa intercept of the line, where $\log[y/(100 - y)] = 0$, is the log dilution

resulting in 50% lysis. The complement level of a serum is normally expressed as the number of CH_{50} units/ml of serum.

TECHNICAL NOTES

- Complement components are highly labile and so fresh serum must be prepared by clotting the blood at 4°C. Preserved guinea-pig serum is available commercially, in which the complement components are stabilized by lyophilization of serum in a hypertonic salt solution.
- The whole assay may be made more sensitive, and use less reagents, if the red cells are radio-labelled with ^{51}Cr for the radioisotopic variant of this assay.
- Instead of erythrocytes, algal cells from *Euglena gracilis* (Stefanski & Ruppel 1991) or fluorescently labelled liposomes (Masaki *et al.* 1989) may be used to increase sensitivity and reproducibility.
- The assay may be modified for use on microlitre plates.

7.5.3 Estimation of CH_{100} by assay in agar

This simple assay, which is analogous to single radial immunodiffusion, may be used on a routine basis with reference to a standard serum. Antibody-sensitized red cells are incorporated into molten agarose and the mixture allowed to set. Wells are cut in the agarose and filled with either the sera under test or dilutions of a standard serum. The complement diffuses into the agarose and reacts with and binds to the antibody-coated red cells. Circles of lysis appear, the size of which depend upon the complement content of the serum.

MATERIALS AND EQUIPMENT

All reagents should be made up in barbitone buffer for complement fixation
Sensitized red cells (made up to 10% v/v)
Agarose, 2% w/v in barbitone buffer
Glass plates (microscope slides are suitable for a small number of estimations)
Gel cutter

METHOD

1 Warm 1.5 ml of the barbitone buffer to 56°C in a water bath.
2 Cool 1.2 ml of molten 2% agarose to 56°C and add to the barbitone buffer.
3 Mix and cool to 45°C in a water bath.
4 Add 0.2 ml of sensitized red-cell suspension and mix gently.
5 Place the glass plate on a level surface; use a spirit level to check.
6 Pour the mixture quickly onto the plate to form a smooth, even surface.
7 When set, place the plate in a box containing moist filter paper and chill to 4°C for a few minutes to harden the agarose.
8 Cut two rows of five wells, approximately 3 mm across using an Ouchterlony gel cutter and remove the agarose plugs with a Pasteur pipette attached to a Venturi pump.
9 Dispense 8 μl samples of the sera under test into separate wells. Similarly, add four doubling dilutions of a standard serum to a series of wells. (For accurate research studies, a larger plate can be used to permit replicate determinations.)
10 Incubate the plate in a moist box overnight at 4°C.

Continued on p. 220

11 Warm the plate, still in the box, to 37°C for 2 h, to allow cell lysis to occur.

12 Measure two diameters at right angles across each well and calculate their mean.

13 Plot the value of the areas (πr^2) of the standard serum dilutions (linear scale) against the log dilution. Determine the concentration of the unknown sera as a percentage of the standard by extrapolation from the standard curve.

TECHNICAL NOTE

This technique is eminently suitable for detecting complement deficiencies both in total and in individual components of complement. Qualitative assay reagents may be prepared in which just one component is missing from the lytic pathway of complement. These reagents are incorporated in agarose and will only lyse the indicator erythrocytes if the missing component is present in the test serum added to the well.

7.6 Detection of antibody or antigen by complement fixation

An antibody, antigen or antigen–antibody complex may be detected by estimating either complement consumption or fixation. Amplifying cascade sequence of complement means a small amount of antigen–antibody complex will cause massive complement fixation or consumption (depending upon whether you assay the complex or the supernatant for complement components). Thus complement fixation reaction is a very sensitive technique for measuring small amounts (< 1 μg) of antigen or antibody.

The disadvantage is that it detects only certain antibody classes. In the human, IgG_1, IgG_2 (weakly), IgG_3 and IgM activate the classical pathway, whereas IgG_4, IgA and IgE cannot. There may, however, be some activation by these three latter classes via the alternative pathway.

In many instances complement fixation has been replaced by other techniques, such as ELISA and radioimmunoassay (see Chapter 5), but it is still used in many microbiological assays. This has the advantage of showing that the reaction measured is capable of activating a biological effector function.

7.6.1 Quantitative complement fixation assay

It is possible to standardize complement activity using antibody-sensitized erythrocytes. If instead of defining the CH_{50} as before, we define the minimum amount of complement required to lyse all of a standard volume of sensitized red cells, i.e. minimum haemolytic dose (MHD), we have an extremely good indicator system for complement consumption tests. In the complement fixation assay a soluble antigen is allowed to react with antibody and so fix complement. When the indicator system of sensitized erythrocytes is added, the degree of lysis observed will be proportional to the amount of complement remaining in the supernatant.

This is widely used in clinical screening procedures, notably in the Wasserman complement fixation test for antitreponemal antibodies in syphilis. The principles of interpretation of this test may be easily appreciated by reference to Fig. 7.4. The assay is made semiquantitative by titrating the test serum to determine the lowest dilution that still gives positive complement fixation.

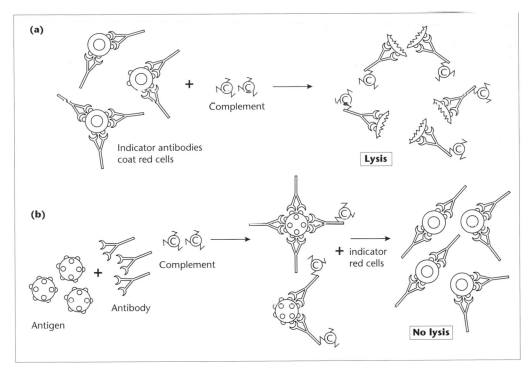

Fig. 7.4 Complement fixation test to detect either antigen or antibody. A detection system of antibody-coated red cells is set up. On the addition of complement the red cells will be lysed (**a**). To test for antibody the mixture of antigen plus test sample is incubated with complement. Indicator antibody-coated red cells are then added to test for free complement. If antibody is present in the test sample, the complement will have been bound by the immune complexes and *no lysis* of red cells will occur. If no antibody is present in the test sample no complexes will be formed and the complement will not be consumed and so will be free to bind to the antibody-coated red cells and lysis will occur (**b**).

MATERIALS AND EQUIPMENT

Human serum albumin (HSA) (1 mg/ml)

Anti-HSA

Sensitized erythrocytes

Barbitone-buffered saline for complement fixation (contains magnesium and calcium ions; use this for all dilutions)

Complement source, e.g. guinea-pig serum (fresh or preserved)

Microtitre apparatus

Microtitre trays—U-shaped wells

Protocol A.

	Tube number						
	1	2	3	4	5	6	7
Barbitone-buffered saline (ml)	0.1	0.2	0.3	0.4	0.5	0.6	0.7
Guinea-pig serum (ml 1 : 10 initial dil.)	0.1————————————————————————————→						
Final complement C dilution	1 : 20	1 : 30	1 : 40	1 : 50	1 : 60	1 : 70	1 : 80

There should not be any complement fixation in either the antigen or antiserum controls, i.e. haemolysis should be complete.

Estimation of minimum haemolytic dose (MHD) of complement

1 Reconstitute the guinea-pig serum if required.
2 Adjust to 1 : 10 dilution.
3 Set up the complement dilutions as in Protocol A.
4 Take 0.1 ml of each complement dilution and add 0.2 ml buffer plus 0.1 ml of sensitized erythrocytes.
5 Incubate for 30 min at 37°C and centrifuge at 100 g for 15 min.

The titre of the first tube in the curve to show a button of erythrocytes is then taken as the MHD. In the assay 2 MHD units are used.

Protocol B.

	Tube number						
	2	3	4	5	6	7	8
Barbitone-buffered saline (ml)	1.0						
HSA (ml, initial conc. mg/ml)	1.0	*mix*	*mix*	etc.			
Final HSA dilution	1 : 2	1 : 4	1 : 8	1 : 16	1 : 32	1 : 64	1 : 128

Antibody and antigen assay

The test is set up as shown in Fig. 7.5. The antiserum is diluted out down the plate (columns) and the antigen is diluted out across the plate (rows).

> **METHOD**
>
> 1 Put 1 drop (25 μl) of buffer in each well. (Hold the dropping pipette vertically.)
> 2 Dilute out the antiserum in the eight columns as for haemagglutination but start at row 2. Row 1 is used as an antigen control.
> 3 Set up antigen dilutions in tubes as in Protocol B.
> 4 Add 1 drop of antigen to each well in columns 2–8: tube number should correspond to column number (see Fig. 7.5). Leave column 1 free of antigen—this is the antiserum control.
> 5 Add 2 MHD units of complement to each well.
> 6 Mix by shaking and incubate at 37°C for 30 min.
> 7 Add 1 drop of sensitized cells to all wells.
> 8 Mix by shaking and incubate at 37°C for 30 min.
> 9 Shake and stand at 4°C for 60 min.
>
> Examine the wells for the presence of unlysed erythrocytes; this indicates previous complement fixation. The end-point titre of this test is usually taken as the first well showing approximately 50% lysis of indicator cells.

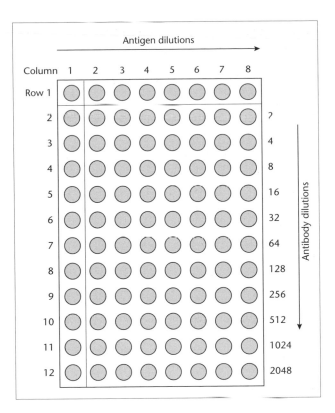

Fig. 7.5 Microtitre plate for quantitative complement fixation assay. Row 1 contains antigen dilutions only and is a control for anticomplementary activity of the antigen. Column 1 contains antibody alone; again this is a control for anticomplementary activity.

TECHNICAL NOTES
- Because IgM has a higher haemolytic efficiency, this antibody class is preferentially detected.
- In the chequer-board design given above, both the antigen and antiserum concentration were varied. For routine use, once the optimum level of either antigen or antibody has been established, a single concentration is usually used for the detection of unknown concentrations of antigen or antibody.
- The final step of settling the indicator cells at 4°C for 60 min may be considerably shortened by gently centrifuging the trays in special microtitre plate holders.
- If any component is anticomplementary the test must be repeated with fresh reagents.

7.7 Assay of complement components with specific antibodies

Most complement components occur in sufficiently large amounts in serum for accurate quantification by a precipitin reaction in gel. The problem with the detection of complement components as antigens is that some antisera do not distinguish between active and inactive complement fragments. However, fragment-specific antisera can be obtained and these can give useful information about the state of complement activation *in vivo*. Some components change their electrophoretic mobility on activation, a qualitative change that may be used to advantage in two-dimensional crossed immunoelectrophoresis to monitor the activation of C3 (see Section 3.9).

A detailed review of available monoclonal antibodies and assay technologies is given by Porcel *et al.* (1993). Most depend on the fine specificity of antibodies for altered complement activation products but care must be taken as not all antibodies have been found to be as specific as the developers have claimed. A clever technique exploits the fact that C4 and C3 are deposited on immune complexes during classical pathway activation and circulate as C4–C3 aggregates.

In this assay, monoclonal antibodies to activated C3 are coated on to microtitre plates, followed by the test samples. The C3–C4 complexes are then detected by adding biotinylated antibodies to C4 (Zwirner *et al.* 1995). This assay illustrates the power of ELISA systems when using two unrelated epitopes for recognition.

TECHNICAL NOTE
Caution is needed when collecting specimens for complement assays as complement is very easily activated during collection. Care must be taken to avoid false results when trying to estimate the activation that has occurred *in vivo*. Therefore collect the blood into ethylene diamine tetra-acetic acid (EDTA), 10 mM, which binds calcium and magnesium and thus will slow activation. The addition of the protease inhibitor nafamostat mesylate will increase the stability.

7.8 Cell lysis

7.8.1 Complement-mediated cytolysis

Antisera directed against cell-surface antigens are used to kill cells carrying these antigens with the aid of complement.

Using erythrocytes as targets is straightforward: haemoglobin released provides a simple measure of cell damage but more often a colourless, nucleated cell is the target of interest. Vital dye exclusion can also be used which is easy to set up without any special equipment but this involves counting live and dead cells, and is time consuming for large numbers of assays.

Radioisotopic methods have proved popular and the release of ^{51}Cr from dead cells is a sensitive indicator. The release of lactate dehydrogenase provides a sensitive assay because of the amplifying affects of the enzyme.

7.8.2 ^{51}Cr-labelled cell lysis

If the cells are labelled with ^{51}Cr it is possible to estimate cell death by the amount of isotope released. In this case it is an advantage to centrifuge the cells after killing to enhance cell dissolution and isotope release.

MATERIALS AND EQUIPMENT
Sodium ^{51}chromate
Inbred mice, 4–6 weeks old
Gamma spectrometer
Antibodies and complement as for the dye exclusion assay

1   Prepare thymus and lymph-node suspensions in tissue culture medium containing HEPES (20 mM) and 5% fetal bovine serum (FBS).

2   Adjust to 5×10^7 lymphocytes/ml and add 37×10^5 Bq of sodium ^{51}chromate to 1 ml of each cell suspension.

3   Incubate at 37°C for 40 min.

4   Wash cells twice with medium and allow to stand on ice for 30 min.

5   Wash cells three times with medium and resuspend to 5×10^6 lymphocytes/ml.

6   Mix 0.1 ml of each cell suspension with antibody and complement and incubate at 37°C for 30 min.

7   After incubation adjust final volume to 0.5 ml, mix well and centrifuge (150 g for 10 min at 4°C).

8   Remove 0.1 ml of supernatant and determine its radioactive content (amount of released isotope) in a γ spectrometer.

TECHNICAL NOTE

Many investigators determine the maximum (100% ^{51}Cr release) by lysing an aliquot of cells, either by freezing and thawing or with 10% saponin. Under the labelling conditions described this is usually 10 000–14 000 c.p.m. (for 5×10^6 cells). For some applications, however, this is not a realistic value. This technique may be used, for example, for quantitative absorption experiments in which the relative amount of cell-surface antigen on different cell types may be compared. A fixed number of cells is used to absorb a fixed concentration of antiserum and the original and absorbed antisera are then assayed on ^{51}Cr-labelled cells. In this case it is advisable to determine the dilutions of original antiserum giving a plateau release value, and to use this as the 100% ^{51}Cr release. Alternatively, one may work more sensitively with the dilution of antiserum required to give 50% of this maximum release. The Technical notes given in Section 7.8.1 also apply to this technique.

7.9 Lactate dehydrogenase assay for cytotoxicity

Lactate dehydrogenase (LDH) release can be determined in a similar assay to the dye exclusion test using an LDH kit (Decker & Lohmann-Matthes 1988). Care must be taken as serum in the medium will contain LDH, and phenol red dye can reduce the sensitivity. A variant assay with adherent target cells works on the principle of washing away dead cells, and then releasing the remaining LDH by lysing the live cells and so estimating the living population as a percentage of the total.

7.10 Further reading

Bajno, L. & Grinstein, S. (1999) Fluorescent proteins: powerful tools in phagocyte biology. *J Immunol Meth* **232**(1–2), 67–75.

Bass, D.A., Parce, J.W., Dechatelet, L.R., Szejda, P., Seeds, M.C. & Thomas, M. (1983) Flow cytometric studies of oxidative product formation by neutrophils: a graded response to membrane stimulation. *J Immunol* **130**, 1910–1917.

Buschmann, H. & Winter, M. (1989) Assessment of phagocytic activity of granulocytes using laser flow cytometry. *J Immunol Meth* **124**, 231–234.

Decker, T. & Lohmann-Matthes, M. (1988) A quick and simple method for the quantification of lactate dehydrogenase release in measurements of cellular cytotoxicity and tumour necrosis factor (TNF) activity. *J Immunol Meth* **15**, 61–69.

Flieger, D., Gruber, R., Schlimok, G., Reiter, C., Pantel, K. & Riethmuller, G. (1995) A novel nonradioactive cellular cytotoxicity test based on the differential assessment of living and killed target and effector cells. *J Immunol Meth* **180**(1), 1–13.

Giamis, J., Lombard, Y., Makaya-Kumba, M., Fonteneau, P. & Poindron, P. (1992) A new and simple method for studying the binding and ingestion steps in the phagocytosis of yeasts. *J Immunol Meth* **154**, 185–193.

Hampton, M.B. & Winterbourn, C.C. (1999) Methods for quantifying phagocytosis and bacterial killing by human neutrophils. *J Immunol Meth* **232**(1–2), 15–22.

Harrison, R.A. & Lachman, P.J. (1997) Complement and complement receptors. In: *Weir's Handbook of Experimental Immunology* (eds L.A. Herzenberg, D.M. Weir, L.A. Herzenberg & C. Blackwell), 5th edn. Blackwell Science, Oxford.

Hartmann, H., Lübbers, B., Casaretto, M., Bautsch, W., Klos, A. & Köhl, J. (1993) Rapid quantification of C3a and C5a using a combination of chromatographic and immunoassay procedures. *J Immunol Meth* **166**, 35–44.

Kipriyanov, S.M., Kupriyanova, O.A., Little, M. & Moldenhauer, G. (1996) Rapid detection of recombinant antibody fragments directed against cell-surface antigens by flow cytometry. *J Immunol Meth* **196**(1), 51–62.

Maillet, F., Fremeaux-Bacchi, V., Uhring-Lambert, B. & Kazatchkine, M.D. (1992) Assessment of complement activation in clinical samples. Comparison of immunochemical and functional measurements of complement components with quantification of activation fragments. *J Immunol Meth* **156**, 171–178.

Masaki, T., Okada, N., Yasuda, R. & Okada, H. (1989) Assay of complement activity in human serum using large unilamellar liposomes. *J Immunol Meth* **123**, 19.

Model, M.A., KuKuruga, M.A. & Todd, III R.F. (1997) A sensitive cytometric method for measuring the oxidative burst. *J Immunol Meth* **202**, 105–111.

Mohanty, J.G., Jaffe, J.S., Schulman, E.S. & Raible, D.G. (1997) A highly sensitive fluorescent microassay of H_2O_2 release from activated human leucocytes using a dihydroxyphenoxazine derivative. *J Immunol Meth* **202**, 133–141.

Montano, R.F. & Morrison, S.L. (1999) A colourimetric-enzymatic microassay for the quantification of antibody-dependent complement activation. *J Immunol Meth* **222**(1–2), 73–82.

Morgan, B.P. (ed.) (2000) *Complement Methods and Protocols: Methods in Molecular Biology*, Vol. 3. Humana Press, New York.

Porcel, J.M., Peakman, M., Senaldi, G. & Vergani, D. (1993) Methods for assessing complement activation in the clinical immunology laboratory. *J Immunol Meth* **157**, 1–9.

Rafnar, B.O., Traustadottir, K.H., Sigfusson, A., Arason, G.J., Valdimarsson, H. & Erlendsson, K. (1998) An enzyme based assay for the measurement of complement mediated binding of immune complexes to red blood cells. *J Immunol Meth* **211**(1–2), 171–181.

Robinson, J.P. & Babcock, G.F. (eds) (1998) *Phagocyte Function: A Guide for Research and Clinical Evaluation (Cytometric Cellular Analysis)*. John Wiley & Sons, New York.

Sepp, A., Binns, R.M. & Lechler, R.I. (1996) Improved protocol for colourimetric detection of complement-mediated cytotoxicity based on the measurement of cytoplasmic lactate dehydrogenase activity. *J Immunol Meth* **196**, 175–180.

Stefanski, V. & Ruppel, H.G. (1991) A new quantitative assay for the determination of complement activity. *Immunol Lett* **30**, 1–5.

Stöve, S., Klos, A., Bautsch, W. & Kohl, J. (1995) Re-evaluation of the storage conditions for blood samples which are used for determination of complement activation. *J Immunol Meth* **182**, 1–5.

van Eeden, S.F., Klut, M.E., Walker, B.A. & Hogg, J.C. (1999) The use of flow cytometry to measure neutrophil function. *J Immunol Meth* **232**, 23–43.

Vuorte, J., Jansson, S.-E. & Repo, H. (1996) Standardization of a flow cytometric assay for phagocyte respiratory burst activity. *Scand J Immunol* **43**, 329–334.

Wan, C.P., Park, C.S. & Lau, B.H.S. (1993) A rapid and simple microfluorometric phagocytosis assay. *J Immunol Meth* **162**, 1–7.

Whaley, K. (ed.) (1988) *Methods In Complement for Clinical Immunologists.* Churchill Livingstone, Edinburgh.

Zahler, S., Kowalski, C., Brosig, A., Kupatt, C., Becker, B.F. & Gerlach, E. (1997) The function of neutrophils isolated by a magnetic antibody cell separation technique is not altered in comparison to a density gradient centrifugation method. *J Immunol Meth* **200**, 173–179.

Zwirner, J., Dobos, G. & Gotze, O. (1995) A novel ELISA for the assessment of classical pathway of complement activation by measurement of C4–C3 complexes. *J Immunol Meth* **186**, 55–63.

Zwirner, J., Wittig, A., Kremmer, E. & Gotze, O. (1998) A novel ELISA for the evaluation of the classical pathway of complement. *J Immunol Meth* **211**(1–2), 183–90.

8 Lymphocyte structure

8.1 Analysis of lymphocyte antigens

Techniques used for the analysis of lymphocyte antigens are: (a) powerful analytical tools for the analysis of complex antigenic systems, including detergent-solubilized cells; and (b) sufficiently flexible and compatible to be capable of improvement and modification to facilitate novel experimental applications.

8.1.1 Radiolabelling of cells and their secreted products

Radiolabelling of cell components (proteins, glycoproteins, phosphoproteins, phospholipids, etc.) can provide convenient markers for analytical and preparative techniques (see Sections 8.1.2 and 8.1.3). Endogenous or biosynthetic labelling of secreted proteins is described in detail for monoclonal antibodies and hybridoma cell lines (see Chapter 2 and Section 8.4). Similar techniques are used for the labelling of other proteins or glycoproteins, e.g. cytokines secreted from cell lines *in vitro* or, indeed, for any constitutive cell protein which undergoes significant turnover during the labelling period (see also Chapter 10).

Chemical or exogenous labelling of the surface of a viable cell is a common starting point for many studies on cell-surface antigens (see Section 8.1.2). Differential exogenous labelling of the surface of intact, viable cells may be compared with labelling of the cells of the same type after detergent solubilization. This can provide valuable information on the relative distribution of an antigen between the cytoplasm and exterior of the surface membrane.

External labelling is usually achieved by confining the chemical coupling reaction to the outer surface of the membrane, e.g. using a molecule too large to cross the membrane (often a protein, as in lactoperoxidase labelling) (see Section 8.1.2), or by binding one of the essential components of the reaction to an insoluble support (the surface of a plastic macrobead or tube, as in Iodogen labelling) (see Section 4.9.3).

Success relies crucially on a population of cells with high (preferably uniform) viability and intact surface membranes.

8.1.2 Cell-surface iodination: lactoperoxidase technique

Lactoperoxidase, in the presence of hydrogen peroxide, catalyses the incorporation of iodine into tyrosine residues. This gentle and efficient method utilizes the action of glucose oxidase on glucose to generate hydrogen peroxide continuously during the reaction. As the enzymes are too big to be able to cross the plasma membrane the addition of iodine is confined to the cell surface.

MATERIALS AND EQUIPMENT

Phosphate-buffered saline (PBS)

Cells for iodination (10^8/ml in PBS)

Lactoperoxidase (0.2 mg/ml in PBS)

Glucose oxidase (2.0 IU/ml in PBS)

50 mM glucose in PBS

Sodium ^{125}I, carrier free

Gamma spectrometer

METHOD

1 Wash the cells three times in PBS by centrifugation (150 *g* for 10 min at room temperature) to remove exogenous material, count and adjust to 10^8 cells/ml.

2 To 100 µl of cell suspension add 10 µl lactoperoxidase (0.2 mg/ml in PBS initial concentration), 10 µl glucose oxidase (2 IU/ml in PBS, initial concentration) and 18.5×10^6 Bq ^{125}I.

3 Initiate the reaction by the addition of 10 µl of 50 mM glucose in PBS and incubate for 10 min at room temperature.

4 Add 10 ml of ice-cold PBS to stop the reaction.

5 Wash the cells three times in PBS by centrifugation (150 *g* for 10 min at 4°C).

6 If required, the cells may be detergent solubilized, and their radioactive incorporation determined.

TECHNICAL NOTES

- Because the lactoperoxidase cannot cross the plasma membrane of viable cells, only surface proteins are iodinated. However, internal and external proteins are labelled if the cells are dead; therefore good cell viability is essential. See Section 6.4 for dead cell removal.
- The method is also useful for soluble proteins, but the enzymes will contaminate the protein preparation. To avoid this, enzymes coupled to a solid phase should be used. Polyacrylamide beads coupled with lactoperoxidase and glucose oxidase are available commercially. The reaction may then be terminated by removal of the beads.
- Lactoperoxidase may be 'poisoned' by the addition of 10 mm sodium azide and the reaction terminated precisely. In addition, be sure that the PBS does not contain sodium azide as a preservative, otherwise the reaction will never start.
- Lactoperoxidase catalyses its own iodination. In some systems, iodination artefacts have been reported due to the adsorption of this material to surface of the cell being labelled. If this is a problem, cells may be iodinated with insolubilized Iodogen but with reduced efficiency.
- Methods using isotopes vary in the harshness (potential for alteration of the conformation of the labelled material) of the reaction required to achieve the desired result.

- It is essential that use of radiolabels is appropriately recorded and safety advice regarding the handling of radioisotopes is followed in accordance with the local guidelines of the institution where the work is carried out.
- For optimum results it is advisable to calculate the half-life decay of the isotopes used. Here are some useful websites that give comprehensive details on radioisotope health and safety procedures as well as useful information regarding detection and half-life:
  http://www.practicingsafescience.org
  http://www.hse.gov.uk

8.1.3 Tritium labelling of cell-surface glycoproteins

Low concentrations of sodium metaperiodate induce specific oxidative cleavage of sialic acids. The aldehydes thus formed can be reduced easily with ^{3}H-sodium borohydride. At 0°C the periodate anion only penetrates the cell membrane very slowly and so oxidation will be restricted mainly to cell-surface sialic acid residues.

MATERIALS
Phosphate-buffered saline (PBS)
Lymphocytes (3×10^7/ml in PBS)
1 M sodium metaperiodate in PBS
0.1 M glycerol in PBS
Tritiated sodium borohydride
Ice
Beta spectrometer

METHOD

1 Wash lymphocytes (3×10^7) twice with PBS by centrifugation (150 *g* for 10 min at 4°C).
2 Resuspend in 1 ml PBS and place on ice.
3 Add 0.1 ml 1 M sodium metaperiodate and incubate on ice for 5 min.
4 Quench the reaction by adding 0.2 ml glycerol (0.1 M).
5 Wash the cells three times with PBS by centrifugation.
6 Resuspend cells in 0.5 ml PBS.
7 Add 18.5×10^6 Bq sodium ^{3}H-borohydride.
8 Incubate for 30 min at room temperature.
9 After washing in cold PBS, the cells may be solubilized in detergent if required and their radioactive incorporation determined.

8.1.4 Specificity of the labelling reaction

Early studies of cell-surface labelling demonstrated that the addition of the radiolabel was indeed limited to the surface membrane, e.g. by electron microscope autoradiography (Fig. 8.1). Techniques are now sufficiently established that, unless you are working with a totally novel or bizarre system, this type of evidence for the localization of labelling is not sought. However, it is necessary to bear in mind that cells can adsorb exogenous proteins (particularly from dead and dying cells) on to their surface and so have a well-developed propensity to trap the unwary.

Fig. 8.1 Electron microscopic autoradiography of ^{125}I-labelled *Trypanosoma cruzi* organisms. Trypomastigotes of the protozoan *Trypanosoma cruzi* were labelled with ^{125}I by the lactoperoxidase technique and processed for ultramicrotome sectioning. Ultrathin sections were dipped in K5 nuclear emulsion, allowed to expose and finally processed photographically before being viewed in a transmission electron microscope. The photograph shows individual silver grains at or near the cell membrane, confirming that the majority of the radioiodine has indeed conjugated to cell-surface residues. Final magnification × 31 000.

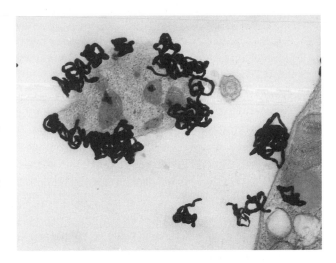

8.2 Lymphocyte surface membrane

In healthy individuals, the majority of the circulating lymphocytes spend their time apparently doing nothing, i.e. as resting or G_0 cells. These dormant cells are specifically activated after contact with antigen. Antigen contact occurs as a specific surface event at the plasma membrane and generates a transduction signal that causes nuclear derepression. The cell enters the cell cycle and divides; it can eventually form a clone of effector and memory cells of the same specificity.

8.2.1 Immunofluorescent staining of lymphocyte membranes

This method is generally applicable to antisera of any specificity used with any viable cell suspension. Antisera dilution used in this experiment should be optimized. Since there is individual variation in antibody affinity and avidity, a wide range of antibody concentrations should be used in the initial standard experiment to ensure reasonable fluorescence. (Obviously cost will, to a certain extent, limit the range used.)

Immunofluorescent staining

MATERIALS AND EQUIPMENT

Lymphoid organs, e.g. lymph node, spleen

Tissue culture medium containing 0.1% w/v bovine serum albumin (BSA) and 20 mM sodium azide

Nylon wool

2-ml syringe barrels

Haemocytometer

Rabbit anti-mouse immunoglobulin (anti-Ig)

Fluorescein-conjugated goat, pig or sheep anti-rabbit immunoglobulin (FITC anti-Ig)

Mounting medium: 70% glycerol, 30% glycine–saline buffer, pH 8.6

Note: Azide is a dangerous chemical—do not discard down the sink.

1 Prepare a lymphocyte suspension from blood or one of the solid lymphoid organs.
2 Filter cell suspensions from lymphoid organs through nylon wool to remove aggregates.
3 Wash all cells three times in tissue culture medium by centrifugation (150 g for 10 min at 4°C).
4 Resuspend the cells in 10 ml of medium and count the number of lymphocytes per ml using a haemocytometer and phase-contrast microscope.
5 Pipette out 2 aliquots of approximately 10^7 lymphocytes of each cell suspension and centrifuge to obtain a pellet (150 g for 10 min at 4°C).
6 Add 0.1 ml of the required dilution of rabbit anti-mouse Ig or normal rabbit serum (NRS) to 1 aliquot of each cell type.
7 Incubate for 30 min on ice.
8 Wash twice by centrifugation (150 g for 10 min at 4°C) to remove unbound protein.
9 Add 0.1 ml of the fluorescein-conjugated anti-rabbit Ig (1 mg/ml total protein) to all cell pellets.
10 Incubate for 30 min on ice.
11 Wash three times by centrifugation (150 g for 10 min at 4°C) to remove the unbound conjugate.
12 Resuspend, add 1 drop of glycerol–glycine mounting medium to the dry cell pellet and mix thoroughly.
13 Put 1 small drop of cell suspension on a microscope slide, add a coverslip and ring with nail varnish.
14 Examine the cell preparations under an incident light UV microscope and identify lymphocytes visible as green rings. This is characteristic of cell-surface staining of viable lymphocytes. In addition, note the homogeneously stained dead cells that will inevitably be present.
15 For each microscope field, count the number of fluorescently stained lymphocytes (green) and then the total viable lymphocytes viewed under phase contrast.
16 Count a total of 200 cells under visible light and calculate the percentage of fluorescing (positive) lymphocytes for each preparation.

TECHNICAL NOTES

- Staining viable cells confines the antibody to the external surface membrane. Staining of internal components can only be accomplished efficiently by cell fixation and membrane permeabilization.
- If required, the method may be abbreviated by exposing the cells to each antibody for 10 min on ice, with only slight loss of sensitivity.
- Precisely the same method may be used to prepare cells for cytofluorimetric analysis.
- Several commercial companies now market an antifade fluorescent mounting medium. It is particularly advantageous to use an antifade compound for photomicroscopy, and also to remember that the quenched fluorochrome slowly recovers. A cheaper but slightly less effective antifade mountant may be prepared as described below.

Antifade mountant

MATERIALS
p-phenylenediamine
Phosphate-buffered saline (PBS)
Glycerol
0.5 M carbonate–bicarbonate buffer, pH 9.0

METHOD

1 Dissolve 100 mg *p*-phenylenediamine in 10 ml of PBS in the dark.
2 Add 90 ml of glycerol and mix thoroughly.
3 Adjust to pH 8.0 with the carbonate–bicarbonate buffer.
4 Store the mixture at –20°C in the dark.
5 Use as glycerol–glycine mountant, step 12 in Method above.
Prepare fresh antifade mountant when the stock solution turns brown.

8.2.2 Antigen-binding lymphocytes

A basic technique is described below by which antigen-binding lymphocytes can be visualized. Applicability of this approach is limited principally by the experimental design to ensure that non-specific binding is avoided. It is difficult in this type of experiment to include a satisfactory specificity control. The approach adopted here is to show that the number of antigen-binding lymphocytes increases after immunization.

Sheep erythrocyte rosettes

A rosette inhibition experiment with anti-mouse immunoglobulin is described at the same time as determining the number of antigen-binding lymphocytes.

Preparation in advance

1 Immunize a mouse 7 days before the experiment with 10^8 sheep erythrocytes (RBC) given intraperitoneally.
2 The anti-mouse immunoglobulin and normal rabbit serum must be absorbed with mouse liver and red blood cells, as well as sheep RBC to be sure they are free of anti-species activity.

MATERIALS AND EQUIPMENT
Sheep erythrocytes (SRBC)
Normal and SRBC-immunized mice
Tissue culture medium
Rabbit anti-mouse immunoglobulin serum (anti-Ig)
Normal rabbit serum (NRS)
Nylon wool
2-ml syringe barrels
2-ml plastic round-bottomed tubes

METHOD

1 Kill both the control and immunized mice and prepare single-cell suspensions from the spleens.
2 Remove phagocytic cells.
3 Wash the cells three times by centrifugation (150 g for 10 min at 4°C).
4 Count the number of viable lymphocytes/ml and adjust to 3×10^7/ml.
5 Label tubes and add 0.1 ml aliquots of the lymphocyte suspensions as shown in the Protocol.

Protocol.

Tube	Lymphocytes from:	Antiserum incubation before rosetting
1	Immune spleen	None
2	Normal spleen	None
3	Immune spleen	Anti-mouse immunoglobulin
4	Immune spleen	NRS

6 Add 0.1 ml of the appropriate sera to tubes 3 and 4. (Use the optimal dilution as determined for immunofluorescence; see Section 8.2.1.) Alternatively a full titration curve of rosette inhibition may be carried out.
7 Incubate tubes 3 and 4 at 4°C for 30 min.
8 Add 0.1 ml SRBC suspension (2.4×10^8 SRBC/ml) to tubes 1 and 2. Mix well.
9 Centrifuge tubes 1 and 2 at 150 g for 10 min at 4°C.
10 Add 0.3 ml of 0.5% acridine orange solution to tubes 1 and 2 if UV microscope is available (otherwise use tissue culture medium) and resuspend the cells on a vertical rotor turning at 8–10 r.p.m. for 5 min. (Alternatively, you may resuspend the cells using a Pasteur pipette. This, however, reduces the number of rosettes because of the shear forces generated.)
11 Repeat the addition of SRBC, centrifugation and resuspension for the cells pretreated with antisera (i.e. tubes 3 and 4). This time, however, add only 0.2 ml of acridine orange solution (or tissue culture medium).
12 Count the number of rosettes in each suspension using a haemocytometer and a microscope. Sample each tube four times and count the rosettes.
If you are using a microscope with UV light, live cells may be seen at the centre of the rosette by their green fluorescence (dead cells are deep red), thus confirming the cell group as a rosette rather than an aggregate of SRBC. If a UV microscope is not used then 0.1% toluidine blue may be used to visualize nucleated cells. Do not count rosettes with more than one lymphocyte, or clumped red cells without lymphocytes. This is shown in Fig. 8.2.

Calculation and evaluation of results

1 Calculate the number of rosettes/ml of suspension and from this the number of rosettes per 10^6 lymphocytes.

(a)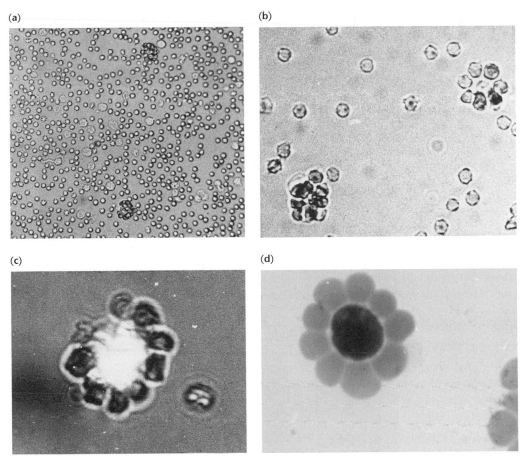

(b)

(c)

(d)

Fig. 8.2 **Mouse lymphocytes showing antigen-specific immunocytoadherence with sheep erythrocytes.**
(a) Antigen-specific lymphocytes will bind sheep erythrocytes to their surface to form rosettes; two are shown
in this field. (b) At 4°C the erythrocytes bind as a single layer. (c) The nucleus of the lymphocyte at the centre
of this rosette has been stained with acridine orange and is visualized under UV and tungsten light. (d) The
morphology of the rosette-forming cell may be seen after Giemsa staining of a cytocentrifuge preparation.
A rosette may be arbitrarily defined as a single lymphocyte binding five or more erythrocytes. If rosettes are
incubated at 37°C, in the absence of metabolic inhibition, erythrocyte 'caps' will form in an analogous
manner to that shown for anti-immunoglobulin.

2   Compare the number of rosettes per 10^6 lymphocytes from the normal and immune animals
     (tubes 1 and 2) and calculate the factor of immunization.
3   You should find that all the rosettes are blocked by the anti-immunoglobulin serum.

8.2.3 Autoradiographic labelling of lymphocytes

The investigation of the surface components of lymphocytes using fluorochrome-labelled
antibodies gives increased sensitivity over that achieved using a radioactive isotope.

Autoradiography is semiquantitative, where the relative number of grains per cell is dependent upon the number of surface determinants detected. The relative distribution of the determinants throughout the cell population may be estimated and, within the same experiment, the

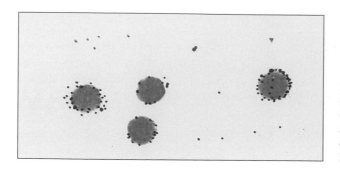

Fig. 8.3 Anti-light-chain (anti-LC) labelling of chicken bursa cells. Cells: 1-day-old white leghorn bursa; antiserum: [125]I anti-LC antibodies; control: ^{125}I-anti-keyhole limpet haemocyanin antibodies.

relative concentration and distribution of determinants between two cell populations. For instance, it has been shown that B cells vary widely in the number of available immunoglobulin molecules on their surface (Fig. 8.3) and that cells differ quantitatively in their membrane content of immunoglobulin. The basic autoradiographic method as described below may be used in any situation where a radioactive isotope is introduced into or onto a cell or tissue.

Example: labelling of chicken lymphocytes

MATERIALS AND EQUIPMENT

1-day-old chickens (see also Section 11.9)

Anti-immunoglobulin antibody: either purified by acid elution, or an IgG fraction

Control: either an irrelevant purified antibody, e.g. anti-keyhole limpet haemocyanin (anti-KLH),
    or normal rabbit IgG (NRIgG)

Chloramine T

Sodium metabisulphite

Sodium [125]I

Sephadex G-25

Glass tubing, internal diameter 6.0 mm

Ilford K5 nuclear emulsion

Although strictly the concentration of antibody used should be titrated until a plateau value of labelled cells is attained, it has been found in practice that 50 μg of pure anti-immunoglobulin per 10^7 lymphocytes is a vast excess.

Specimen experimental protocol

Anti-immunoglobulin labelling of bursa cells from six 1-day-old chicks: antiserum, rabbit anti-chicken light chain (anti-LC) purified by acid elution from immunoadsorbent of chicken IgG; control serum, rabbit anti-KLH antibody prepared in a similar manner.

Calculation of initial concentration of reagents for protein iodination

Oxidation conditions: use 37×10^6 Bq of ^{125}I per 200 μg of protein in 100 μg chloramine T (final concentration). The protein concentration must be at or above 5 mg/ml to avoid excessive denaturation.

Specimen calculation

Rabbit anti-LC and anti-KLH at 20 mg/ml initial concentration. To label 6 aliquots of bursa cells at 50 µg of antibody per aliquot = 300 µg protein, use 55.5×10^6 Bq ^{125}I. To maintain 5 mg/ml protein concentration calculate permissible volume of chloramine T as follows:

protein used – 15 µl at 20 mg/ml,

maximum permissible oxidation volume = 60 µl at 5 mg/ml.

Final oxidation mixture

15 µl protein + 15 µl ^{125}I + 20 µl chloramine T (total volume = 50 µl, protein concentration = 6 mg/ml).

Chloramine T used at 100 µg/ml final concentration, therefore initial concentration must be 250 µg/ml, i.e. prepare an initial solution of 25 mg chloramine T in 100 ml PBS.

Reaction stopped by a two-fold excess, by weight, of sodium metabisulphite.

Final mixture

15 µl protein + 15 µl ^{125}I + 20 µl chloramine T + 50 µl sodium metabisulphite. Total volume = 100 µl.

Final concentration of metabisulphite = 200 µg/ml; initial concentration must be 400 µg/ml, i.e. prepare an initial solution of 40 mg sodium metabisulphite in 100 ml PBS.

METHOD

1 Partially seal the end of two pieces of glass tubing, length 30 cm, internal diameter 0.6 cm, and plug with cotton wool.
2 Pour two columns of Sephadex G-25, height 10 cm.
3 Determine void volume and expanded sample volume of each column using 0.3 ml blue dextran (initial sample volume). Equilibrate columns with PBS.
4 Pipette out protein for iodination into pointed glass tubes.
5 Add calculated volume of sodium ^{125}I (carefully).
6 Add chloramine T and oxidize for 3 min at room temperature.
7 Terminate reaction by addition of sodium metabisulphite.
8 Adjust final volume to 0.3 ml with PBS.
9 Pass the iodination mixture through the Sephadex G-25 column.
10 Monitor the column effluent for the first appearance of radioactivity. (This should be just after the void volume has left the column.)
11 Collect the labelled protein in the expanded sample volume.
   The radioactively labelled protein may be stored overnight at 4°C before use.

Cell labelling

1 Add 50 µg of iodinated protein (either anti-LC or anti-KLH) to aliquots of 10^7 bursal lymphocytes.
2 Incubate at 4°C for 30 min.
3 Centrifuge each aliquot of cells through a 2-ml discontinuous gradient of 50% and 100% fetal bovine serum (FBS) in tissue culture medium at 225 *g* for 15 min at 4°C.

4 Suck off the supernatant and resuspend the cells in 1 ml tissue culture medium.

5 Layer the cells onto a second gradient and centrifuge.

6 Finally resuspend the cell pellet in a few drops of FBS and prepare smears.

7 Check that the smears are adequate using a phase-contrast microscope, and adjust the cell concentration in the original suspension with FBS if required.

8 Prepare at least six smears per cell aliquot, and label the slides for identification.

9 Fix the slides, wash with running tap water for 30 min and finally air dry.

10 Dip the slides in a 1 : 5 solution v/v of Ilford K5 nuclear emulsion and dry slides in front of a fan or over silica gel overnight (in a photographic dark room).

11 Leave slides to expose in light-tight containers at 4°C. (Do not store near radioactive materials.)

Exposure time

1 Under the conditions described, one sample slide should be removed from each group after 4–5 days.

2 Develop, fix and wash the sample autoradiographs and then stain in May–Grünwald/ Giemsa.

3 Examine the slides under oil immersion. If the autoradiographs in the control groups show more than eight to 10 grains per cell, develop all the slides. If, however, the control staining is low, examine the anti-LC-treated cells. If the grain counts are clearly above the control values, develop all the slides.

4 Sample the autoradiographs at least every 4 days until satisfactory positive labelling is achieved with a low number of grains on the control cells.

5 At the end of the exposure period (usually 10–14 days under the conditions described), select at least two slides per group for grain counting. Use the following criteria:
   (a) the cells must be sufficiently spread so that the grains between two adjacent cells do not overlap;
   (b) the cell density must be similar on anti-LC and control slides within each group;
   (c) the emulsion over the cells must be free from 'fogging' of any source.

6 Count the number of grains over at least 200 cells per group (Fig. 8.3). Record and rank the grain counts as shown in Fig. 8.4.

7 Calculate the frequency of cells within each ranked group.

Calculation of percentage of positive cells

The proportion of cells showing positive labelling, i.e. grains above those expected by the non-specific binding of labelled protein and for other non-specific reasons, may be calculated by the following equation.

For each grain-count category:

$$C_p = (C_a - C_c) \times \frac{1}{1 - C_c} 100$$

where C_p is percentage of positively labelled cells, C_a is proportion of cells labelled with antiserum and C_c is proportion of cells labelled with control serum.

Calculate the percentage positive cells in each category for each group. Plot a graph of cell frequency against grain counts. A specimen result and calculation is shown in Fig. 8.4.

Proportion of labelled cells											
Number of grains	0 5	6 11	12 17	18 23	24 29	30 25	36 41	42 47	48 53	54 59	>60
Anti-LC	0.08	0.15	0.17	0.17	0.10	0.10	0.08	0.06	0.02	0.03	0.04
Anti-KLH	0.95	0.05									
% positive cells	0	11	17	17	10	10	8	6	2	3	4

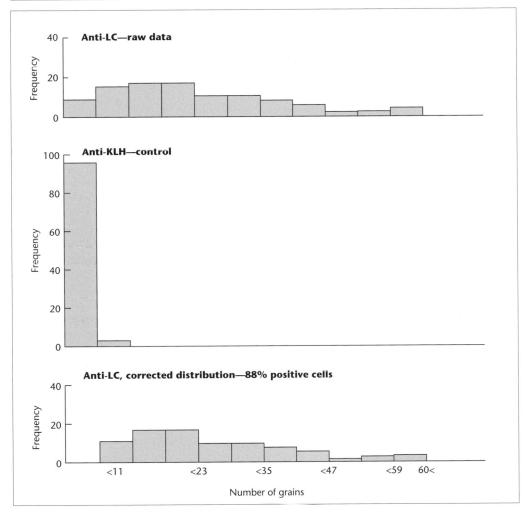

Fig. 8.4 Histograms of grain counts from autoradiographs of ^{125}I anti-light chain (anti-LC) and anti-keyhole limpet haemocyanin (anti-KLH) labelling of chicken B lymphocytes.

8.3 Fc and complement receptors (binding sites)

Cells that possess Fc receptors include mast cells, monocytes, neutrophils, lymphocytes, platelets and placental syncytiotrophoblasts.

Although there is a weak, easily reversible binding of native (monomeric) IgG to such cells, the strength of binding is greater with IgG antibody either complexed with antigen or aggregated by heat. This is in direct contrast to the high affinity shown by mast-cell Fc receptors for monomeric IgE (affinity constant around 10^9–10^{10}/M). It is also possible to demonstrate a site for the binding of the activation products of C3 (presumably *in vivo* in the form of antigen–antibody–complement complexes) to many cells, including B lymphocytes. In many cases the function of the Fc or C3 receptors is clear, For example, both are involved in promoting the phagocytic activity of macrophages.

8.3.1 Detection of Fc receptors on lymphocytes

MATERIALS

Mice

Sheep erythrocytes (SRBC)

Anti-SRBC serum, mouse or rabbit

Saline

Tissue culture medium

Tris(hydroxymethyl)-aminomethane (Tris)–ammonium chloride (see Appendix A)

METHOD

1 Wash SRBC three times in saline by centrifugation (300 g for 5 min).
2 Resuspend pellet to 2×10^8 cells/ml (approximately 1% v/v) in tissue culture medium.
3 Incubate aliquots of the erythrocytes with the antiserum dilutions in a total volume of 0.5 ml (shown in the Protocol) for 30 min at 37°C.

Protocol.

	Tube number			
	1	2	3	4
SRBC (2×10^8/ml)	0.5 ml————————————→			
Final antiserum dilution	1 : 5	1 : 10	1 : 20	1 : 40

4 Wash each aliquot of SRBC three times in tissue culture medium by centrifugation and resuspend to 1 ml.
5 Take a sample from each aliquot of SRBC and examine under a microscope. Discard all aliquots showing visible agglutination.
6 Prepare cell suspensions from thymus, lymph nodes and spleen and wash three times in tissue culture medium by centrifugation (150 g for 10 min at 4°C).
7 Count lymphocytes and adjust to 5×10^6 cells/ml.
8 Mix 0.1 ml of each lymphocyte suspension with 0.2 ml of sensitized SRBC. Use SRBC suspension with the lowest antiserum dilution not giving agglutination.
9 Incubate at room temperature for 60–90 min.

Continued

10 Add acridine orange or toluidine blue dye.
11 Determine the number of rosettes/ml.
12 Count the number of viable lymphocytes/ml.
13 Calculate the percentage of lymphocytes forming Fc rosettes.

8.4 Plasma cells and intracellular immunoglobulin

Preparation in advance

Prime mice 7–8 days before the experiment with 400 µg of alum-precipitated DNP–FγG (dinitrophenyl–fowl γ-globulin) plus *Bordetella pertussis*.

8.4.1 Demonstration of plasma cells

This can be done either on spleen sections or with single-cell suspensions smeared on microscope slides.

Frozen sections

MATERIALS AND EQUIPMENT

Immune mouse (immunized, see Section 11.2.2)
Acetone
Solid carbon dioxide (dry ice)
OCT (optimal cutting temperature) compound, Tissue Tek II
Freezing microtome

METHOD

1 Add small pieces of solid CO_2 to acetone in an insulated metal container until bubbling stops.
2 Kill the mouse, remove the spleen and chop it transversely into about five pieces.
3 Drop the spleen fragments into the freezing mixture.
4 Mount one of the fragments on a microtome chuck using OTC compound and cut 5-µm sections. These must be air-dried and can then be stored at −70°C for up to 3 months.

Isolated cells

MATERIALS AND EQUIPMENT

Immune mouse
Tissue culture medium at 4°C
Fetal bovine serum (FBS)
Cytocentrifuge

1   Kill the mouse, remove the spleen and prepare a single-cell suspension in tissue culture medium.

2   Allow the aggregates to settle for 10 min at 1 *g*. Do not filter the cells through nylon wool because you are going to look at large cells which are easily damaged and trapped in nylon wool.

3   Wash the cells twice with medium by centrifugation (150 *g* for 10 min at 4°C).

4   Count the cells and adjust to 2×10^7/ml.

5   Add an equal volume of FBS to the cell suspension.

6   Prepare cell smears on a cytocentrifuge. Spin at 100–150 *g* for 20 min. It will be necessary to vary the number of drops of cell suspension used to obtain a good smear; however, the total volume of liquid should be maintained at 4 drops per well (see also Section 11.6.3).

7   Dry the smears thoroughly and fix in 95% methanol.

It is possible to prepare these smears as described for small lymphocytes, but the plasma cells are large and fragile, so you must not use a 'spreader' slide. Simply shake the slide to spread out the drop and air dry before methanol fixation.

8.4.2 Staining of sections or cytosmears for antibody-producing cells

Here it is demonstrated that there are antibody-producing cells present, and many of these cells are specific for antigenic determinants on the immunizing antigen, either carrier (FγG) or hapten (DNP).

MATERIALS
Frozen section or smears from immunized mice
Fluorescein isothiocyanate (FITC)-conjugated rabbit anti-mouse immunoglobulin
Guinea-pig or pig-liver powder
Phosphate-buffered saline (PBS)

There is a serious problem of non-specific adsorption of conjugated antisera to fixed material, in contrast to the very low background associated with viable cell immunofluorescence. You should use antisera with a low substitution ratio and in addition absorb the antiserum with liver powder as follows.

1   Dilute the antiserum 1 : 5 with PBS and absorb 1 ml with 100 mg of pig-liver powder (use pro rata).

2   Mix for 30 min at 4°C and spin off the liver powder (500 *g* for 20 min at 4°C).

This absorption must be done at the beginning of each staining session.

8.4.3 Detection of intracellular immunoglobulin

1   Dilute 2 aliquots of the absorbed antiserum to a final dilution of 1 : 10, 1 : 20 and 1 : 40 with PBS.

2   Apply 1 drop of each FITC conjugate dilution to separate spleen sections or cytosmears.

3   Incubate for 20 min at room temperature.

4   Wash off the excess antiserum. This can be done by putting the slides in a tray (face up!) and flooding them with PBS. Washing can be made more effective by placing the tray over a magnetic stirring platform with the mixing bar at the extreme end of the tray from the slides. Mix slowly for 5 min.

5   Change the PBS and mix for a further 5 min.

6   Add 1 drop of mounting medium and add a coverslip. Ring with nail varnish.

7   Examine the slides under a UV microscope.

Plasma cells should be easily visualized as shown in Fig. 4.2.

TECHNICAL NOTES

- You may see a high background reaction when staining spleen sections for immunoglobulin because of secreted antibody entrapment. This should not be a problem with cytosmears.

- Slides of tissue sections may be stored at –20°C for several weeks after drying. Remove from the deep freeze and dry before use.

- The antigen detected above (immunoglobulin) is relatively insensitive to drying-induced denaturation. For long-term storage, cells may be fixed after smearing.

- Sometimes antigen reactivity can be lost if cells are allowed to dry out before or after fixation (Fig. 4.3a,b). In this case, apply a concentrated suspension of cells to a slide pretreated with 1% w/v solution of poly L-lysine (to aid adhesion), allow them to settle at room temperature in a humid chamber for 5–10 min and then add an aqueous fixative.

- An essentially similar technique can be used for staining paraffin-embedded tissue sections with monoclonal antibodies, thus gaining additional information from the better preservation of histological structure.

We have described a direct immunofluorescence technique as this usually gives sufficient sensitivity to detect the relatively large amount of immunoglobulin in the average plasma cell.

An indirect technique may be used if the antigen is scarce or poorly immunogenic. The first antibody, in this case rabbit anti-mouse immunoglobulin, is unconjugated. Its binding is visualized by a second antibody, e.g. FITC-conjugated goat anti-rabbit immunoglobulin (as illustrated in Fig. 4.2). The indirect technique gives a significant gain in sensitivity (up to eight second antibodies may bind for each first antibody), with only a marginal increase in the background of non-specific fluorescence. It also has the added convenience of having to prepare only a single conjugate of an antiserum from a large animal rather than a series of direct conjugates. For example, a FITC-conjugated IgG fraction of goat or sheep anti-rabbit immunoglobulin may be used to visualize a range of rabbit antisera to different antigens.

However, the technique is time-consuming and can be cumbersome if used for the simultaneous detection of different antigenic determinants in two-colour immunofluorescence. If using indirect immunofluorescence to stain tissue sections, only the fluorescent conjugate need be absorbed with liver powder.

8.4.4 Detection of specific antibody using fluorescent probes

To demonstrate the antigen-binding specificity of intracellular antibody, incubate spleen sections or cell preparations with fluorescein-conjugated FγG or unconjugated FγG visualized by

FITC-conjugated rabbit anti-FγG antibody. We have described the indirect technique, which is more sensitive.

MATERIALS

Frozen sections or smears from mice immunized with fowl γ-globulin

Fowl γ-globulin (FγG)

Fluorescein-conjugated anti-FγG

METHOD

Again you should absorb the fluorescent conjugate with liver powder and, in addition, absorb or ultracentrifuge the FγG as this is also 'sticky'.

1 Dilute FγG to 1 mg/ml and put 1 drop onto each of three sections or cytosmears of FγG-immune spleen.
2 Incubate for 20 min at room temperature.
3 Wash away the unbound antigen with PBS (see Section 8.4.3).
4 Add 1 drop of 1 : 5, 1 : 10 and 1 : 20 fluorescein-conjugated anti-FγG to each slide, respectively, and incubate for 20 min at room temperature.
5 Wash away the excess conjugate, blot dry and mount.
6 Examine the preparations under a UV microscope.

TECHNICAL NOTE

It is important to ensure that the FITC-conjugated rabbit anti-FγG does not cross-react with mouse immunoglobulin, i.e. it does not bind directly to the contents of the murine plasma cells. If it does, absorb with glutaraldehyde-insolubilized mouse γ-globulin.

8.4.5 Detection of plasma cells with hapten–enzyme conjugates

This technique is similar in principle to that used for anticarrier antibodies (see Chapter 4). However, in this instance the detection molecule (enzyme) is much bigger than the antigen (the hapten, DNP).

Preparation in advance

This method works equally well using horseradish peroxidase (HRP) or alkaline phosphatase (AP). Conjugate the enzymes with DNP according to the method in Chapter 4. Although AP may be conjugated at room temperature (optimum substitution ratio DNP_{10-15} AP), HRP should be conjugated at 4°C to slow the rate of reaction and so obtain the necessary low substitution ratio (optimum DNP_{1-2} HRP). Enzyme activity is lost if HRP is oversubstituted, probably because of the addition of DNP groups into the catalytic site. The technique is designed to detect intracellular anti-DNP antibodies (see also Section 4.8.1).

TECHNICAL NOTE

Determine the 280 and 360 nm absorbance values before conjugation as HRP has significant absorbance up to 403 nm. It is necessary to subtract the initial absorbance reading at 360 nm from that obtained after conjugation, to calculate the true degree of dinitrophenylation.

Cryostat sections (or cytosmears) from mouse immunized with DNP on a carrier protein

Acetone

Methanol

Hydrogen peroxide

Hapten–enzyme conjugate, e.g. dinitrophenyl–horseradish peroxidase (DNP–HRP)

Diaminobenzidine (DAB) (*Take care—this is a carcinogen*)

Phosphate-buffered saline (PBS)

Bovine serum albumin (BSA)

METHOD

1. Air dry the cryostat sections and fix for 30 min in acetone containing 0.2% v/v hydrogen peroxide at room temperature to inactivate any endogenous peroxidase.

2. Rinse three times in PBS and wipe the slide around the section.

3. Overlay with DNP–HRP diluted to 0.5 mg/ml in PBS containing 0.1% w/v BSA. Leave for 30 min at room temperature in a humid atmosphere.

4. Wash in PBS and finally wipe the slide around the section.

5. Prepare the DAB substrate by adding 4 μl hydrogen peroxide to 10 ml PBS containing 6 mg DAB; filter and use immediately.

6. Add a few drops of DAB solution to each section and allow the colour reaction to develop for 20 min at room temperature in a humid chamber.

7. Wash carefully under tap water and counterstain, e.g. with Harris haematoxylin.

8. If permanent mounts are required, the sections may be dehydrated through graded alcohols, treated with xylene and mounted in DePeX.

9. Observe the sections under bright-field illumination; cell nuclei should be blue while plasma cells containing anti-DNP antibody should have blue cytoplasm.

8.5 Flow cytometry

Fluorescence is the emission of photons by molecules that have absorbed light. Electrons move from a ground to an excited state, and on return to the ground state, a photon is emitted, of lower energy than the excitation light, which is represented by an increase in wavelength. The excitation of a fluorescent material, e.g. fluorescein by blue light, leads to an emission of green light, but the reverse is not possible. The shift in wavelength is an important and useful feature, since it is possible to excite several fluorescent dyes (used to label proteins, etc.) simultaneously by a single excitation wavelength, in, say, the 'blue' region, yet by choosing dyes with different emission wavelengths. It enables separate information to be retrieved from the emissions from each dye, using selective filters for different wavelengths (see Fig. 8.5).

In flow cytometry, cells are channelled into a thin liquid stream through the passage of a narrow beam of light, these days normally a blue (488 nm) laser beam. As individual cells pass through the laser beam photomultipliers situated around the plane of the laser, two types of information may be derived: (i) scattering of the excitation (488 nm) laser beam; and (ii) photons

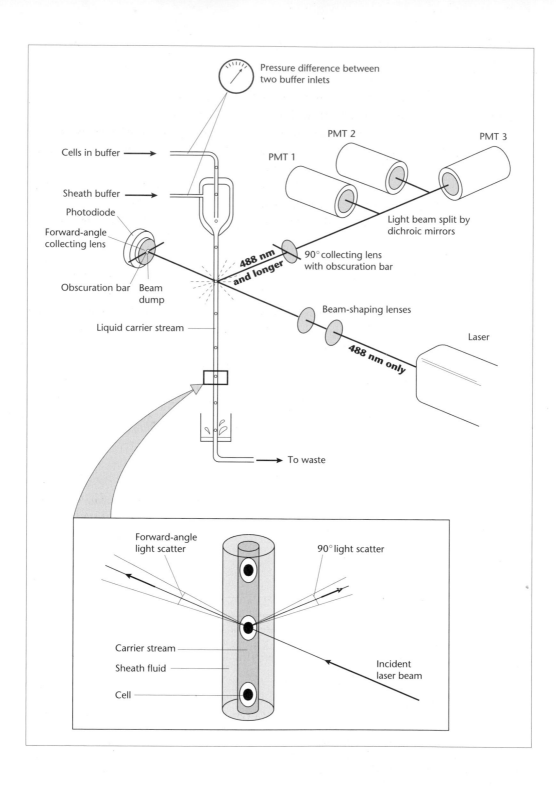

Pressure difference between two buffer inlets

Cells in buffer →

Sheath buffer →

Photodiode

Forward-angle collecting lens

Obscuration bar   Beam dump

Liquid carrier stream

PMT 1

PMT 2

PMT 3

Light beam split by dichroic mirrors

488 nm and longer

90° collecting lens with obscuration bar

Beam-shaping lenses

488 nm only

Laser

To waste

Forward-angle light scatter

90° light scatter

Carrier stream

Sheath fluid

Cell

Incident laser beam

of different wavelengths emitted by fluorescent dyes used to label molecules on or within the cell (see Figs 8.6 and 8.7).

There are two types of light scattering:

1 forward scatter (Fsc), the degree of which is related to cell size; and
2 side scatter (Ssc) which is related to granularity.

These scatter characteristics may be utilized to display and define the cell type being investigated in a mixed population of cells. Such cells can be selected or gated to specifically examine the fluorescence on the surface of the chosen population.

The flow cytometer can analyse the distribution of antigen expression on mixed cell phenotypes to provide discrete information on each population (see Fig. 8.8). Information from up to three fluorescent dyes can be monitored in selected cell populations, usually green-, orange- and red-emitting dyes.

In flow cytometry, generally directly labelled monoclonal antibodies to a particular antigen are used (but this is a relatively insensitive method of labelling). Sensitive photomultipliers are used to detect the light emitted by the entire cell. It allows the simultaneous analysis of three cellular molecules using different labels. Under these circumstances the three labelled antibodies can be incubated simultaneously with the cell. The green-emitting label is fluorescein or some close derivative. The orange-red is phycoerythrin, although in common use it is described as red. The third colour is more difficult and examples are PerCP (Becton-Dickinson) and Badshaw's Tricolour. Some of these stains are relatively simple to couple in the laboratory, e.g. fluorescein, others are not. Usually the development of dyes for flow cytometry is designed around an assumption that the most commonly used laser for excitation is the blue 488 nm.

Fig. 8.5 (*opposite*) **The continuous-flow cytometer.** Cells, in dilute suspension, are injected into the centre of a plastic nozzle through which a stream of sheath fluid flows continuously. As the cell and sheath buffer inlets are at different pressures, the concentric buffer streams emerging from the nozzle run at different rates and therefore do not mix; the cells are thus constrained at the centre of the carrier stream. Under stable conditions, each cell should follow virtually the same path.

Laser light, usually from an argon ion laser, is passed through a set of shaping lenses to produce a beam with an elliptical cross-section, which is aimed at the buffer stream falling to waste. The buffer stream acts as a vertical cylindrical lens and disperses a small proportion of the laser light in the same horizontal plane as the beam. However, the majority of the light continues forward through the buffer stream and is absorbed harmlessly by the cylindrical beam dump. The optical system is aligned so that, provided the laser beam does not hit a cell, no light signal is recorded by the instrument; the horizontally dispersed light is absorbed by obscuration bars placed across the front face of the collecting lenses in the forward angle and at 90° to the incident beam.

Any cell interacting with the laser beam acts as a spherical lens and disperses the light in all directions out of the horizontal plane (shown in the inset). Light is collected by detector systems placed in the direction of travel of the beam (forward-angle light scatter) and at right angles to the direction of travel (90° light scatter). The cell is labelled with one or more fluorochromes. The emitted light that is shifted to a longer wavelength, is resolved from the original exciting wavelength of the laser (for example, 488 nm for the laser and fluorochrome combinations most frequently used) by a combination of dichroic mirrors and long- and short-pass filters. The filters direct the light to a series of photomultiplier tubes (PMT 2 and PMT 3 in the figure). PMT 1 is being used in this case for the detection of the 90° light scatter signal. The integral of the electrical impulse thus generated is digitized and stored or analysed in a computer.

Although the laser beam can be of sufficient intensity to burn a hole in a piece of card, the high thermal capacity of water protects the cells from harm. Viable cells can be sorted using this instrument.

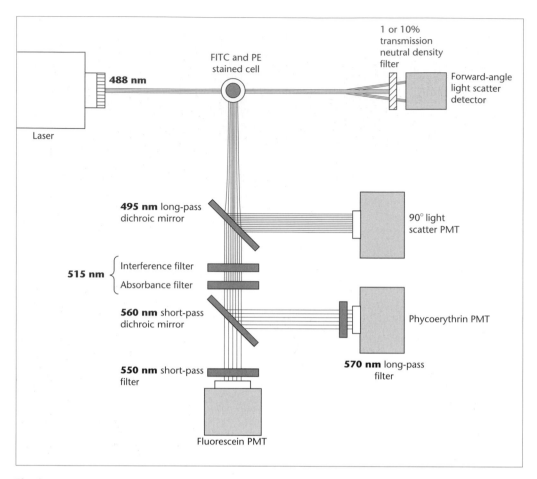

Fig. 8.6 Lens and mirror combinations used to resolve the signals emitted by stained cells. Laser light is monochromatic, stable and very powerful. Thus even subtle shifts of wavelength and minor changes of direction caused by refraction through a single cell can be detected by judicious selection of filters and dichroic mirrors. In principle, light near the original exciting wavelength is used to measure forward-angle light scatter (FALS) (using a photodiode placed in the forward angle) and 90° light scatter (a weaker signal so it is detected using a photomultiplier). Thereafter, light of the exciting wavelength is stripped off using a pair of 515-nm filters which pass only longer (emitted) wavelengths. The dichroic mirror placed at an angle of 45° to the light beam, and after the stripping filters, directs long wavelength light to the photomultiplier set to detect red light (phycoerythrin PMT). Shorter wavelengths are not interrupted in their passage to the photomultiplier set to detect green light (fluorescein PMT). As the mirror does not split the wavelength perfectly, it is 'backed-up' by long- and short-pass absorbance filters, as shown in the diagram. The final traces of 'breakthrough' between the red and green channels can be removed by electronic processing of the photomultiplier signals.

Fig. 8.7 (*opposite*) **Multiparameter cytometry.** (**a**) and (**b**) show an isometric (three-dimensional) and planar (two-dimensional) projection of the same data. Whole blood was stained with fluorescein- and phycoerythrin-conjugated antibodies, the erythrocytes lysed by osmotic shock and the resulting cell suspension washed by centrifugation. (**a**) In this histogram, forward-angle light scatter (FALS) is plotted along the *y*- (rear) axis; 90° light scatter (90°-CLS) along the *x*- (left) axis and frequency on the *z*- (vertical axis). Although the relative numbers of cells in the different populations may be easily appreciated from this type of display, the nature of the populations (in terms of the parameters being measured) is more easily appreciated from a planar view, as in (**b**). (**b**) An approximation to the relative abundance of the different populations is achieved in the two-dimensional display by different pixel densities, representing three selected 'levels' in the frequency data. The four populations of cells marked in the figure have the following characteristics and identity:

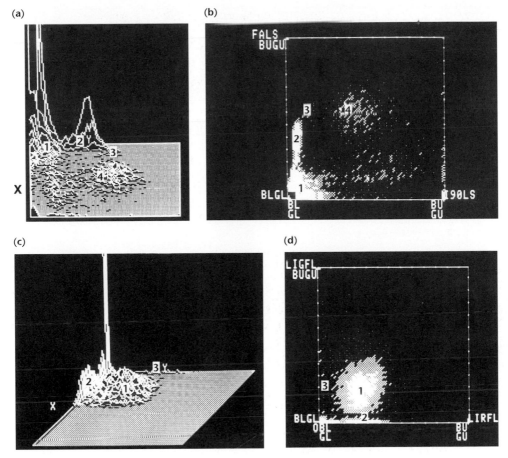

(a)   (b)

(c)   (d)

1   low FALS and 90°-CLS—red-cell ghosts and platelets;
2   medium FALS and low 90°-CLS—lymphocytes;
3   high FALS and low 90°-CLS (also low abundance)—monocytes;
4   high FALS and high 90°-CLS—granulocytes.

Electronic gates were set around the 'lymphocyte' population which was then analysed for the presence of T- and B-lymphocyte markers. Even though other cells are present, both stained and unstained, they are now 'gated out' from further analysis.

Histograms (c) and (d) show three- and two-dimensional plots of fluorescent emissions of the cells examined in (a) and (b). (c) It is possible to discern three distinct populations: one massive population in the centre of the distribution (1), and more minor populations on the x- (2) and y- (3) axes. The x-axis corresponds to the red fluorescence associated with an antibody against a T-cell marker; whereas the y-axis corresponds to the green fluorescence associated with an antibody against a B-cell marker. The three cell populations, more easily seen in (d), have the following characteristics and identities:

1   high red and high green fluorescence—this is a population of B lymphocytes (see below) expressing a
    T-cell marker;
2   high red, low green—this is the staining pattern of the normal blood T-lymphocyte population;
3   low red, high green—this is the staining pattern of the normal B-lymphocyte population in the blood;
    however, in this patient, it is a very minor population.

These cells are derived from a patient with B-cell chronic lymphocytic leukaemia and so contain a monoclonally expanded population of aberrant B lymphocytes. The residual normal B lymphocytes—on the y-axis in (c)—have been virtually replaced by leukaemic cells, whereas the T-lymphocyte population is virtually unchanged. This type of qualitative and quantitative analysis can provide crucial data for haematological diagnosis of disease.

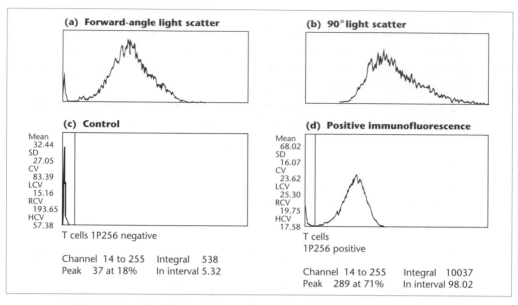

(a) Forward-angle light scatter

(b) 90° light scatter

(c) Control

Mean	32.44
SD	27.05
CV	83.39
LCV	15.16
RCV	193.65
HCV	57.38

T cells 1P256 negative

Channel 14 to 255   Integral   538
Peak   37 at 18%   In interval 5.32

(d) Positive immunofluorescence

Mean	68.02
SD	16.07
CV	23.62
LCV	25.30
RCV	19.75
HCV	17.58

T cells
1P256 positive

Channel 14 to 255   Integral   10037
Peak   289 at 71%   In interval 98.02

Fig. 8.8 Flow cytometry parameters. The data in the figure were derived from the analysis of the T-cell line CEM, in each case analysing 10 000 events. Forward-angle light scatter, 90° light scatter and fluorescent data are plotted as frequency histograms using an ascending logarithmic horizontal scale divided into 256 channels. (**a**) Forward-angle light scatter (FALS). The intensity of the FALS signal is directly proportional to the volume of the cell being measured. The data have a clear bimodal distribution. There is a minor population of particles with a very low FALS signal (extreme left of distribution), probably due to cell debris and inorganic particles (described in flow cytometry jargon by a variety of epithets of Anglo-Saxon derivation), and a major population with a peak value just midway along the axis—these are the viable CEM cells. Although the standard polystyrene beads used to set up the instrument would have given a FALS distribution with a very low coefficient of variation, living cells—even from a cloned cell line—show marked variation in cell size. It is possible to examine a proportion of the above population only by setting an electronic 'gate'. In this instance the lower gate would be set to the right of the minor population, and the upper gate to the extreme right of the major population. It is then possible to confine the measurement of a second parameter purely to those cells falling within the preset FALS values: they are 'gated in'.

(**b**) 90° light scatter (90°-CLS). This signal is proportional to the volume of the cell, but is also affected by other parameters such as granularity, surface topography, etc. Although in this instance, where we are using a tumour-cell line with a homogeneous cytoplasm, this parameter yields little additional information over FALS alone, its true value may be appreciated with reference to Fig. 8.7(**a,b**).

Histograms (**c**) and (**d**) show the relative fluorescent intensity of cell populations stained with a directly conjugated irrelevant monoclonal antibody (**c**) or a pan-T monoclonal antibody (**d**). In each case, we are examining the fluorescence associated with the FALS 'gated-in' population alone. (**c**) The majority of the signals given by the cells in this population could not be detected above the electronic 'noise' of the instrument. In order to set the fluorescent intensity limits for this negative control, it is convenient to set the lower cursor (depicted as vertical line) to a channel number which excludes (to the left) about 95% of the population in the example shown. Around 5.3% of the cells fall in the interval between channels 14 and 255 (to the right of the cursor). (**d**) This population of cells has been analysed with the same instrument settings as in (**c**), and 98% of the 10 000 cells analysed gave a fluorescent signal falling in the channel interval defined in (**c**). They are the specifically stained population. The computing software used on this instrument can use much more precise definitions of the positive and negative populations and carry out a 'channel-by-channel' analysis to obtain full information from the data.

In examples (**c**) and (**d**) we have used electronic cursors to define the fluorescent population only for analysis and integration. It is possible, however, to define a 'gated-in' population, either alone or with reference to the FALS gates already set from histogram (**a**). One may then examine a third parameter in relation to cells of a certain size (perhaps lymphocytes rather than platelets) and with a certain fluorescent attribute (for example, pan-T-positive lymphocytes in a population of peripheral blood mononuclear cells). The ability to measure using correlated parameters on a per cell basis provides these instruments with exquisite analytical and preparative capabilities.

The emergence of flow cytometry as an important research and diagnostic tool is the result of three major developments: (i) the generation of monoclonal antibodies to a variety of cell antigens, used for the cell phenotyping; (ii) characterization and analysis of the functional significance of cell subsets and cell receptors; and (iii) the development of instrumentation which is relatively cheap, reliable and simple to use.

Typically, cells may be analysed at a rate of several hundred/second, but flow rates an order of magnitude higher are within the capabilities of the instruments.

MATERIALS

Cells to be investigated

Labelled antibody

2% paraformaldehyde in phosphate-buffered saline (PBS)

METHOD

1 Centrifuge 2×10^5 cells at 250 g for 5 min at 4°C. Discard the supernatant and agitate the pelleted cells.

2 Add 10 µl of each labelled antibody and incubate at 4°C for 30 min.

3 Centrifuge the mixture of cells and antibody at 250 g for 5 min at 4°C. Discard the supernatant and agitate the pelleted cells.

4 Fix cells with 2% paraformaldehyde in PBS.

5 Cells may be stored in the dark at 4°C for up to 1 week.

Technical applications

Clinical uses: immunophenotyping, cellular deficiencies, tumour-cell detection and tumour progression, cell kinetics, chromosomal analysis, and the analysis of ploidy.

Research interest: analysis of receptor distribution, cell surface and intracellular molecules (see Section 4.5.1 for methods on permeabilization of cells in preparation for flow cytometry), changes in expression, functional analysis of receptor behaviour.

8.6 Modification of cell-surface antigens

Continuous flow cytometry is used to quantify antibody binding to cell surfaces after various manipulations designed to yield information about the nature and distribution of the target molecule. The technique relies on efficient detection of the maximum number of cell-surface epitopes at all times. The antibody must be titrated for saturation binding (shown by plateau staining as in Fig. 4.1) with minimum non-specific binding, both before and after each treatment. Few of the treatments are totally devoid of side reactions; for example, enzymes often contain other contaminating enzymes. For maximum reliability, link a degradation experiment with resynthesis in the presence of specific inhibitors. Resynthesis experiments are not limited to permanent cell lines grown *in vitro*; even normal cells are capable of extensive short-term resynthesis of membrane components *in vitro*. The connectivity pathways shown in the flow chart (Fig. 8.9) should give useful and related information; however, not all the assays are necessary for each monoclonal antibody. The information to be gained from this general approach could be increased by

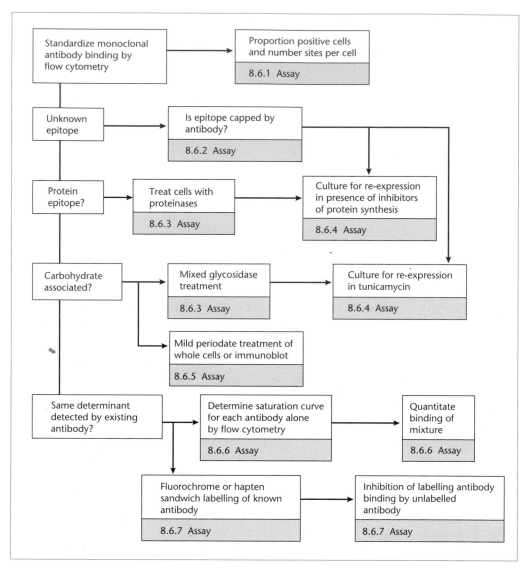

Fig. 8.9 **Determination of the chemical nature of unknown monoclonal antibody-defined epitope using flow cytometry.** The assay numbers refer to the technique in Section 8.6 for the measurement of antibody binding following the indicated treatment. The applicability of this general approach could be extended, where appropriate, by the inclusion of lipases and glycosidases or inhibition of antibody binding by mono- or oligosaccharides.

extending the range of useful reagents; for example, by inclusion of specific glycosidases, inhibition of antibody binding by mono- or oligosaccharides, lipases, etc.

8.6.1 Binding site distribution

To determine the distribution of antibody-binding sites on the cell population of interest with respect to: (i) proportion of total cells carrying the epitope; and (ii) the relative distribution of

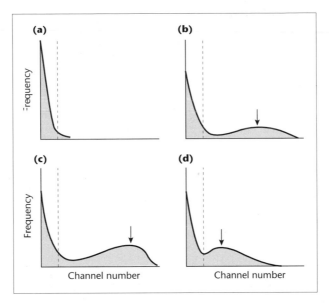

Fig. 8.10 **Distribution of fluorescence intensity in lymphocytes stained with monoclonal antibodies.**
Four illustrative histograms of flow cytometry data are shown; the horizontal logarithmic scale is divided into intervals of increasing fluorescence intensity, the vertical scale shows the frequency of cells at each level of relative fluorescence.

(a) When cells are reacted with an irrelevant monoclonal antibody, about 95% of the total population sampled (usually 10 000 cells) should fall within the first few channel numbers (to the left of the vertical line) and so define the proportion of lymphocytes that bind the irrelevant monoclonal antibody and fluorescent conjugate (if an indirect staining technique is used) non-specifically.

(b) Lymphocytes in this sample have been stained with a monoclonal antibody that binds to their surface membrane. To analyse the distribution, it is arbitrarily divided into two by placing the cursor (vertical line) in the same position as in histogram (a). Channels to the left of the line contain the 'non-specifically' stained population, whereas channels to the right contain 'specifically' stained cells, in this case about 50% of the total population sampled (value obtained by integrating the area under the curve). The modal or peak relative fluorescence, indicated by the arrow, is that showing the greatest frequency in any one channel.

(c) and (d) These histograms show different populations of lymphocytes stained with the same monoclonal antibody as in (b). Although approximately the same proportion of lymphocytes are positively stained, the population in (c) is brightly stained (modal fluorescence shifted to the right) whereas the population in (d) is weakly stained (modal fluorescence shifted to the left). If the antibody defined a lymphocyte receptor, then 50% of both populations in (c) and (d) would have this receptor but cells more frequently have receptors in (c) than in (d).

binding sites per cell in the positive population, it is most convenient to use a continuous-flow cytometer. An illustrative example is shown in Fig. 8.10.

8.6.2 Antibody-induced capping

This is a useful technique because: (i) the antibody can induce capping showing that the antigen is mobile in the membrane (or not!), which in turn can be informative; and (ii) it is a gentle and highly selective way to initiate resynthesis of the molecule of interest (e.g. compared to pro-teinase treatment).

Table 8.1 Enzymes for modification of cell-surface antigens on viable cells

Enzyme	Working concentration	Specificity
Proteinases		
Pronase	0.5 mg/ml ⎱	Multiple sites of hydrolysis
Papain*	0.3 mg/ml ⎰	along the polypeptide chain
Glycosidases†		
Neuraminidase	0.5 iu/ml	N-terminal sialic acid
Endoglycosidase H	5.0 iu/ml	Linkage between
		oligosaccharide and protein

* Add also 5 mg/ml cysteine–HCl to activate the enzyme.
† Use preparations of mixed glycosidases with caution, lack of modification of staining might be due to an insufficient concentration of a crucial glycosidase. In any case, endoglycosidase H has now largely replaced crude mixtures of glycosidases for this treatment, because the latter is frequently contaminated with proteinases.

Briefly, it involves the incubation of the cell population with antibody at 37°C for varying time periods. If modulation is incomplete or absent with the monoclonal antibody alone, then add an anti-immunoglobulin antibody as well as the monoclonal in a parallel assay. Even so, modulation of surface-antigen expression does not occur with all monoclonal antibodies.

8.6.3 Proteinase- or glycosidase-sensitive epitopes

MATERIALS
As in Section 8.2, but in addition:
Cells carrying the antigen of interest
Proteinases or glycosidases, as Table 8.1
Tissue culture medium
Fetal bovine serum (FBS)
Phosphate-buffered saline (PBS), containing 10 mM sodium azide

Note: *Azide is a dangerous chemical—do not discard down the sink.*

METHOD

1 Count cells and determine their viability by dye exclusion. Adjust to 5×10^6/ml in serum-free tissue culture medium. If necessary remove dead cells.
2 For each time point of the assay, mix 1 ml cell suspension with 1 ml enzyme (see Table 8.1), or 1 ml serum-free medium alone.
3 Incubate for 60 min in 37°C water bath with occasional mixing.
4 Add 8 ml ice-cold tissue culture medium containing 10% FBS to stop the reaction.
5 Wash twice by centrifugation (150 *g* for 10 min at 4°C) and label by indirect immunofluorescence for flow cytometry.

TECHNICAL NOTE
Always purchase the enzyme in its purest available form; this limits the number of contaminating enzymes and therefore the number of confusing side reactions.

Table 8.2 Inhibitors of protein synthesis, glycosylation and secretion

Inhibitor	Stock solution	Working concentration	Specificity
Paramycin dihydrochloride	1.0 mg/ml in water	1.5 µg/ml	Disrupts RNA. Forms amino acyl puromycin resulting in premature chain termination
Cyclohexamide	1.0 mg/ml in water	20 µg/ml	Blocks peptide synthesis by interfering with the ribosomes
Tunicamycin	1.0 mg/ml in DMSO*	1.0 µg/ml	Prevents addition of sugars to hydroxyl and amino groups of polypeptides
Monensin	1 mM in water	100 nM	Blocks processing of polypeptides by the Golgi apparatus, thus preventing secretion

* This inhibitor is dissolved in dimethyl sulphoxide (DMSO); add an equal volume of DMSO alone to a parallel cell culture to control for potential non-specific inhibition of resynthesis.

8.6.4 Inhibition of resynthesis

MATERIALS

As 8.6.3 above, but in addition:
Inhibitors as Table 8.2
Bovine serum albumin (BSA)

METHOD

1. After enzyme or antibody treatment, wash cell suspensions three times by centrifugation (150 g for 10 min at room temperature) in tissue culture medium containing 10% FBS.
2. Determine cell viability by dye exclusion and adjust to 10^6 cells/ml.
3. Prepare separate aliquots of enzyme-treated cells alone, enzyme-treated cells plus appropriate inhibitor (Table 8.2) and, where necessary, enzyme-treated cells plus solvent used to dissolve the enzyme inhibitor.
4. Culture overnight at 37°C in a humidified atmosphere containing 5% CO_2 in air.
5. Harvest the cells and wash twice by centrifugation using PBS containing 1% w/v BSA and 10 mM sodium azide.
6. Label by indirect immunofluorescence for flow cytometry.

8.6.5 Periodate treatment

MATERIALS

As 8.6.3 above, but in addition:
Sodium metaperiodate
Phosphate-buffered saline (PBS)

1　Dissolve sodium metaperiodate in PBS to 0.1 M, use fresh and keep in the dark.

2　Determine cell viability and adjust to 10^6 cells/ml.

3　For each time point, allow 2×1 ml aliquots of cells.

4　Add 10 µl stock periodate solution to 1 aliquot; the other will serve as untreated control.

5　Incubate at 4°C between 30 min and overnight.

6　Recover and wash cells by centrifugation (150 g for 10 min at room temperature) in PBS containing 10 mM sodium azide and 1% w/v BSA.

7　Label by indirect immunofluorescence for flow cytometry.

TECHNICAL NOTE

Under the mild conditions described here, cell-surface sialic acid residues are specifically oxidized and cell viability should be virtually unaffected. However, the reaction is relatively inefficient. If you are still in doubt, having obtained a negative result, we recommend that you use low-pH periodate pretreatment of an immunoblot, thus permitting the efficient oxidation of *cis*-vicindal diol groups.

8.6.6　Double antibody binding

For a proper assessment of additive or competitive binding, both antibodies should be used under saturating (plateau) conditions, and so must have been titrated. Aliquots of cells carrying the antigen of interest should be reacted either with antibody alone or with the two as a 1 : 1 mixture (label by indirect immunofluorescence for flow cytometry). Non-competitive binding of the two antibodies should result in a positive displacement of modal fluorescence intensity (peak staining shifted right). Competitive binding should result in the antibody mixture having a peak intensity equal to the peak of the brighter of the two antibodies alone.

It should be noted that it is desirable to label with each antibody at a consistent dilution, whether it is used alone or used in an antibody mixture, and yet maintain an equivalent protein concentration in each case. This may be achieved by diluting the monoclonal antibodies into an irrelevant protein solution, e.g. 0.1% fetal bovine serum. It is not a valid way of comparing different isotypes: IgM and IgG antibodies with precisely the same variable regions would not react with the same binding avidity or permit the same specificity and sensitivity of detection.

8.6.7　Competition with labelled standard

Label a reference monoclonal antibody by direct conjugation to a fluorochrome or by hapten conjugation for hapten sandwich labelling, then carry out a more precise assessment of competitive or non-competitive binding using different concentrations of the monoclonal as required for proper immunoassay. Where one is trying to compile a reference set of new monoclonal antibodies, it is desirable to avoid reselection of commonly occurring monoclonal antibodies. It is often possible to incorporate recurring antibodies into the primary screen and so favour the detection of less immunodominant clones. For example, a binding assay designed to detect IgG monoclonals by the use of a labelled anti-IgG Fc reagent could be 'spiked' by the addition of the F(ab')$_2$ fragment of an already banked monoclonal.

- The use of a control for non-specific binding (fluorescein-conjugated irrelevant monoclonal antibody of the same isotype) is crucial throughout all the manipulations described above. Chemical or enzyme treatment of a cell population might increase or decrease non-specific binding in an unpredictable manner.

- Results from these assays must be interpreted with the same caution as any data using these highly sensitive antibody probes. For example, lack of binding to a test-cell population might mean that the epitope is absent or merely inaccessible. Similarly, enzyme treatment of a cell surface could increase or decrease antibody binding by changing the accessibility of the binding site rather than through a direct effect on the epitope.

It is recommended that you optimize the staining protocol used in flow cytometry for the individual experiments and cells to be investigated.

8.7 Laser scanning confocal microscopy

8.7.1 Principles of laser scanning confocal microscopy

In this technique a focused laser beam is scanned across a specimen and light emitted from the specimen is collected point by point through a pinhole in front of a photomultiplier. The pinhole ensures that as the laser scans, information is only collected from one particular focal plane, i.e. it removes the out-of-focus information observed in conventional microscopy. An 'optical slice' through a specimen is produced, resolving detail within that particular slice and eliminating focus glare. Multiple wavelengths can be collected simultaneously, using filtering systems to direct light to separate photomultipliers. Although in flow cytometry a single 488-nm argon ion laser is used for most purposes, in confocal microscopy it is more common to have two or more lasers, most frequently a 'blue' and a 'green' laser (see Fig. 8.11). There is a difference in the dyes used. For flow cytometry, dyes are based on the 488-nm excitation laser used. But since the cell spends less than a millisecond in the laser beam, the dyes do not need to be as resistant to quenching as those used in confocal microscopy. Consequently, although fluorescein is suitable for both applications, because phycoerythrin quenches rapidly, other orange-red dyes such as Texas Red and rhodamine are more commonly used in confocal microscopy, i.e. the traditional dyes of the microscopist. Direct labelling of primary antibodies is a less sensitive process than flow cytometry, i.e. a system in which a single measurement is obtained for emission from the entire cell.

For most purposes, more sensitive indirect staining techniques are used. However, use of two monoclonal antibodies simultaneously for direct labelling creates a dilemma, since the indirect anti-mouse Ig labels could react with either of the primary antibodies. Some of the ways around this problem include the use of:

- one directly conjugated antibody for the highest-expressing of the two antigens being detected, combined with one indirect assay. The indirect technique is used first to detect one primary monoclonal antibody and then the directly conjugated primary antibody is used last; a normal-mouse-serum 'blocking' step is used between the two;

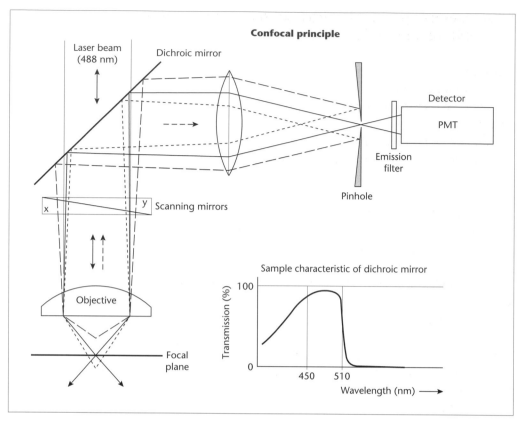

Fig. 8.11 Principles of confocal microscopy.

- different monoclonal immunoglobulin classes or isotypes for the primary antibodies, and then isotype-specific second antibodies, e.g. a combination of IgG and IgM, or an IgG_1 and IgG_{2a};
- two different species of primary antibody, e.g. one mouse monoclonal and one rabbit polyclonal, and the appropriate species-specific antibody.

Typically, staining is performed on either cryostat tissue sections or fixed cells on conventional slides. Tissues and cells may be fixed with solvents, such as: (i) cold acetone (generally good for preservation of antigenic sites); (ii) methanol; (iii) conventional agents of insolubilization such as paraformaldehyde; or (iv) cross-linking agents such as glutaraldehyde (poor for antigen preservation). Techniques are available that allow the recovery of antigens inactivated by paraffin embedding. Antibodies have been developed that will react with tissue that has been treated in this way. Antiquenching agents are normally used, to reduce quenching under the laser light, e.g. Vectashield (Vector Labs). A typical double-staining assay is illustrated below. This is used on tissue sections for detecting two molecules, using one primary monoclonal antibody and one primary rabbit (polyclonal) antibody. Incubation with free biotin and avidin is performed to neutralize natural avidin-binding activity in some tissues, but is not essential for all purposes, even when using avidin–biotin staining assays. Incubation volumes depend on the size of the area containing the tissue, but 30 μl is frequently enough.

8.7.2 Example protocol using laser scanning confocal microscopy as detection

MATERIALS

Cells to be investigated

Microscope slides and coverslips

Acetone

Phosphate-buffered saline (PBS)

0.5% w/v bovine serum albumin (BSA) in PBS

Avidin D

Biotin

Primary monoclonal antibody

Biotinylated anti-mouse antibody (secondary antibody)

Steptavidin–fluorescein isothiocyanate (FITC)

Primary rabbit antibody

Anti-rabbit antibody tetramethyl rhodamine isothiocyanate (TRITC)

Varnish

Antiquenching agent

METHOD

  1 Air-dry sections for 20 min in a fume hood, then fix with cold acetone for 10 min.
  2 Perform serial washes with:

   $1 \times$ PBS for 1 min;

   $3 \times 0.5\%$ BSA in PBS for 5 min.
  3 Add one drop of avidin D (Vectashield) to the section and incubate for 15 min.
  4 Wash in $3 \times 0.5\%$ BSA in PBS for 5 min.
  5 Add 1 drop of biotin to the section and incubate for 15 min.
  6 Wash in $3 \times 0.5\%$ BSA/PBS for 5 min.
  7 Incubate with 30 µl monoclonal antibody.
  8 Wash in 0.5% BSA in PBS for 5 min.
  9 Incubate with biotinylated anti-mouse antibody for 30 min.
 10 Wash in 0.5% BSA in PBS for 5 min.
 11 Incubate with streptavidin–FITC for 30 min.
 12 Wash in 0.5% BSA in PBS for 5 min.
 13 Incubate with rabbit primary antibody for 30 min.
 14 Wash in 0.5% BSA in PBS for 5 min.
 15 Incubate with pig anti-rabbit TRITC for 30 min.
 16 Wash in $2 \times 0.5\%$ BSA/PBS three times for 5 min.
 17 Rinse in PBS (this may improve life of antiquencher).
 18 Mount in antiquenching agent, and varnish.

It is recommended that the labelling protocol used in laser confocal microscopy is optimized for the individual experiments and cells being investigated.

8.8 Further reading

Allan, V.J. (2000) *Protein Localization by Fluorescence Microscopy: A Practical Approach.* Oxford University Press, Oxford.

Baumgarth, N. & Roederer, M. (2000) A practical approach to multicolor flow cytometry for immunophenotyping. *J Immunol Meth* **243**(1–2), 77–97.

De Jong, M.O., Rozemuller, H., Bauman, J.G.J. & Visser, J.W.M. (1995) Biotinylation of interleukin-2(IL-2) for flow cytometric analysis of IL-2 receptor expression. *J Immunol Meth* **184**, 101–112.

Griwatz, C., Brandt, B., Assmann, G. & Zanker, K.S. (1995) An immunological enrichment method for epithelial cells from peripheral blood. *J Immunol Meth* **183**(2), 251–65.

Haugland, R.P. (2001) *Handbook of Fluorescent Probes and Research Chemicals,* 8th edn. Molecular Probes Inc.

Kerr, M.A. & Thorpe, R. (1994) *Immunochemistry LABFAX BIOS* Blackwell Science, Oxford.

Lacey, A.J. (1999) *Light Microscopy in Biology—A Practical Approach,* 2nd edn. Oxford University Press, Oxford.

Ling, N.R. (2000) Immunoglobulin production by culture human lymphocytes [Review]. *J Immunol Meth* **238**, 3–15.

Lyons, A.B. (2000) Analysing cell division *in vivo* and *in vitro* using flow cytometric measurement of CFSE dye dilution. *J Immunol Meth* **243**(1–2), 147–154.

Marquez, M.G., Galeano, A., Olmos, S. & Roux, M.E. (2000) Flow cytometric analysis of intestinal intraepithelial lymphocytes in a model of immunodeficiency in Wistar rats. *Cytometry* **41**(2), 115–122.

Ormerod, M. (2000) *Flow Cytometry—A Practical Approach,* 3rd edn. Oxford University Press, Oxford.

Phillips, T.M. & Dickens, B.F.(2000) *Affinity and Immunoaffinity Purification Techniques.* Eaton Pub Co, Biotechniques Press, Westborough MA.

Robinson, J.P., Darzynkiewicz, Z., Rabinovitch, P. *et al.* (eds) (1997) *Current Protocols in Cytometry.* John Wiley & Sons, New York.

Roden, M.M., Lee, K.H., Panelli, M.C. & Marincola, F.M. (1999) A novel cytolysis assay using fluorescent labelling and quantitative fluorescent scanning technology *J Immunol Meth* **226**, 29–41.

Rowland-Jones, S.L. & McMichael, A. (2000) *Lymphocytes: A Practical Approach.* Oxford University Press, Oxford.

Sabri, S., Richelme, F., Pierres, A., Benoliel, M. & Bongrand, P. (1997) Interest of image processing in cell biology and immunology. *J Immunol Meth* **208**, 1–27.

Shapiro, H.M. (1994) *Practical Flow Cytometry*, 3rd edn. Alan R Liss, New York.

Steiner, G.E., Ecker, R.C., Kramer, G., Stockenhuber, F. & Marberger, M.J. (2000) Automated data acquisition by confocal laser scanning microscopy and image analysis of triple stained immuno-fluorescent leucocytes in tissue. *J Immunol Meth* **237**, 39–50.

Steyger, P. (1999) Assessing confocal microscopy systems for purchase. *Methods* **18**, 435–446.

Todd, D., Singh, A.J., Greiner, D.L., Mordes, J.P., Rossini, A.A. & Bortell, R. (1999) A new isolation method for rat intraepithelial lymphocytes. *J Immunol Meth* **224**, 111–27.

Wouters, C., Bossuyt, X., Ceuppens, J. & Stevens, E.A. (2000) Comparative study of two cytofluorometric methods of analysis. *J Immunol Meth* **234**, 89–98.

Lymphocyte function

9.1 Enumeration of antibody-secreting cells *in vitro*

Before even contemplating biological assay it is essential to be aware that biological materials do not behave in an exactly similar manner between laboratories and so each system must be standardized for research purposes.

Plasma cells synthesize antibody for secretion and this can be used to quantify the number of antibody-producing cells in an organ. The basic assay developed by Jerne and Nordin can be used to detect cells producing antibody against erythrocyte antigens. Spleen cells from immune mice are incubated in an agar gel with the immunizing erythrocytes. After the addition of complement, the erythrocytes in the locality of the plasma cells are lysed, producing macroscopic holes or plaques in the erythrocyte suspension. This relatively simple and robust assay has undergone several modifications to improve its convenience and application range.

9.1.1 Enumeration of total plasma cells by reverse Jerne plaque assay

This technique is useful for the enumeration of total immunoglobulin-secreting cells. Secreted immunoglobulin is captured by protein A coated onto indicator erythrocytes, which are then lysed by the addition of a developing anti-immunoglobulin serum plus complement.

Preparation in advance—coating of sheep erythrocytes with protein A

MATERIALS AND EQUIPMENT
Sheep red blood cells (SRBC) in Alsever's solution
0.14 M sodium chloride in distilled water (saline)
Protein A (2 mg/ml in saline)

Chromic chloride (0.1 mg/ml in saline)
Phosphate-buffered saline (PBS)

METHOD

1 Wash SRBC six times in saline by centrifugation (300 *g* for 10 min at room temperature).
2 Add 1 ml of protein A solution (2 mg/ml initial concentration) to 1 ml of packed erythrocytes.
3 Add 6 ml of chromic chloride solution (0.1 mg/ml) dropwise. After mixing add 10 ml saline and incubate overnight at 4°C.
4 Wash the erythrocytes three times by centrifugation (300 *g* for 10 min at room temperature) and resuspend to 10% v/v in PBS.

Coated erythrocytes may be stored at 4°C and should be used within 1 week.

Assay

MATERIALS AND EQUIPMENT

Cell suspension for assay, e.g. spleen from immunized mouse
Protein A-coated erythrocytes (prepared as above)
Phosphate-buffered saline (PBS)
Agarose, 1.8% w/v in distilled water
Tissue culture medium (three times concentrated)
Bovine serum albumin (BSA) 7% w/v in PBS
Anti-mouse immunoglobulin, developing serum
Guinea-pig serum, as complement source
Plastic Petri dishes, 50 mm

METHOD

1 Mix 14 ml agarose solution with 5.5 ml of tissue culture medium, which has been concentrated three times, and add 1.5 ml of BSA solution.
2 Dispense 0.7 ml volumes of agarose mixture into glass test tubes in a water bath at 45°C.
3 For each assay dish add 0.2 ml of lymphoid cell suspension, 0.1 ml of anti-immunoglobulin serum and 0.05 ml of protein A-coated sheep erythrocytes to each tube containing 0.7 ml agarose mixture. Mix thoroughly and pour into a plastic Petri dish. Swirl the dish to ensure an even covering of agarose–cell suspension.
4 Incubate for 1–1.5 h in a humid 37°C incubator gassed with 5% CO_2 in air.
5 Add 1 ml of diluted guinea-pig serum, as a complement source (the dilution must be predetermined empirically) and continue incubation at 37°C until haemolytic plaques are visible (within 30–60 min).
6 Count the number of haemolytic plaques and calculate the number of antibody-secreting cells in the original cell suspension.

TECHNICAL NOTES

• The optimal dilution of anti-immunoglobulin serum and complement source must be determined.
• Illuminate the assay dish with light at a low angle of incidence to aid visualization of the plaques. They will appear as uniform dark holes in a light, birefringent layer of erythrocytes.

- The cell suspension for assay should be used at a concentration to give not more than 100–200 plaques per assay dish.

9.1.2 Enumeration of antigen-specific plasma cells by Jerne plaque assay

The Jerne haemolytic plaque-forming cell technique uses the original immunogen, sheep erythrocytes (SRBC), in an antibody–antigen binding reaction to detect antibody-secreting plasma cells. In this case, the addition of complement results in the formation of a lytic halo associated only with SRBC antigen-secreting plasma cells.

Preparation in advance

- Immunize two mice with 2×10^8 SRBC given intraperitoneally 5 days before the experiment.
- *Agar underlay.* Make up 1.4% Difco Bacto Agar in Hanks' saline. Melt the agar in a microwave oven and then directly over a bunsen flame to get rid of all of the lumps if necessary. Take care to swirl the agar gently to avoid charring. Add enough of the agar solution to a 5-cm plastic Petri dish to just cover its base. An underlay is used to ensure that the base of the assay dish is reasonably flat, so pouring must be done on a levelled surface.
- *Agar overlay.* Prepare 0.7% agar solution in Hanks' saline containing 0.5 mg/ml of diethylaminoethyl (DEAE)–dextran (final concentration). DEAE–dextran is used to prevent anti-complementary activity of the agar. Alternatively, use the more expensive agarose as in the previous section.

MATERIALS AND EQUIPMENT
SRBC-immunized mice
2–4-week-old sheep blood in Alsever's solution
Agar overlay
Petri dishes containing agar underlay
Hank's saline, without phenol red indicator dye
Water bath, 45°C
Guinea-pig serum, as complement source

METHOD

1 Wash SRBC three times in Hank's saline by centrifugation (300 g for 10 min at room temperature). Adjust to 20% v/v after resuspension in Hank's saline.
2 Remove spleens from mice and prepare a single-cell suspension by teasing them apart with forceps into ice-cold saline. Discard the fibrous connective tissue that remains.
3 Suck suspension in and out of a Pasteur pipette to disperse the cells; it is not usually necessary to let the cells stand to settle out the small aggregates. (To avoid loss and damage to the plasma cells do not filter cells through nylon wool and do not use a syringe and needle for cell dispersion.)
4 Adjust to a total volume of 2.5 ml in Hank's saline.
5 Dilute 1 ml of the spleen-cell suspension 1 : 10 and 1 : 100 with Hank's saline.
6 Pipette out 0.8 ml of overlay into small test tubes in a 45°C water bath. Use a warm pipette.
7 Add 0.25 ml of the original or diluted spleen-cell suspensions to each assay dish according to the Protocol.

Continued on p. 264

	Dish number		
	1	2	3
Spleen-cell suspension (ml)	0.25	0.25	0.25
(initial dilution)	(neat)	(1 : 10)	(1 : 100)
Agar overlay (ml) ⎫	⎧ 0.80 ml ⎫		
SRBC (20%) (ml) ⎭	⎩ 0.15 ml ⎭	⟶	
Fraction of spleen assayed	1/10	1/100	1/1000

8 Place dish on a levelled surface.

9 Add 0.15 ml SRBC suspension to each overlay tube just before use. Mix well by flicking the end of the tube.

10 Add overlay to dish and mix thoroughly with spleen cells.

11 Allow agar to set and add 1.0 ml of a 1 : 10 dilution of guinea-pig serum as a source of complement.

12 Incubate dishes at 37°C for 1–1.5 h. If the plaques are not clear when the dishes are removed from the incubator, allow them to stand at room temperature for about 30 min before counting.

Plaques can be seen by holding the Petri dish up to the light (without its lid), but counting is easier and more accurate if you use a low-power binocular microscope and draw lines on the bottom of the dish. Only direct plaques (mainly IgM antibody) are detected by the method described above because of the high haemolytic efficiency of this antibody class. In theory, a single molecule of IgM can initiate the complement cascade and cause SRBC lysis. To detect IgG plaques increase the number of molecules binding to any one site (two adjacent molecules of IgG are required to activate the complement sequence via the classical pathway); plaques must therefore be developed with an antiserum against mouse immunoglobulin. This method of detecting so-called 'indirect' plaques can be used to assay each of the mouse IgG subclasses using appropriate subclass-specific antisera.

Indirect plaques

MATERIALS AND EQUIPMENT

As preceding method, plus rabbit anti-mouse immunoglobulin (anti-Ig)

METHOD

1 Prepare a plaquing mixture as in the preceding method (steps 1–10) but instead of adding complement, add 0.1 ml of a 1 : 10 dilution of rabbit anti-mouse Ig and incubate at 37°C for 45 min.

2 Wash away the developing antiserum by flooding the plate twice with Hank's saline.

3 Add l ml of 1 : 10 dilution of guinea-pig serum. Incubate for 45 min at 37°C.

Plaques may be clearer if the plates are left at room temperature for 30 min before counting. Under experimental conditions it is necessary to titrate the developing antiserum until the maximum number of plaques are obtained. The direct, or 'IgM', plaques are then subtracted from the total to give the number of 'IgG' plaques. The technique as described can be used to enumerate antibody-producing cells in any species. In the case of chicken antibody-producing cells you must use an homologous serum as a source of complement. Chicken antibody does not fix the first component of mammalian complement (C1q). Alternatively, develop both IgM and IgG plaques using rabbit anti-chicken immunoglobulin class-specific antisera and guinea-pig complement.

TECHNICAL NOTES
- If large numbers of SRBC are used for immunization (10^6–10^9 per mouse) the peak of the direct plaque-forming-cell (PFC) response is 4 days; at lower doses (10^4–10^5 per mouse) the peak of the direct response is day 5. However, the numbers of indirect plaques peak at day 5–6 after immunization. Day 5 is usually an acceptable compromise for measuring both the direct and indirect PFC response to SRBC. Other antigens may show different kinetics.
- At doses of SRBC of 10^4 and below, the route of immunization is important: intravenous injection gives more PFCs than intraperitoneal injection. Above 10^5 SRBC per mouse both routes of administration give approximately the same number of plaques.
- Use a spleen dilution giving approximately 200–300 plaques per assay plate. As cell density increases plaque size decreases and PFC number is not linear.
- Some anti-immunoglobulin developing sera suppress IgM direct plaques while revealing IgG indirect plaques. Once the optimum dilution for plaque development has been determined, it is necessary to test for suppression of direct plaques by the serum, using PFC response, 3 days after SRBC immunization. The response is low but virtually all are IgM direct plaques.

The haemolytic plaque method can be extended using antigen coupled to erythrocyte-indicator cells. This, of course, allows more widespread application of the technique, especially in the technically more convenient Cunningham modification.

9.2 Cunningham plaque assay

9.2.1 Cunningham assay for plaque-forming cells

This assay was modified by Cunningham from the Jerne haemolytic plaque assay (Section 9.1) and can be used to enumerate antibody-forming cells against soluble antigens (haptens) conjugated to the surface of indicator erythrocytes, e.g. dinitrophenol (DNP) or trinitrophenol (TNP).

9.2.2 Preparation of DNP- or TNP-conjugated erythrocytes

There are three methods of sensitizing the indicator erythrocytes (e.g. sheep or horse RBC):
1 *Chemical.* TNP coupled directly to the erythrocytes—a more gentle reaction than dinitrophenylation, and TNP cross-reacts strongly with DNP.

2 *Dinitrophenylated, non-complement fixing antibodies.* As chicken antibodies do not fix mammalian complement, DNP–chicken anti-erythrocyte antibodies may be used to sensitize indicator cells at subagglutinating doses. Using this assay method for DNP plaques, fowl γ-globulin (FγG) cannot then be used as a carrier molecule.

3 *Dinitrophenylated fragments of mammalian anti-erythrocyte antibodies.* Addition of whole DNP–rabbit IgG anti-SRBC to the SRBC indicator cells would cause haemolysis, so the dinitrophenylated non-complement-fixing Fab fragment must be used to sensitize erythrocytes. DNP–Fab will still bind to the erythrocytes but cannot induce agglutination or fix complement.

9.2.3 Trinitrophenylation of erythrocytes

MATERIALS AND EQUIPMENT

Erythrocytes, horse or sheep
2,4,6-trinitrobenzene sulphonic acid (TNP)
Glycyl glycine
Phosphate-buffered saline (PBS)

METHOD

1 Prepare a phosphate buffer solution by dissolving 5.62 g sodium dihydrogen phosphate dihydrate and 16.19 g disodium hydrogen phosphate in 1 l water. This solution is pH 7.2 and isotonic with sheep erythrocytes (SRBC) (289 mosmol) and so causes less SRBC lysis than the original method which used 0.28 M cacodylate buffer, pH 6.9.

2 Wash erythrocytes three times with PBS by centrifugation at 300 g for 10 min at room temperature.

3 Resuspend 4 ml of packed cells in 16 ml phosphate buffer, and react with trinitrobenzene sulphonic acid according to the Protocol.

4 Mix TNP solution with cells for 30 min on a magnetic stirrer at room temperature.

5 Add 50 ml of a solution of glycyl glycine (initial concentration of 2 mg/ml) in phosphate buffer to each aliquot to react the free TNP sulphonate.

6 Wash three times in PBS by centrifugation (300 g for 10 min) and store at 4°C.

Determine the optimum conditions for sensitization according to Section 9.2.7.

	Tube number				Protocol.
	1	2	3	4	
TNP in 2 ml buffer (mg)	25	30	35	40	
20% suspension SRBC (ml)	5———————————→				

9.2.4 DNP–Fab' anti-sheep erythrocyte (SRBC) sensilization

Preparation of Fab anti-SRBC

The antiserum prepared in Section 3.11 is suitable for this purpose. This method described works well but it is not the only route that may be used to prepare Fab or Fab'.

MATERIALS AND EQUIPMENT
Rabbit anti-sheep erythrocyte (anti-SRBC) hyperimmune serum
Other materials and equipment required—see the following sections: Sections 1.3, 1.7, 2.12, 3.11, 4.8, 7.5 and Appendix B.1.2.

METHOD

1 Isolate the IgG fraction of the antiserum by diethylaminoethyl (DEAE)–cellulose ion-exchange chromatography (see Section 1.3).

2 After concentration, dialyse the IgG anti-SRBC against 0.1 M sodium acetate and digest with pepsin to obtain the $F(ab')_2$ fragment (see Sections 1.7 and 2.12).

3 Apply the digest to a Sephacryl S-200 column equilibrated with PBS, recover the $F(ab')_2$ peak, concentrate and dialyse against PBS (see Appendix B.1.2).
   Store a small sample at –20°C for testing later.

4 Reduce the $F(ab')_2$ fragments with 0.02 M dithiothreitol for 30 min at 37°C.

5 Alkylate with 0.05 M iodoacetamide for 10 min at room temperature.

6 Dialyse Fab' mixture overnight against PBS.
   Reduction and alkylation of the $F(ab')_2$ is usually sufficient to prevent haemagglutination and so it is not necessary to fractionate the mixture any further.

7 Dinitrophenylate the Fab' anti-SRBC, and determine the average number of DNP groups per Fab' molecule (see Section 4.8).

8 Test each preparation by haemagglutination (see Section 3.11) and haemolysis (see Section 7.5) according to the Protocol (see below).

Protocol.

Preparation number	Description	Haemagglutinin titre	Haemolysin titre
1	Rabbit anti-SRBC whole serum		
2	IgG anti-SRBC		
3	$F(ab')_2$ anti-SRBC		
4	Fab' anti-SRBC		
5	Fab' anti-SRBC + goat or sheep anti-rabbit immunoglobulin		
6	DNP–Fab' anti-SRBC		
7	DNP–Fab' anti-SRBC + goat or sheep anti-rabbit immunoglobulin		

The haemagglutination and haemolysis test should be carried out after each stage of the procedure, and the procedure continued only if the results of the tests are satisfactory.

9.2.5 Sensitization of indicator cells

MATERIALS AND EQUIPMENT
Sheep erythrocytes
DNP–Fab' anti-SRBC
Phosphate-buffered saline (PBS)

METHOD

1 Wash SRBC three times in PBS by centrifugation (300 *g* for 10 min at room temperature) and adjust to a final concentration of 40% v/v.
2 Sensitize aliquots of SRBC according to the Protocol.

Protocol.

	Aliquot number					
	1	2	3	4	5	6
DNP–Fab' anti-SRBC added (µl) (initial conc. 1 mg/ml)	1	5	10	20	40	100
SRBC 40% v/v suspension (ml)	1——————————————————→					

3 Incubate at 37°C for 30 min, mixing occasionally.
4 Wash five times with PBS by centrifugation (300 *g* for 10 min at room temperature) to remove unbound protein.
5 Adjust cell concentration to 20% v/v and store at 4°C.
Determine the optimum conditions for sensitization as described in Section 9.2.7.

TECHNICAL NOTES
• Use 2–3-week-old SRBC, but fresh horse RBC.
• The sensitized erythrocytes are stable for 1 week at 4°C. It is, however, advisable to wash the cells each time before use.

9.2.6 Preparation of assay chambers

MATERIALS AND EQUIPMENT
Glass microscope slides
Adhesive tape, double-sided
Photographic roller

METHOD

1 Wash slides overnight in a strong solution of a free rinsing detergent and rinse thoroughly in distilled water. Soak overnight in absolute ethanol. Air dry the slides. Clean slides are absolutely essential to allow bubble-free filling of the assay chambers.
2 Place 20 slides in a line with their long edges adjacent and stick double-sided tape along each edge and along the centre of the row (see Fig. 9.1).

Continued

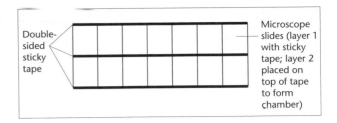

Fig. 9.1 Double layer of slides held together with double-sided tape.
Slides are then cut apart, giving two culture compartments for each slide pair.

3 Remove the backing from the tape and add a second row of slides to complete the sandwich.
4 Roll the slides firmly with a photographic roller to seal the chambers.
5 Separate adjacent slides.

9.2.7 Anti-DNP assay

Direct plaque detection

MATERIALS AND EQUIPMENT

Dinitrophenyl–fowl γ-globulin (DNP–FγG)-, or DNP–keyhole limpet haemocyanin (DNP–KLH)-primed mice

Trinitrophenyl (TNP)-, or dinitrophenyl (DNP)-sensitized sheep erythrocytes (SRBC)

Tissue culture medium

Fetal bovine serum (FBS)

Guinea-pig serum, as complement source (fresh or preserved serum)

Assay chambers

50 : 50 mixture of paraffin wax and petroleum jelly on hot plate

Micro-titre tray, U-shaped

Dropping pipettes (18-gauge needle with end cut square attached to a 1-ml syringe barrel delivers a constant but approximate 25 µl) or automatic pipette

METHOD

1 Remove the spleens from two or three mice and prepare a single-cell suspension as described in Section 6.3.
2 Adjust to 10^7 lymphocytes/ml.
3 Place 25 µl of medium into each well of the microtitre tray to be used.
4 Add 25 µl of 20% sensitized erythrocyte suspension.
5 Add 100 µl of spleen-cell suspension.
6 Add 25 µl of neat guinea-pig serum absorbed with SRBC (see Section 11.10.2, Technical notes).
7 Mix the suspension in each well of the tray and load into an assay chamber with a Pasteur pipette.
8 When both chambers are full, seal edges by dipping into paraffin wax–petroleum jelly mixture.
9 Incubate at 37°C and examine at 30, 45, 60 and 90 min.

Continued on p. 270

10 Remove all the assay chambers as soon as plaques are clearly visible to the naked eye.

11 Count the number of plaques per chamber using a low-power binocular microscope.

12 Calculate the number of plaques per total spleen for each group, and plot a graph of plaque-forming cells (PFCs) against volume or concentration of sensitizing agent, as shown in Fig. 9.2.

Use this optimum volume or concentration of sensitizing agent in all future assays.

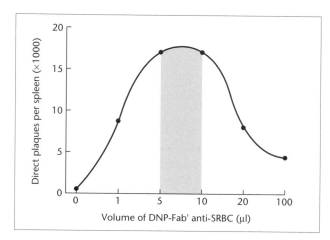

Fig. 9.2 Relationship between number of anti-DNP plaques and volume of DNP-Fab' anti-SRBC used to sensitize indicator cells. The optimal volume for sensitization within the tinted area would be used in routine assays.

TECHNICAL NOTES

- It is technically more convenient to remove clumps from the spleen suspensions by settling them through 1 ml of fetal bovine serum instead of filtering through nylon wool.
- It is not necessary to perform replicates of each assay point; the major source of experimental variation is the likely difference between mice receiving the same immunogen or similar numbers of transferred cells. Immunization relies upon cell proliferation and so the experimental error arises exponentially.
- Use a 37°C incubator without forced air circulation: any vibration will prevent uniform settling of the erythrocytes.
- Use a low angle of incidence for the light when counting the plaques under the microscope. The plaques will appear as dark holes in the birefringent layer of erythrocytes.

In the assay described above, direct (mainly IgM) plaques were detected; indirect (mainly IgG) plaques may be detected by the addition of a developing serum, e.g. anti-mouse immunoglobulin, as described below.

Indirect plaque detection

MATERIALS AND EQUIPMENT

Optimally sensitized erythrocytes (see Direct plaque detection above and Fig. 9.2)

Rabbit anti-mouse immunoglobulin

Other materials and equipment as given for previous section

1   Dilute the anti-immunoglobulin serum with PBS as shown in the Protocol.

Protocol.

	Tube number				
	1	2	3	4	5
PBS (ml)	0.8	0.5			
Antiserum (ml)	0.2				
Dilution	1 : 10	1 : 20	1 : 40	1 : 80	1 : 160

mix | *mix* | etc.

0.5 ml   0.5 ml

2   Add 25 µl of each dilution to corresponding wells of the microtitre tray.
3   Repeat the assay as in previous section, but omit the 25 µl of medium from each well of the tray; this has been replaced by the anti-immunoglobulin serum.
4   Determine the dilution of developing serum giving the maximum number of plaques.

TECHNICAL NOTES

- The IgG plaques are taken to be the difference between the total number of developed plaques and the number of direct plaques.
- Some anti-Ig sera inhibit IgM plaques while developing IgG plaques. If this is found to be the case in your system, then no correction of the number of developed plaques is required.
- Test for the inhibition of direct plaque formation as follows. Determine IgM (direct) plaques with and without anti-Ig using either: (a) spleen cells from an animal 4 days after antigen priming; or (b) spleen cells from an animal primed with a highly substituted carrier. This will prime for an IgM response but not allow IgG switching.

Although a great deal of time is spent standardizing reagents, application of the assay to an experimental situation is extremely rapid.

9.3 Organ culture for studying antibody production

Most studies of *in vitro* immune responses use isolated preparations of cells rather than organized structural arrangements as found within lymphoid organs. Hoffmann *et al.* (1995) describe a straightforward technique in which explants of spleen may be successfully cultured *in vitro* with little loss of cell viability over a 7-day culture. Tissue slices 5–8 mm in diameter and 400 µm thick are cut from cores of human spleen and cultured on nucleopore membranes resting on gel sponges immersed in tissue culture medium. Studies have shown that the spontaneous production of immunoglobulin can be more rapid and reach higher levels than that found with isolated cell preparations from the same tissue. Cells can be cultured with substances, e.g. mitogens, to manipulate the response, but larger doses are needed than for isolated cell culture.

9.3.1 Solid-phase detection of antibody-forming cells

ELISPOT (enzyme-linked immunospot)

This is an alternative to the Jerne and Nordin plaque technique for antibody-forming cells that is similar in principle to an ELISA, except that the antibody to be assayed is generated by secreting cells cultured in antigen-coated wells. In the assay cells are allowed to settle on the antigen-coated surface and secreted antibody binds to the antigen in the immediate vicinity of the cell. Cells are then washed away and bound antibody is revealed by the addition of an enzyme-linked second antibody. The substrate is added in agarose to allow only limited diffusion of the coloured products so that visible 'spots', corresponding to plasma cells, can be counted.

MATERIALS AND EQUIPMENT
Nunc-Linbro 24-well plates
Antigen, e.g. human serum albumin (HSA)
Phosphate-buffered saline (PBS)
PBS with 0.05% v/v Tween 20
Mouse immunized with HSA
Horseradish peroxidase-conjugated anti-mouse immunoglobulin in PBS with 0.05% Tween 20 containing 1% w/v bovine serum albumin (BSA)
ELISA conjugate buffer (PBS with 0.05% Tween 20 containing 1% w/v bovine serum albumin (BSA))
3-amino-9-ethylcarbazole in 0.1 M sodium acetate, pH 5.0
Agarose

METHOD

1 Coat each well of a 24-well plate with 500 µl of a 10 µg/ml solution of antigen in PBS.
2 Leave to incubate at 4°C overnight.
3 Wash plate with PBS containing 0.05% Tween.
4 Wash plate twice with PBS alone.
5 Prepare a single-cell suspension from the spleen of the immunized mouse.
6 After washing in tissue culture medium containing 5% fetal bovine serum, prepare a series of dilutions of spleen cells (between 2×10^4 and 2×10^6 lymphocytes/ml) and add 500 µl of each spleen-cell suspension to different antigen-coated wells.
7 Incubate the plate, without disturbance, for 1 h at 37°C in a humid atmosphere containing 5% CO_2 in air.
8 Wash plates with cold PBS–Tween until all adherent cells are removed.
9 Add 500 µl of appropriate dilution (usually 1 : 500–1 : 2000) of horseradish peroxidase-conjugated anti-mouse immunoglobulin in conjugate buffer.
10 Incubate at 37°C for 1 h.
11 Wash three times with PBS–Tween.

Continued

12 Mix 4 volumes ELISPOT substrate (3-amino-9-ethylcarbazole) with 1 volume molten 3% agarose in 0.1 M sodium acetate buffer, pH 5.0, and, before it sets, add 500 μl to each well.

13 Allow the agarose to set on a levelling table and then incubate at 37°C for 1 h.

14 Coloured spots should be seen, which correspond to the former positions of individual antibody-secreting cells. They are most easily counted with a microscope using low-power magnification (× 6.4).

9.4 Lymphocyte circulation

Lymphocytes do not circulate in a random manner—there is a functional division of lymphocytes into the so-called recirculating and non-recirculating pools. A full knowledge of the parameters affecting the passage of cells from one pool to the other during the immune response is essential. Cells show set migration patterns during ontogeny, moving, for example, from the central to the peripheral lymphoid organs. The traffic pattern of lymphocytes may be followed using radioisotope- or fluorescein-labelled cells as detailed below.

9.4.1 Ontogenic migration patterns

Dividing cells in the primary lymphoid organs may be labelled by an intraorgan infusion of ^{3}H-thymidine or ^{131}I-iododeoxyuridine.

Caution: It is essential to minimize the effect of 'spill-over' of the labelled material into the peripheral tissues, and so the animal is 'flooded' by an intravenous injection of non-radioactive DNA analogue.

Isotopically labelled cells in the peripheral lymphoid organs may then be identified by auto-radiography of tissue sections as described in Section 8.2.3. Please refer to the following websites for comprehensive details on radioisotope health and safety procedures as well as useful information regarding detection and half-life:

http://www.practicingsafescience.org
http://www.hse.gov.uk

9.4.2 Lymphocyte 'homing'

If lymphocytes are removed from an animal, isotopically labelled *in vitro* and returned to a syngeneic recipient, they show definite migration patterns, localizing within different organs at different times.

MATERIALS AND EQUIPMENT
Inbred mice
Sodium ^{51}chromate (Na^{51}CrO$_4$)
Gamma spectrometer

1 Prepare a lymph-node suspension from two to four donor mice (Section 6.3).

2 Count and adjust the suspension to 10^8 viable lymphocytes/ml.

3 Incubate 1 ml of cells with 11.1×10^5 Bq Na^{51}CrO$_4$ for 30 min at 37°C in tissue culture medium buffered with HEPES (20 mM) and containing 5% fetal bovine serum.

4 Wash the cells five times by centrifugation and resuspend in 2 ml of medium.

5 Inject 5×10^6 cells intravenously into each of 12 recipients, and retain an aliquot of 5×10^6 cells for γ counting.

6 Kill three recipient mice at 4, 24, 48 and 72 h postinjection.

7 Remove the thymus, spleen, mesenteric lymph nodes and liver from each recipient and count the amount of isotope in each organ. (^{51}Cr is a high-energy γ emitter and therefore whole-organ counting is possible.) Count also the aliquot of 5×10^6 original cells.

8 Calculate the amount of radioactivity in each organ as a percentage of the original counts injected.

9 Plot a graph of percentage radioactivity against time for each organ.

TECHNICAL NOTES

- Indium-111 is an alternative label for cells.
- The technique may also use fluorescently-labelled cells and confocal microscopy to identify the trafficking of cells to other organs (see Section 9.4.4).

Interpretation of results

The percentage radioactivity per organ is an estimate of the proportion of lymphocytes localizing in that organ.

The ratio of counts localizing in the spleen relative to the liver is a good estimate of the viability of the original lymphocyte suspension. If the suspension has a high viability the index is high, and vice versa. The ratio of spleen : liver localization also changes if cells are coated, but not necessarily killed, with anti-membrane antibodies.

Lymphocyte suspensions with high viability pass from the blood and localize predominantly in the spleen. Eventually cells leave the spleen and enter the lymph nodes, as shown by the change in radioactivity of each organ with time. No re-injected cells were detected in the thymus; the thymus is virtually excluded from the recirculation pathway of immunocompetent lymphocytes once they have left the thymic cortex. The mature T lymphocytes in the thymic medulla seem to be a long-term resident population, members of which recirculate only rarely. These data were obtained with thoracic-duct lymphocytes which have almost 100% viability. It is necessary to combine dead-cell removal (Section 6.4) with the method outlined in the text to obtain comparable results.

9.4.3 Intraorgan distribution of cells

It is necessary to use a different isotope as high-energy γ emissions cannot be efficiently captured by a photographic emulsion.

MATERIALS AND EQUIPMENT
Inbred mice

Tritiated uridine

Materials for autoradiography (see Section 8.2.3)

METHOD

1   Prepare a lymph-node suspension from two or three donor mice.

2   Count cells and adjust to 5×10^7 cells/ml in tissue culture medium buffered with HEPES (20 mM) and containing 5% fetal bovine serum.

3   Add ^{3}H-uridine to a final concentration of 92.5×10^4 Bq/ml and incubate at 37°C for 30 min.

4   Wash the cells three times by centrifugation and inject 1×10^7 cells intravenously into each of four recipients.

5   Kill recipients at 0.5, 4, 8 and 24 h postinjection.

6   Remove the spleen and mesenteric lymph nodes from each recipient and fix for histological sectioning.

7   Prepare sections of each organ and dip in photographic emulsion for autoradiography (see Section 8.2.3).

8   After development of the autoradiographs, stain the tissue sections in haematoxylin and eosin.

Labelled cells may be identified by the presence of black grains of silver over their nucleus and cytoplasm. Examine the slides at low power and determine the change in distribution of labelled cells within the spleen and lymph node with time.

This technique can be used to determine the differential localization of any pure cell-line populations.

9.4.4 Fluorescent label for *in vivo* studies

Radioisotopes and autoradiography may be avoided by using intensely fluorescing dyes that bind to the cytoplasmic proteins (e.g. carboxy-fluorescein diacetate) or DNA (e.g. the bis benzimide H33342) of viable cells. These dyes do not impair the migration or localization pattern of cells and are diluted only at cell division (small lymphocytes divide only rarely). Moreover, they can be visualized under the fluorescent microscope in viable cell suspensions or histological sections, either frozen or after formaldehyde fixation.

MATERIALS AND EQUIPMENT
Inbred mice

H33342 dye

METHOD

1   Prepare a stock solution of the dye at 600 μg/ml in distilled water at 4°C.

2   Prepare a lymph-node suspension from two to three donor mice as in Section 6.3.

3   Count cells and adjust to 5×10^7 cells/ml in tissue culture medium buffered with HEPES (20 mM) and containing 5% fetal bovine serum.

Continued on p. 276

4 Dilute the stock solution of the dye 1 : 100 into the cell suspension, final dye concentration 6 μg/ml.

5 Incubate for 15 min at 37°C in a water bath.

6 Dilute in tissue culture medium and wash twice by centrifugation, then use as part of *in vivo* assays as appropriate. Cells may be visualized by confocal microscopy of sections from target organs.

9.4.5 T–B lymphocyte cooperation

In the intact immune response the production of antibody by B cells depends not only on an interaction with antigen-presenting cells but also on an interaction with T cells, i.e. cooperation. Cooperation involving T and B cells cannot be easily demonstrated using thymus and bursa cells from the chicken as they are essentially immunoincompetent cells, and the experiment would require the use of relatively rare inbred chickens. In the mouse the bone marrow behaves as though it were a source of B cells devoid of T cells and it is therefore operationally equivalent to the avian bursa.

MATERIALS AND EQUIPMENT

6-month-old inbred mice for X-irradiation

3–4-week-old inbred mice as thymus and bone marrow donors

Sheep erythrocytes

X-ray machine or γ source

Materials for haemolytic plaques (see Section 9.1)

We will use X-irradiated (immunosuppressed) mice as a suitable vehicle to examine the response of T and B cells, separately and together, to sheep erythrocytes.

Protocol.

Group	Number of mice*	Cells for transfer	No. ml i.v.	Sheep-cell challenge
A	3	Bone marrow	0.1	10^8 i.p.
B	3	Thymocytes	0.1	10^8 i.p.
C	3	Bone marrow + thymocytes	0.1 + 0.1	10^8 i.p.

* For experimental purposes it is better to use five or more mice per group.
i.p., intraperitoneally; i.v., intravenously.

METHOD

1 Give nine mice 8 Gy of irradiation.

2 Remove the femurs from six untreated donor mice.

3 Cut each end off the bones and 'blow out' the marrow with tissue culture medium using a hypodermic syringe with an 18-gauge needle.

4 Disperse the cells gently with a Pasteur pipette.

Continued

5   Count the cells and adjust to 2×10^8/ml.

6   Remove the thymus from each of four donors and tease the cells into medium.

7   Wash the cells twice by centrifugation (150 g for 10 min at 4°C), count and adjust the cells to 10^9/ml.

Reconstitute and challenge the X-Irradiated recipient mice as shown in the Protocol.

8   After 8 days assay the recipient spleens for direct haemolytic plaques as described in Section 9.1.2.

9   Calculate and tabulate the number of plaque-forming cells per spleen for each group of mice.

TECHNICAL NOTES

• No control group is included to show that the X-irradiation was successful in suppressing the immune response of the recipient mice.

• Bone marrow is a relatively poor source of B cells. In the regime described you will obtain a maximum of $4.0–6.0 \times 10^3$ plaques per spleen. More satisfactory results may be obtained using 'B' spleens, prepared either by reconstitution of X-irradiated, thymectomized recipients, nude mice (T-lymphocyte deficient) (see Appendix B) or, more conveniently, by anti-Thy-1 treatment of normal spleen (Sections 6.3 and 11.10.2). Using 2×10^7 'B' spleen cells $+ 10^8$ thymus cells you can expect at least 3×10^4 plaques per spleen.

9.5 **Mitogenic response**

When lymphocytes meet their specific antigen they are stimulated to undergo division. This mitogenic response is usually accompanied by a morphological change to a blast cell. The degree of lymphocyte activation may be assayed by either determining the percentage of blast cells in the culture, or measuring the amount of radioactive DNA analogue incorporated into newly synthesized DNA. It is important to note, however, that blast transformation, DNA synthesis and cell proliferation are not necessarily synonymous. Several instances have been reported where incorporation of DNA analogue has occurred without cell division. The *in vitro* mitotic response has been shown to have an approximate correlation with the *in vivo* situation, e.g. a normal individual would have a lower mitotic response to PPD (purified protein derivative of tubercle bacilli) than a Mantoux-positive individual. In addition, an immunodeficient individual with poor Mantoux reactivity would have a low *in vitro* mitotic response to PPD.

Lectins or phytomitogens, that are derived from plants, have the ability to induce blast-cell transformation and mitosis in a manner similar to antigen. The mitogen binds to a specific cell-surface receptor, as does antigen, the signal generated causes the nucleus to be derepressed and the lymphocyte enters the cell cycle. However, unlike antigens, the mitogen can stimulate a large proportion of lymphocytes. Again, as for antigen stimulation of lymphocytes *in vitro*, it has been possible to show an approximate correlation between the *in vitro* response to mitogens and the immune status of the individual. Phytohaemagglutinin (PHA) is the most extensively studied of the phytomitogens. Evidence suggests that soluble PHA stimulates only T cells, although the activated T lymphocytes secrete cytokines that in turn activate B lymphocytes. Mitogens have been identified that stimulate both T and B cells (pokeweed mitogen) or B cells alone (lipopolysaccharides, such as *Escherichia coli* endotoxin). The ability of mitogens to stimulate T and/or B cells selectively varies not only with species but also with the cell source, suggesting that only a subpopulation of T and/or B cells are capable of responding to mitogen stimulation.

We describe two *in vitro* techniques for the assay of the response of human peripheral blood to PHA: (i) a 'low-tech' tube-based macro-assay that uses a lot of cells and is not convenient for large numbers of experimental groups but requires very little specialized equipment; and (ii) the microassay based upon microculture wells which uses very small quantities of cells and reagents and has been semiautomated, thus enabling many experimental groups with three to five replicates per group to be tested.

9.5.1 Tube radioassay for cell proliferation

MATERIALS AND EQUIPMENT
Human peripheral blood
Phytohaemagglutinin (PHA)
Density gradient for lymphocyte isolation
Tissue culture medium containing antibiotics
Fetal bovine serum
^{3}H-thymidine
5 ml plastic tubes, Falcon
37°C incubator
Cylinder of 5% CO_2 in air

All procedures must be carried out under sterile conditions.

METHOD

1 Mix the blood with an equal volume of serum-free tissue culture medium.
2 Layer an equal volume of defibrinated blood onto the density gradient and centrifuge at 400 *g* for 20 min at 4°C. (For economy, it is possible to use a 2 : 1 ratio of diluted blood to density gradient.)
3 Most of the leucocytes will be found as a fuzzy white band at the serum–density gradient interface. Insert a Pasteur pipette into this band and aspirate the cells.
4 Wash the cells once with serum-free medium (250 *g* for 15 min at room temperature) and twice with medium containing 5% fetal bovine serum (150 *g* for 10 min at room temperature) by centrifugation.
5 Count lymphocytes and adjust to 2×10^6/ml.
6 Set up lymphocyte cultures with PHA according to the Protocol.
7 Incubate the tubes in a 37°C CO_2 incubator.
   The maximum uptake of ^{3}H-thymidine occurs about 72 h after PHA stimulation. If you intend to conduct a complete experiment, it is essential that you investigate both the full dose–response curve and the kinetics of the response in your own culture system.
8 Four hours before harvesting, add 37×10^3 Bq of ^{3}H-thymidine to each culture.

Continued

Protocol.

	Tube number (3–5 replicates of each tube)				
	1	2	3	4	5
1 ml PHA diluted to:	0	1 : 10	1 : 20	1 : 40	1 : 80
Volume of lymphocytes (ml) (2×10^6/ml initial conc.)	1 $\longrightarrow$				
Final PHA concentration	0	1 : 20	1 : 40	1 : 80	1 : 160

TECHNICAL NOTE

Anti-CD3 may also be used as a polyclonal activator.

Cell harvesting and counting

MATERIALS AND EQUIPMENT

Filter papers, Whatman 3 MM, 2.1-cm circle

Phosphate-buffered saline (PBS)

Chloroform

Trichloroacetic acid (TCA), 10% w/v aqueous solution

Scintillation fluid

Scintillation vials

Beta spectrometer

METHOD

1 Wash cells two to three times in PBS by centrifugation.
2 Resuspend cell pellet in 0.4 ml PBS.
3 Support filter discs (one for each culture tube and numbered in pencil) on a pin in a cork board.
4 Place 0.2 ml of cell suspension onto the corresponding disc.
5 Air dry discs with a fan.
6 Wash all discs in 10% cold TCA to precipitate the protein. (At this stage all the discs may be combined.)
7 Wash discs in PBS and then absolute alcohol.
8 Rinse in the chloroform and allow to dry.
9 Place each disc in a scintillation vial containing scintillation fluid and count emissions in a scintillation counter.

Assessment of results

Calculate the geometric mean c.p.m. for each group of replicates (because the researcher is considering cell doubling in populations). There are basically two ways of recording data:

1 by simply giving the mean c.p.m. for stimulated and unstimulated cultures or their difference (Δ c.p.m.);

2   as an index of stimulation. This is calculated by the following equation:

$$\text{Index of stimulation} = \frac{\text{c.p.m. PHA cultures}}{\text{c.p.m. unstimulated cultures}}$$

To compare different types of cells, each having their own unstimulated control, the situation is more complex. Cells from different tissues may have varying numbers of cells undergoing spontaneous division and often the serum supplement used for culture is itself mitogenic, sometimes more on some tissues than others. Unstimulated (i.e. not PHA stimulated, in this case) or 'background' radioisotope incorporation may be abnormally high in some cultures but not others. Spleen cultures, for example, show a much higher background incorporation than blood lymphocyte cultures. In this case an index of stimulation would not be a useful way in which to present the data as the background variation would be hidden.

TECHNICAL NOTES
- It may be necessary to test several batches of fetal bovine serum as they vary in their ability to 'support' *in vitro* cultures.
- ^{131}Iodo-deoxyuridine may be used instead of ^{3}H- or ^{14}C-thymidine. This DNA analogue has the advantage that it is not re-utilized in a culture and so is a measure of incorporation alone, without the complication of turnover. In addition, as it is a γ emitter, it does not require scintillation fluid for counting.
- In the experiment above, we used only a 4-h pulse with ^{3}H-thymidine instead of the 16–20 h (overnight) pulse used by some investigators. We do this not only to shorten the time in culture after isotope addition, thus reducing any effect of bacterial infection, but also to avoid re-utilization of isotope released from cells. This latter consideration is, however, of minimal importance under these conditions as there is a vast excess of free thymidine.
- Occasionally a high 'background' incorporation may be encountered when culturing cells from penicillin-sensitive individuals due to the antibiotic in the culture medium. Under these conditions use gentamycin alone.
- The potency of the mitogen needs to be considered and this may be deduced by initially performing a dose–response curve to assess mitogen stimulation.

9.5.2 Colorimetric microassay for cell proliferation

This is an alternative method for measuring cell proliferation that does not require a radioisotope and counting equipment.

MATERIALS AND EQUIPMENT
IL-2-dependent T-cell line or mitogen-induced T-cell blasts
Tissue culture medium
Fetal bovine serum (FBS)
Phenol red-free tissue culture medium
Phosphate-buffered saline (PBS)
3-(4,5-dimethylthiazol-2-yl)-2,5-diphenyl tetrazolium bromide (MTT), stock solution at 5 mg/ml in PBS (stored in the dark)
Isopropyl alcohol

96-well microtitre plates, flat wells
Centrifuge carriers for microplates
ELISA reader

1. Wash the cells three times by centrifugation to remove residual mitogen or IL-2 and resuspend at 1×10^5/ml in complete tissue culture medium (plus 10% FBS).
2. Dispense 100 μl aliquots into individual wells of a microtitre plate.
3. Add 100 μl aliquots of the IL-2 test samples to individual culture wells and incubate the plates at 37°C for 48 h.
   Controls should include cells, alone and with a positive standard IL-2 preparation.
4. After 48 h incubation, centrifuge the plates at 90 g for 10 min and remove the medium by rapidly inverting the plates with a firm flick.
5. Add 100 μl of MTT (1 mg/ml in tissue culture medium without phenol red) and incubate the plates for a further 3–4 h. Centrifuge the plate and remove medium as before.
6. Add 100 μl of isopropyl alcohol to each well to solubilize the formazan dye.
7. Read the plates on an ELISA reader using the following settings: test wavelength 570 nm, reference wavelength 630 nm.

Plot a curve of concentration versus optical density (equivalent to cell proliferation) for the standard preparation of IL-2 and use this to determine your unknown samples by interpolation. If a standard preparation of IL-2 is not available, arbitrary units should be assigned to the dilution of IL-2 that gives 50% maximal stimulation.

9.6 Microculture technique and response to non-recall antigens (primary immune response *in vitro*)

This technique uses a maximum of only 10^5 responding cells per culture. The reduced cell number allows a greater number of variables to be tested per experiment. The introduction of semi-automated procedures has greatly reduced the time required for plating out and harvesting.

MATERIALS AND EQUIPMENT
Blood, containing heparin (10 IU/ml). The heparin must be preservative free
Tissue culture medium
Lymphoprep
^{3}H-thymidine (^{3}H-TdR)—use at 37×10^4 Bq/ml in tissue culture medium
Scintillation fluid
Microculture trays, 96 wells, flat bases
Eppendorf multidispenser
Cell-harvesting machine
Beta scintillation counter

1 Mix the blood with an equal volume of serum-free tissue culture medium.

2 Carefully layer 6 ml of diluted blood onto 3 ml Lymphoprep or similar separation medium to obtain PBMC (will contain lymphocytes and antigen-presenting cells).

3 Centrifuge at 400 g (interface force) for 20 min at room temperature. A misty layer of lymphocytes will be visible at the plasma–density gradient interface.

4 Remove lymphocytes using a Pasteur pipette and mix with an equal volume of tissue culture medium.

5 Centrifuge at 250 g for 15 min at room temperature and remove the supernatant.

6 Wash twice in tissue culture medium by centrifugation (150 g for l0 min at room temperature).

7 Remove an aliquot of cells and determine the number of viable lymphocytes/ml. Adjust to 2×10^6 lymphocytes/ml.

8 Prepare cultures in microwells according to the following Protocol.

Protocol.

Control wells	Stimulated wells
100 µl tissue culture medium	50 µl tissue culture medium
	50 µl stimulant*
50 µl lymphocyte suspension	50 µl lymphocyte suspension
50 µl autologous plasma	50 µl autologous plasma
200 µl total volume	*200 µl total volume*

* Mitogen, antigen or allogeneic cells, at optimum concentration.

9 Set up three to five replicate cultures of each treatment using an Eppendorf multidispensing pipette.

10 Replace the lid and place the culture tray in a humidified incubator gassed with 5% CO_2 in air.

11 The magnitude of the mitotic response is determined by the addition of 50 µl of ^{3}H-TdR to each well before harvesting.

As an approximate guide:

(a) For PHA cultures add ^{3}H-TdR 40–48 h after the initiation of culture; incubate for 4 h at 37°C before harvesting.

(b) For mixed lymphocyte or antigen-stimulated (e.g. *Candida* or PPD) cultures add ^{3}H-TdR 5 days after the initiation of culture; incubate for 6 or 18 h at 37°C before harvesting, depending on the sensitivity of the assays in your hands. Once the assay is highly reproducible, you will need fewer counts to detect a significant difference between experimental groups so a shorter 'pulse' time will be possible.

(c) Primary responses may be studied in this microculture system with harvesting around day 6–7 rather than the 4–5 days that are optimal for recall antigens (Young *et al.* 1995).

Continued

12 Harvest the cultures using a semi-automatic cell-harvesting procedure.

13 Dry filter strips from harvesting machine at 37°C for at least 3 h.

14 Remove discs from the filter strips and place each disc in a counting vial containing scintillation fluid.

15 Count β emissions in a scintillation counter; assess the results as in Section 9.5.1.

TECHNICAL NOTES

- The volume of PBMC may be usefully increased to 200 ml for non-recall antigens to increase the chances of responding cells being present.
- Autologous plasma gives low backgrounds but for convenience this can be replaced with human AB serum. Make up the medium to 5% serum.
- Addition of dendritic cells has been reported to increase the sensitivity for detecting responses to non-recall antigens (Macatonia *et al.* 1989).

9.6.1 Dye-monitored lymphocyte proliferation

Lymphocyte proliferation monitored by the incorporation of ^{3}H-thymidine is very sensitive but its measurement involves the lysis of the proliferating cells and their harvesting, so no further characterization is possible of the same cell population. Alamar Blue dye changes its colour from blue to red in the presence of proliferating cells. This was originally thought to be brought about by the release of metabolites into the medium that then acted upon the dye. It is now known that the colour change is dependent on the presence of activated cells interacting directly with the dye. The dye is added to cell cultures, in microtitre plates, 24–48 h before measurement. Plates are then monitored in an ELISA reader at 600 nm (oxidized dye) and 570 nm (reduced dye). This is subtracted from the reading at 570 nm to give a measure of proliferation (Zhi-Jun *et al.* 1997). As there is no interference with the cells, plates may be read again at various time points. The cells may also be washed and further studied in other systems, for instance in the fluorescence-activated cell sorter after labelling with appropriate antibodies. The assay correlates very closely with the ^{3}H-thymidine incorporation system. See also the use of 3-(4,5-dimethylthiazol-2-yl)-2,5-diphenyl tetrazolium bromide (MTT) described in Sections 10.2.2 and 10.3.

9.6.2 Mixed-lymphocyte reaction

The mitotic response obtained when cells taken from two inbred strains or from two outbred individuals of any species are mixed in *in vitro* culture is known as the mixed-lymphocyte reaction (MLR). It is an *in vitro* counterpart of the host versus graft (HvG) or graft versus host (GvH) reactions examined later. Like the GvH reaction: (i) the majority of the responsive (as opposed to responding) cells are T lymphocytes; (ii) it has not been possible to demonstrate unequivocally an effect of previous immunization on the magnitude of the response between strains with a 'strong' H-2 difference; and (iii) it is possible to increase the magnitude of the response by previous sensitization across 'weak' H-2 differences.

It is important to distinguish between responsive and responding cells because of the phenomenon known as back stimulation; it was found that F_1 cells gave a mitotic response when mixed with X-irradiated or mitomycin-treated parental cells. According to MLR genetics the F_1 should not recognize the parent cells as being foreign. The mechanism proposed to explain this back stimulation was that the blocked parental cells recognize the F_1 cells as foreign and produce 'mitogenic factors' (previously cytokines) which non-specifically induce proliferation in the immunologically unresponsive F_1 cells. MLR cultures may be performed using culture conditions similar to those described for PHA but mixing 10^6 cells from each of two donors to yield the total of 2×10^6 per culture. A two-way MLR will result, i.e. donor A will recognize B and vice versa. In many situations it is an advantage to have a unidirectional response and so parent and F_1 mixtures can be used, or, more simply, the proliferation of either cell type may be blocked with X-irradiation or mitomycin C treatment.

A suggested experimental protocol is given below; these cultures are then used as a source of cytotoxic effector cells. Activation and expansion of T-lymphocyte populations on a clonal basis by antigenic stimulation and culture in interleukin 2 (see Section 6.7) has provided a much more sensitive and precise method of quantification of antigen-reactive T lymphocytes by limiting dilution analysis (see below).

9.6.3 Whole blood assay for T-cell responses

Purification of lymphocytes is (i) time consuming and expensive and involves collecting reasonably large volumes of blood, and (ii) difficult when working with patients where large samples are not available, or where such demands would discourage participation in experiments. A technique for assaying responses in whole blood has been developed which gives comparable results to the conventional technique with separated cells.

MATERIALS AND EQUIPMENT
Blood—with preservative-free heparin as anticoagulant
Microtitre, 96 U-shaped well plates
Antigen or mitogen
Methyl ^{3}H-thymidine
Tissue culture medium
Cell-harvesting apparatus
Beta scintillation or plate counter

METHOD

1 Dilute blood 1 : 10 with tissue culture medium.
2 Place 200 μl samples in triplicate, in multiwell plate.
3 Add antigen (see Technical notes).
4 Incubate at 37°C in humidified incubator with 5% CO_2.
5 On day 6 (or follow time course) add 37×10^3 Bq ^{3}H-thymidine to each well.
6 Incubate for 18 h at 37°C.
7 Harvest cells, e.g. onto glass-fibre filter paper strips (as above).
8 Count in scintillation counter.

- The response to mycobacterial antigens was found to be optimal at around 1–10 µg/ml, but this will need to be retested for different antigens.
- Sensitive estimates of T-cell responsiveness can be obtained by determining cytokine secretion following antigen stimulation. Supernatant (100 µl) samples can be taken on day 6 and estimated for interferon-γ concentration by ELISA
- It is necessary to eliminate interference in the scintillation count with haemoglobin by removal of red blood cells at the harvesting stage (see also Sewell *et al.* 1997).

9.7 Cell-mediated cytotoxicity

T lymphocytes will respond to foreign cell-surface antigens by blastogenesis. Later in this response, effector cells are generated that will specifically lyse relevant target cells *in vitro*. This *in vitro* killing is generally regarded as being analogous to one type of cell-initiated tissue damage *in vivo*. T-cell-mediated cytotoxicity was elucidated using lymphocytes sensitized to DBA/2 alloantigens and assayed on ^{51}Cr-labelled P815Y (DBA/2) mastocytoma cells. A similar system can be used to investigate T-cell killing against any system of alloantigens using PHA-transformed blast cells labelled with ^{51}CrO$_4$. Alternatively, cytotoxicity may be monitored by the production of cytotoxic cell-specific enzymes, or through changed physical behaviour of cytotoxic cells.

9.8 Mixed-lymphocyte reaction (MLR) and cell-mediated cytolysis (CMC)

MATERIALS AND EQUIPMENT
CBA or C3H and DBA/2 mice
P815Y mastocytoma cells
Sodium ^{51}chromate
X-ray machine or γ source
Gamma spectrometer

9.8.1 Mixed-lymphocyte reaction

METHOD

1 Prepare spleen-cell suspensions from C3H and DBA/2 mice.
2 Irradiate DBA/2 cells (30 Gy); these will be used as MLR-stimulator cells. Irradiate immediately before putting into culture. The stimulatory capacity of irradiated cells falls within a few hours if they are allowed to stand at 4°C.
3 Prepare MLR cultures using irradiated DBA/2 and C3H cells. Mix 10^6 of each cell type and culture in 3 ml of medium in 5 ml Falcon plastic tubes as in Protocol A.

Continued on p. 286

Prepare sufficient replicates of each tube to provide cells for the CMC assay on the 4th day of MLR culture (see Protocol B) (viability of MLR cultures varies—this must be standardized for each laboratory) and, in addition, prepare three replicates of tubes 1–3 for the assay of DNA synthesis in the MLR culture.

4 On the 4th day of the MLR culture collect cells for the CMC assay (Protocol B).
5 On the 5th day of the MLR culture add ^{3}H-thymidine to three replicates of tubes 1–3 to assay for DNA synthesis.

We have given absolute numbers of MLR cells rather than the usual lymphocyte : target ratio. In fact, the efficiency of target-cell killing is not ratio dependent over a wide range.

A MLR protocol.

	Tube number		
	1	2	3*
X-irradiated cells	2×10^6 DBA/2	10^6 DBA/2	10^6 C3H or CBA
C3H- or CBA-responder cells	0	10^6	10^6

* This is a better control than unirradiated cells alone as irradiated cells might exert a slight inhibitory activity upon the generation of possible CMC cells.

B CMC protocol.

	Tube number (three replicates)					
	1	2	3	4	5	6
^{51}Cr-labelled mastocytoma cells	10^5———————————————→					
MLR lymphocytes from tube number:						
1	50×10^5–	–	–	–	–	–
2	–	50×10^5	20×10^5	10×10^5	–	–
3	–	–	–	–	50×10^5	–

9.8.2 Cell-mediated cytolysis

METHOD

1 Label mastocytoma cells with ^{51}CrO$_4$.
2 Count number of viable lymphocytes recovered from MLR (Protocol A).
3 Prepare cell mixtures in 2 ml of medium as shown in Protocol B.
4 Culture for 6 h at 37°C in a CO$_2$ incubator.
5 Resuspend the cells after culture and centrifuge (150 g for 10 min at 4°C).
6 Remove 1 ml of the supernatant from each tube for γ counting.

9.8.3 Calculation of isotope release (equivalent to target-cell destruction)

METHOD

1   Lyse an aliquot of 10^5 original ^{51}Cr-labelled mastocytoma cells either by freezing and thawing (three times at 37°C and –20°C) or with 10% w/v saponin.

2   Spin down insoluble material from the lysate and count radioactivity in the supernatant. Use this value as the maximum (100%) isotope release.

3   Calculate spontaneous release from the labelled mastocytoma (tube 6 in triplicate) as a percentage of the total counts released by saponin. The mean of these three determinations will be used to correct the release observed in lymphocyte–target mixtures (tubes 1–5).

4   Calculate experimental release for each lymphocyte–target mixture as a percentage of the total counts released by saponin (tubes 1–5, in triplicate).

5   Calculate specific release as follows:

$$\% \text{ specific release} = \frac{10[R_e - R_s]}{100 - R_s}$$

where R_e is mean percentage experimental release and R_s is mean percentage spontaneous release.

6   Plot a graph of percentage specific release for each group against the number of MLR-derived cells used to lyse the mastocytoma cells. Calculate also the standard deviation of each group.

TECHNICAL NOTE

In experimental determinations of CMC it is advisable to assay at 4, 6 and 8 h to determine the optimum under your conditions, rather than at the single time point as suggested here.

9.8.4 CMC with PHA blasts

The applicability of CMC may be extended to any system of alloantigens using ^{51}Cr-labelled PHA blasts as target cells. PHA blasts may be produced en masse as follows.

MATERIALS AND EQUIPMENT

As Section 9.5 (mitogenic response), but in addition:

Inbred mice

Tissue culture medium containing fetal bovine serum and antibiotics

Plastic tissue culture flasks

METHOD

1   Prepare cell suspension from mouse lymph nodes.

2   Count cells and adjust to $3–5 \times 10^6$/ml.

3   Add optimal concentration of PHA (see methods in Section 9.5).

4   Add 20 ml of cell suspension to each bottle and gas for 60 s with 5% CO_2 in air.

Continued on p. 288

---

5 Place bottles on their sides in a 37°C incubator.

The kinetics of the response are essentially similar to those seen in Section 9.5.

6 After 72 h, pool cells, wash three times in tissue culture medium and label with $^{51}CrO_4$.

7 Use for CMC as above in Section 9.8.2.

TECHNICAL NOTES

- The protocols above are technically less demanding when carried out with human peripheral blood lymphocytes (PBL). In general, PBL, even from the mouse, are much easier cells to culture and give a very low spontaneous background.

- The ability to expand T lymphocytes to form large clonal populations using antigen stimulation and the cytokine interleukin 2 (IL-2) means that cytotoxic effector cells may be generated from even a single progenitor cell grown in limiting dilution culture. Although the implications of this powerful cell technology are enormous, such refinements are natural developments of the techniques described here.

9.9 Production of granzyme B as a marker of cell-mediated cytotoxicity

Cytotoxicity is generally measured using death of target cells as the indicator. The killing process is mediated by the transfer of granzymes, from granules in cytotoxic cells, to the target cells. The expression of granzymes correlates well with the activation of the killing process. Granzyme B specifically hydrolyses *tert*-butyloxycarbony-Ala-Ala-Asp-thiobenzyl ester and this has been used to form the basis for a cytotoxic assay that gives similar results to the ^{51}Cr release assay (McElhaney *et al.* 1996). Following activation the cells are lysed and the enzyme assayed to give the cytotoxic activity.

9.10 Cytotoxic T-lymphocyte assay for recognition of peptide major histocompatibility complex class I complexes

This is a very simple assay for screening cytotoxic T-lymphocyte cell lines for recognition of peptide epitopes (Leggatt *et al.* 1997) which allows many different peptides to be tested against a cytotoxic T-cell line to allow efficient epitope mapping. It is based on the settling pattern of cytotoxic cells in the presence or absence of cognate peptide. Cell lines fall to the bottom of round-bottomed microtitre wells in the absence of cognate peptide. In the presence of specific peptide the cells adhere to the plastic as they fall and form a disperse layer of cells.

9.11 Estimation of antigen-specific lymphocyte-precursor frequency

One factor that determines the magnitude of an immune response is the number of antigen-specific lymphocytes available to respond at the time of antigenic challenge. The effector cell assays described earlier in the chapter only give an overall impression of the quality of the immune response and have inherently poor quantification.

The principle of the theoretical basis of such assays assumes that one in 5000 T lymphocytes responds to any particular foreign major histocompatibility complex (MHC) gene product in a mixed-lymphocyte culture. In a pool of 10^5 T lymphocytes on average 20 antigen-specific lymphocytes could be expected, so if we dispersed our lymphocyte pool into 50 microcultures, each containing 2×10^7 lymphocytes, some of the wells would contain no antigen-specific lymphocytes, whereas others would receive one, two or more antigen-specific precursor cells. The frequency with which the wells containing zero, one, two or more responsive cells occur within the microplate follows the Poisson distribution (Fig. 9.3), and so can be described by the equation:

$$F_x = \frac{u^x \cdot e^{-u}}{x!}$$

where F_x is the fraction of wells containing x cells ($x = 0,1,2$, etc.), x is the number of antigen-specific precursor cells per well, u is the average number of antigen-responsive precursor cells per well and e is the base of the natural logarithm.

If we were to set up a series of such mixed-lymphocyte microcultures and assay them 10–12 days later, when the proliferation of a single cell would have been sufficient to permit its clonal progeny to be detected, we would find that some cultures had responded whereas others had not. Because we are dealing with a cell suspension in liquid culture we cannot tell whether a responding culture had received one, two, three or more precursor lymphocytes; indeed, all that is known with confidence is the fraction of negative (non-responding) cultures which must have effectively received no antigen-specific lymphocytes.

Fig. 9.3 The Poisson distribution. The Poisson distribution describes the relative frequency of occurrence of numbers of rare elements in each sample of a randomly sampled population. Where $u = 1$, there is a relatively high frequency of samples containing 0 or 1 element; thereafter the frequency of samples containing 2 or more elements declines steeply.

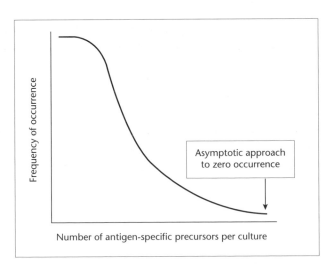

Asymptotic approach to zero occurrence

frequency of occurrence

Number of antigen-specific precursors per culture

The above equation can be applied to predict the expected fraction of negative wells for any frequency of responding cells: Substituting for the zero-term:

$$F_0 = \frac{u^0 \cdot e^{-u}}{0!}$$

$$F_0 = e^{-u}$$

where F_0 is the fraction of negative wells and other terms are as above.

Thus, we can calculate the frequency of responding cells from the observed fraction of negative cultures, as below.

Clearly, if we added too many responsive lymphocytes to each well all cultures would be positive, and the converse would apply if too few lymphocytes were added. As the frequency of responsive cells is the unknown we wish to measure, we cannot know how many cells to add to ensure that the assay is on the correct part of the 'information curve'. In practical terms, it is necessary to set up a titration series of assays with different numbers of total lymphocytes (only some of which can respond) and then record the fraction of negative cultures at different cell input numbers. These data can be used to calculate precursor frequency using the logarithmic transformation of the zero-term equation:

$$u = -\ln F_0$$

where symbols are defined as above.

In other words, the mean number of antigen-specific precursors is proportional to the negative value of the natural logarithm of the fraction of negative wells. The data can be represented and analysed graphically as a semilog plot, as in Fig. 9.4. Provided the data lie along a straight line the assay is said to show 'single-hit kinetics' and can be analysed to yield a frequency estimate. If the data show significant deviation from linearity (calculated by X-square statistics and confidence limits for the slope; see Technical notes of Section 9.11.1) then more than just the

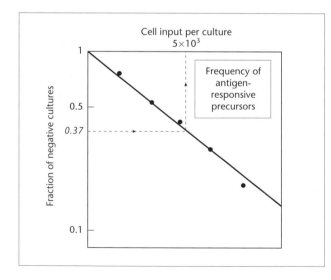

Fig. 9.4 Semilog plot of cell input data and proportion of non-responding cultures from a limiting dilution assay. If only one element is limiting, in this case the specific antigen-reactive T lymphocytes, then data should approximate to a straight line. When there is, on average, one responsive lymphocyte in the volume dispensed into each culture, 0.37 of the cultures should be negative. Interpolation from the point on the x-axis (dashed line) to cell input numbers allows the frequency of antigen-responsive lymphocytes in the total population to be estimated.

number of responding cells is limiting (e.g. two cells may need to act together to give a response, culture conditions may be suboptimal, or many other things) and the calculated frequency would be meaningless.

Assuming that our curve was linear, then when we had on average one respond cell per culture ($u = 1$), 37% of the cultures would be negative by random chance. To confirm this, substitute $u = 1$ into the zero term of the Poisson formula:

$$F_0 = e^{-u}$$

If $u = 1$ then

$$F_0 = e^{-1}$$

Fraction of non-responding cultures $F_0 = 0.37$ (or 37%).

Interpolation from the y-axis at 0.37 (Fig. 9.4) onto the x-axis gives an estimate of the numbers of normal human T lymphocytes that must be added to have, on average, one responding cell per culture; in this case, 1 : 5000. (Remember, that the immune response to MHC antigens is special as it involves complex antigens recognized by a large number of precommitted lymphocytes and shows little increase following deliberate immunization. Frequencies to more 'conventional' antigens such as keyhole limpet haemocyanin or dinitrophenylated foreign protein antigens would show much lower frequencies—between 1 : 20 000 and 1 : 50 000—which increase significantly after immunization.)

The limiting dilution assay can be used to estimate the frequency of antigen-specific lymphocytes which undergo or mediate a wide range of immune transformations *in vitro*: proliferation, antibody production, B- and T-lymphocyte cooperation, suppression and cytotoxicity.

The utility of the assay as a route to functional quantification of the immune response is constrained only by the experimenter's ingenuity in designing appropriate assays. We will describe a technique based upon the estimation of the frequency of cytotoxic effector cells reacting to MHC antigens.

9.11.1 Limiting dilution analysis (LDA) assay

This is an assay to estimate the frequency of lymphocytes from the peripheral blood of one individual (responder) capable of differentiating into cytotoxic effector cells specific for the MHC antigens of a second individual (stimulator). In principle, a one-way mixed-lymphocyte reaction (MLR), with different numbers of responding cells, may provide the necessary data. The main practical attribute required to make these assays work reproducibly is the ability to dispense large numbers of replicates of very small volumes of cell suspensions accurately: remember to mix intermittently while dispensing.

Mixed-lymphocyte culture

MATERIALS AND EQUIPMENT
Prepare lymphocytes (see Chapter 6) using microculture technique (see above), and in addition:
Interleukin 2 (IL-2) as recombinant protein. Material should be pretitrated for its ability to support the growth of T lymphocytes.

1 Prepare lymphocytes from heparinized whole blood taken from the 'stimulator' and 'responder' donors (assign status arbitrarily at the beginning of the experiment).

2 Irradiate 30×10^6 stimulator cells in 10 ml tissue culture medium with 35 Gy of γ or X-irradiation to prevent their proliferation in culture.

3 Wash the irradiated stimulator cells once by centrifugation and resuspend them to 4.0×10^6 lymphocytes/ml in complete tissue culture medium.

4 Add an equal volume of IL-2-containing medium, units/ml previously standardized for ability to support lymphoblast proliferation *in vitro*.

5 While the stimulator cells are being irradiated, prepare a suspension of responder cells at 8.0×10^4 lymphocytes/ml and dilute with complete tissue culture medium to obtain a 1 : 2 titration series according to the Protocol.

Protocol.

	Tube number				
	1	2	3	4	5
Tissue culture medium (ml)	0	2.25			
Lymphocyte suspension (ml)	2.25	2.25			
Cells/ml	8×10^4	4×10^4	2×10^4	1×10^4	0.5×10^4

mix $\xrightarrow{\quad 2.25 \text{ ml} \quad}$ mix $\xrightarrow{\quad 2.25 \text{ ml} \quad}$ etc.

6 Dispense 100 μl volumes of the cell suspensions into microcultures (Fig. 9.5), and incubate at 37°C in a humidified incubator gassed with 5% CO_2 in air for 7 days.

7 Examine the culture plate from below by eye to determine the degree of proliferation, visible as small white clumps (compare wells containing responding and stimulator cells with those containing stimulators alone).

8 If the medium has turned yellow at 7 days, add 50 μl of fresh tissue culture medium containing IL-2 to each well.

TECHNICAL NOTE

It is preferable to use recombinant IL-2 for technical convenience: titrate the units of activity to determine the optimum concentration in your system. This is likely to be around 2000 U/ml. Alternatively, IL-2-containing supernatants can be prepared from T-lymphocyte lines (MLA-144 (gibbon line) for use with human cells or EL4 for use with murine cells) or from normal lymphocytes (e.g. rat spleen) stimulated in bulk with concanavalin A (mitogenic stimulation as for phytohaemag-glutinin (PHA) in Section 9.8.4). IL-2 is constitutively produced by the cell lines; however, its production may be maximized by growing the cells to their plateau density, washing them into serum-free medium and incubating overnight at 37°C in a humidified atmosphere containing 5% CO_2 in air.

IL-2 from any of these sources will maintain murine T lymphocytes, but human T lymphocytes need primate IL-2.

Left plate

	1	2	3	4	5	6	7	8	9	10	11	12
A	100 µl serum-free tissue culture medium in each border well											
B	100 µl complete tissue culture medium											
C	100 µl 0.5 × 10^4 responders/ml											
D	100 µl 0.5 × 10^4 responders/ml											
E	100 µl 1.0 × 10^4 responders/ml											
F	100 µl 1.0 × 10^4 responders/ml											
G	100 µl 2.0 × 10^4 responders/ml											
H												

Right plate

	1	2	3	4	5	6	7	8	9	10	11	12
A	100 µl serum-free tissue culture medium in each border well											
B	100 µl complete tissue culture medium											
C	100 µl 2.0 × 10^4 responders/ml											
D	100 µl 1.0 × 10^4 responders/ml											
E	100 µl 4.0 × 10^4 responders/ml											
F	100 µl 8.0 × 10^4 responders/ml											
G	100 µl 8.0 × 10^4 responders/ml											
H												

Each well, except those in the borders, also receives 100 µl stimulator cell suspension containing IL-2.

Fig. 9.5 Experimental design of a limiting dilution assay (LDA) plate. Suggested layout of LDA assay plates for estimation of the frequency of MHC-reactive lymphocyte precursors in paired samples of human peripheral blood. The numbering and lettering correspond to that of conventional 96-well microculture plates. The border wells are filled with tissue culture medium and are not used for cultures in order to improve humidification, and therefore observed reproducibility, across the plate. In the cell-mediated cytolytic assay, which will be carried out on the clonal products of these microcultures, rows B of each plate provide the data for the calculation of the mean ± standard deviation of the spontaneous leakage of isotope from intact target cells. In assays employing conventional, rather than cell-based, antigens, row B should also receive irradiated 'filler' cells as explained in the Technical note to Section 9.11.1 (cell-mediated cytolysis) (see over page).

Cell-mediated cytolysis

MATERIALS AND EQUIPMENT

As for Sections 9.5 (mitogenic responses) and 9.8 (MLR), but use heparinized human peripheral blood.

METHOD

1 Prepare PHA lymphoblasts from each of the 'stimulator' donors 3 days before the CMC assay with PHA blasts (see above).

2 Harvest the lymphocytes and wash twice in serum-free tissue culture medium by centrifugation (150 g for 10 min at room temperature). You will need about 4×10^5 lymphoblasts as targets.

3 Resuspend the cell pellet in 150 µl of medium containing 11.1×10^6 Bq of $^{51}CrO_4$ and incubate in a 37°C water bath for 90 min with regular shaking.

4 Wash cells three times by centrifugation in tissue culture medium containing 10% fetal bovine serum and resuspend in 5 ml of medium for a haemocytometer count. (Take care, the cells should now be radioactive.)

5 Prepare a 15-ml suspension containing 2.5×10^4 target cells/ml from each original donor.

6 Remove 100 µl of supernatant from each of the culture wells of the limiting dilution assay plates and add 100 µl of the target-cell suspension.

7 Incubate for 4 h at 37°C in a humidified incubator gassed with 5% CO_2 in air.

8 Remove 100 µl of supernatant medium from each well for counting in the γ counter. Take care not to disturb the cell pellet during aspiration of the supernatant sample.

Continued on p. 294

9 In order to determine an acceptable maximum for spontaneous $^{51}CrO_4$ release, calculate the mean and standard deviation of the radioactive content of the supernatant in rows B of plates 1 and 2 (Fig. 9.5).

10 Set the minimum threshold for a positive culture at the sum of the mean plus 3 standard deviations of the spontaneous release.

11 Score cultures as positive or negative according to this threshold, and determine the fraction of negative cultures at each input number of responder cells.

12 Plot the fraction of negative cultures on a log scale against the cell input, as in Fig. 9.4, and determine the cell input number giving 37% (0.37) negative cultures.

This corresponds to the input number required to give, on average, one responder lymphocyte per well which is able to recognize the stimulator MHC molecules.

TECHNICAL NOTES

- The Protocol above has been designed to provide a simple robust assay by which to illustrate the important principles of limiting dilution analysis. Previous experiments have shown that the frequency of precursor cytolytic cells in human blood sample pairs lies in the range 1 : 500–1 : 5000, hence our ability to choose an arithmetic dilution series and so gain maximum information for the construction of the semilogarithmic plot. In addition, the efficient generation of cytotoxic effectors by these antigens results in a high effector : target-cell ratio, thus increasing the sensitivity of the cytolytic assay by maximizing the difference between the ^{51}Cr released spontaneously from intact target cells and that released by specific lysis. It therefore provides an excellent assay for teaching purposes.

  In experimental situations with less favourable antigens, it is usual to perform an LDA in two cycles. In the first the cell input numbers vary logarithmically, and so only a fraction will show a useful proportion of negative cultures. The LDA should then be repeated with an arithmetic series of cell input numbers around the optimum of the logarithmic series.

- The efficiency of the *in vitro* response of lymphocytes is cell-density dependent. If the density is too high, nutrients and culture conditions become limiting. More importantly, if the cell density falls too low then the linear relationship between cell numbers and observed effector function is lost. In the assay described above, we added a standard number of irradiated stimulator lymphocytes (4×10^5 per culture); these also acted as 'filler' cells to maintain optimum cell numbers. This 40-fold excess of filler stimulator cells renders the variations due to the fourfold change in responder numbers insignificant. If an LDA assay is performed on a single lymphocyte population responding to a 'conventional' antigen then irradiated autologous 'filler' cells should be added, both to counteract the variation in cell number in the dilution series and also to provide sufficient antigen-presenting cells.

- Computer programmes have been published for statistical analysis of the curve and calculation of the precursor frequency.

9.12 Apoptosis

Cell death may occur as a result of necrosis (accidental cell death) or apoptosis (programmed cell death). An evaluation of the structural changes in the chromatin which arise before membrane lysis is one way of ascertaining the nature of the cell death. This may be achieved by *either*:

(a) microscopic examination of nuclear material following uptake of fluorescent dyes (ethidium bromide and or acridium orange; see 9.12.1); or *alternatively*

(b) detection and quantification using (i) flow cytometry, or (ii) *in situ* histological examination of tissue sections, using the TUNEL technique (see Section 9.12.2). This involves the terminal deoxynucleotide transferase-mediated labelling of fragmented double-stranded DNA with dUTP(2′-deoxyuridine 5′-triphosphate)–biotin, for the qualitative and quantitative analysis of chromatin. Equipment and solutions that are in direct contact with cells should be sterile, and appropriate sterile laboratory techniques employed.

9.12.1 Quantification of cell viability and apoptotic index

The isolated cells are mixed with a fluorescent dye that binds to DNA, and the cells subsequently visualized and counted using fluorescent microscopy. The two dyes used are ethidium bromide and acridine orange. The differential uptake of these two stains permits the identification of viable and non-viable cells.

MATERIALS

Dye 1: Acridine orange in phosphate-buffered saline (PBS) at a concentration of 100 µg/ml

Dye 2: Acridine orange in PBS at a concentration of 100 µg/ml containing 100 µg/ml of ethidium bromide

Glass test tube

Microscope slide

Coverslips

Fluorescence microscope

Cells of interest, e.g. lymphocytes

Caution: Ethidium bromide and acridine orange are potential carcinogens.

METHOD

1. Adjust the number of cells in suspension to around 5×10^6 cells per ml.
2. Mix 25 µl of cell suspension with either (a) 1 µl of dye 1 or (b) 1 µl of dye 2.
3. Drop a 10 µl aliquot onto a microscope slide, cover with a coverslip and examine using a fluorescent microscope.
4. Dye 1 (acridine orange only): Evaluate 500 cells, counting the number of cells with normal nuclei and cells with apoptotic nuclei.

$$\text{Apoptotic index} = \frac{\text{Number of cells with nuclei which demonstrate apoptosis} \times 100}{\text{Total number of cells counted}}$$

5. Dye 2 (acridine orange and ethidium bromide): Evaluate 500 cells, counting the number of (i) viable (*A*) and non-viable cells (*B*) with normal nuclei and (ii) viable (*C*) and non-viable cells (*D*) with apoptotic nuclei.

Calculation of the apoptotic index and necrotic index

$$\text{Apoptotic index} = \frac{C+D}{A+B+C+D} \times 100$$

$$\text{Necrotic index} = \frac{B}{A+B+C+D} \times 100$$

TECHNICAL NOTES
- Staining with acridine orange alone. Nuclei of non-apoptotic cells look fluorescent green of variable intensity, depending on the distribution of nuclear chromatin, whereas the nuclei of apoptotic cells have dense uniform staining. In the cells exhibiting advanced apoptosis the fluorescence is diminished for they will have lost their DNA, or it may have become fragmented into apoptotic bodies.
- Staining with acridine orange and ethidium bromide.
  A: Viable cells with normal nuclei: organized cellular structure with vivid green chromatin.
  B: Non-viable cells with normal nuclei: organized cellular structure with vivid orange chromatin.
  C: Viable cells with apoptotic nuclei: dense chromatin which may be fragmented and stained vivid green.
  D: Non-viable cells with apoptotic nuclei: dense chromatin which may be fragmented and stained vivid orange.

9.12.2 **TUNEL technique**

(TUNEL: terminal deoxynucleotide transferase-mediated dUTP–biotin nick-end labelling (Gavrieli *et al.* 1992; Gorczyca *et al.* 1993.)

TUNEL is a technique which may be employed for the detection of fragmented DNA within apoptotic cells. It relies on the labelling of broken ends of the double-stranded DNA with biotinylated dUTP, catalysed by the enzyme terminal deoxynucleotide transferase (TdT).

Apoptotic cells may be quantified using flow cytometry, or *in situ* on histological tissue sections.

Quantifying apoptotic cells by flow cytometry

MATERIALS
Cells of interest to be analysed
Paraformaldehyde solution (1% w/v paraformaldehyde in phosphate-buffered saline (PBS) and containing 0.01% v/v Tween 20)
PBS
95% v/v ethanol (ice cold)
TdT reaction buffer (0.5 M sodium cacodylate, pH 6.8, containing 1 mM $CoCl_2$, 0.5 mM dithiothreitol (DTT), 0.15 M NaCl and 0.05% w/v bovine serum albumin—BSA)
TdT/biotin–dUTP mixture (TdT reaction buffer containing 1 µM biotin–dUTP and 3 U TdT; see Technical notes)
Fluorescein (FITC)-conjugated streptavidin (see Technical notes)
Centrifuge tubes

METHOD

1 Count cells, then transfer 5×10^5 cells into a centrifuge tube containing 2 ml PBS, then centrifuge at 300 *g* for 10 min at 4°C.

2 Remove the supernatant and then resuspend the pelleted cells in 250 µl of ice-cold PBS.

3 With care gently vortex the cells and at the same time slowly add 750 µl of the ice-cold 95% v/v ethanol, then incubate on ice for 20 min.

4 Add 3 ml PBS and centrifuge at 450 *g* for 10 min at 4°C, then discard the supernatant.

5 Resuspend the cells in around 50 µl PBS using flicking action on the centrifuge tube.

6 Whilst gently vortexing the cells, *very slowly* add 1 ml of paraformaldehyde, then incubate at room temperature for about 30 min. Then repeat step 4.

7 Wash cells with 500 µl of reaction buffer, decant the supernatant and remove the residual supernatant by blotting the rim of the centrifuge tube with tissue paper.

8 Add 50 µl of TdT–biotin/dUTP mixture and gently resuspend the cells using flicking action on the centrifuge tube. Incubate for about 40–50 min at 37°C.

9 Repeat step 4.

10 Incubate the washed cells with FITC-conjugated streptavidin at room temperature for 30 min.

11 Repeat step 4.

12 Analyse the cells by flow cytometry (see Chapter 8)—a characteristic pattern for dead cells, FITC-stained cells and unstained cells will be produced.

TECHNICAL NOTES

- Stir the paraformaldehyde solution at 70°C to dissolve the paraformaldehyde, then pass through a 0.2 µm filter prior to use.
- During the fixation of the cells, the slow addition of the ethanol/paraformaldehyde whilst vortexing helps to prevent excess clumping of the cells.
- When the fixed cells (from step 6) have been washed three times in PBS, they may be stored in the dark at 4°C for up to 3 days.
- Fixation with 95% ethanol causes the cells to shrink.
- Fixation with paraformaldehyde augments the sensitivity of the TUNEL technique by allowing greater accessibility to the intracellular contents.
- Biotin–dUTP, TdT and other reagents may be obtained from Boehringer Mannheim, and the concentrations need to be optimized for the experiment. The manufacturer provides indicative optimum working concentrations. Solutions must be prepared immediately prior to use.
- Dilution of the FITC-conjugated streptavidin needs to be optimized; manufacturers provide the indicative optimum working concentration.

Detection of apoptotic cells in frozen histological tissue sections using the TUNEL reaction

MATERIALS

Frozen cells or tissue sections for TUNEL analysis

1% w/v paraformaldehyde in phosphate-buffered saline (PBS) (see first Technical note of previous Section)

Tris(hydroxymethyl)-aminomethane (Tris)-buffered saline (TBS)

0.1% v/v hydrogen peroxide in TBS

2% v/v fetal bovine serum in TBS

TdT reaction buffer (0.5 M sodium cacodylate, pH 6.8, containing 1 mM CoCl$_2$, 0.5 mM dithiothreitol (DTT), 0.15 M NaCl and 0.05% w/v bovine serum albumin—BSA)

TdT/digoxigenin–dUTP mixture (TdT reaction buffer containing 2 µM digoxigenin-11–dUTP and 3 U TdT; see first Technical note)

Primary antibody solution (sheep antidigoxigenin Fab antibody in TBS containing 2% v/v fetal bovine serum; see second Technical note)

Secondary antibody solution (horseradish peroxidase-conjugated F(ab')$_2$ fragment of donkey anti-sheep IgG in TBS containing 2% v/v fetal bovine serum; see second Technical note)

AEC solution: 25 µl 3-amino-9-ethylcarbazole (AEC) stock solution containing 1 ml 0.17 M sodium acetate, pH 5.2, and 1 µl 30% hydrogen peroxide (see third Technical note)

Haematoxylin solution

Crystal mount medium

PAP pen (for drawing hydrophobic boundary on glass slide)

Coplin jars for staining

Humidifier container

METHOD

1 Using a PAP pen, draw a hydrophobic boundary on the glass microscope slide around the frozen tissue section.

2 To fix the section, cover with the 1% paraformaldehyde solution, and leave in container (with a secure lid) at room temperature for 30 min.

3 Gently pour the 1% paraformaldehyde solution off the section.

4 Wash for about 5 min in a Coplin jar containing TBS, occasionally dipping the slide in and out of the jar.

5 Cover the tissue section with the solution of 0.1% hydrogen peroxide in TBS, then place in a container with a secure lid and incubate at room temperature for 30 min.

6 Repeat step 4.

7 Remove the TBS and cover the section with the TdT reaction buffer (see Technical notes).

8 Remove the TdT reaction buffer and gently add 25 ml TdT/digoxigenin–dUTP mixture and incubate in the humidified chamber at 37°C for 60 min.

9 Using the same dipping technique as in step 4, perform serial 5-min washes:
   1 × TBS
   1 × TBS containing 2% v/v fetal bovine serum.

10 Remove the solution (TBS containing 2% v/v fetal bovine serum) from the slide, then cover the section with the primary antibody solution and incubate in a closed container at room temperature for 60 min.

11 Repeat step 9.

12 Remove the solution (TBS containing 2% fetal bovine serum) from the slide, then cover the slide with the secondary antibody solution and incubate in a closed container at room temperature for 60 min.

13 Repeat step 9.

Continued

14 Cover the section with the working AEC solution and incubate in a closed container at room temperature for 20 min.
15 Repeat step 9.
16 Counterstain the tissue section by incubating the slide in a Coplin jar of haematoxylin for 1 min, then transfer the slide to another Coplin jar and wash under running tap water for 5 min.
17 Remove from the Coplin jar and clear excess water from the slide, then mount with Crystal Mount and a coverslip (see Technical notes).

TECHNICAL NOTES

- TdT/digoxigenin–dUTP mixture must be prepared immediately prior to use. Reagents may be obtained from Boehringer Mannheim, and the concentrations need to be optimized for the experiment. The manufacturer provides indicative optimum working concentrations.
- The concentrations of the sheep anti-digoxigenin Fab antibody and anti-sheep antibodies need to be optimized for the experiment.
- AEC stock solution: 4 mg/ml of 3-amino-9-ethylcarbazole (AEC) in dimethyl sulphoxide (DMSO), to be stored at 20°C in the dark. This stock solution is viable for about 2–3 weeks, but the working solution must be prepared immediately prior to use.
- The initial incubation of the section with TdT reaction buffer is essential as the TdT enzyme is very sensitive to changes in buffer conditions.
- Counterstaining can give rise to fading with the AEC staining, therefore step 16 is optional. If step 16 is to be omitted, then the tissue section may be mounted after step 15.

9.13 **Further reading**

Ahmed, S.A., Gogal, R.M. & Walsh, J.E. (1994) A new rapid and simple nonradioactive assay to monitor and determine the proliferation of lymphocytes: an alternative to [^{3}H] thymidine incorporation assay. *J Immunol Meth* **170**, 211–224.

Borrebaeck, C.A.K. & Hagen, I. (1993) *Electromanipulation in Hybridoma Technology: A Laboratory Manual*. Oxford University Press, Oxford.

Dolzhanskiy, A. & Basch, R.S. (1995) Flow cytometric determination of apoptosis in heterogeneous cell populations. *J Immunol Meth* **180**, 131–140.

Fazekas da St. Groth, S. (1982) The evaluation of limiting dilution assays. *J Immunol Meth* **49**, 11–23.

Fujihashi, K., McGhee, J.R., Beagley, K.W. *et al*. (1993) Cytokine-specific ELISPOT assay: Single cell analysis of IL-2, Il-4 and IL-6 producing cells. *J Immunol Meth* **160**, 180–189.

Gao, L.-Y. & Kwaik, Y.A. (2000) The modulation of host cell apoptosis by intracellular bacterial pathogens [Review]. *Trends in Microbiol* **7**, 306–313.

Gavrieli, Y., Sherman, Y & Ben-Sasson, S.A. (1992) Identification of programmed cell death *in situ* via specific labelling of nuclear DNA fragments. *J Cell Biol* **119**, 493–501.

Gorczyca, W., Gong, J. & Darzynkiewicz, Z. (1993) Detection of DNA strand breaks in individual apoptotic cells by the *in situ* terminal deoxynucleotidyl transferase and nick transplantation assays. *Cancer Res* **53**, 1945–1951.

Gupta, S. & Cohn, J.J. (eds) (1996) *Mechanisms of Lymphocyte Activation and Immune Regulation*. Plenum, London.

Herberman, R.B., Reynolds, C.W. & Ortaldo, J. (1986) Mechanisms of cytotoxicity by NK cells. *Annu Rev Immunol* **4**, 651–674.

Hoffmann, P., Skibinski, G. & James, K. (1995) Organ culture of human lymphoid tissue I. Characteristics of the system. *J Immunol Meth* **179**, 37–49.

Lakew, M., Nordstrom, I., Czerkinsley, C. & Quiding-Jarbrink, M. (1997) Combined immunomagnetic cell sorting and ELISPOT assay for the phenotypic characterization of specific antibody-forming cells. *J Immunol Meth* **203**, 193–198.

Lefkovitz, I. & Waldmann, H. (1979) *Limiting Dilution Analysis of the Immune System.* Cambridge University Press, Cambridge.

Leggatt, G.R., Alexander-Miller, M.A., Kumar, A., Hoffmann, S.L. & Berzofsky, J.A. (1997) Cytotoxic T lymphocyte (CTL) adherence assay (CAA): a nonradioactive assay for murine CTL recognition of peptide–MHC class I complexes. *J Immunol Meth* **201**, 1–10.

Macatonia, S.E., Taylor, P.M., Knight, S.C. & Askonas, B.A. (1989) Primary stimulation by dendritic cells induces antiviral proliferative and cytotoxic T cell responses *in vitro*. *J Exp Med* **169**, 1255–1264.

McElhaney, J.E., Pinkoski, M.J., Upshaw, C.M. & Bleackley, R.C. (1996) The cell-mediated cytotoxic response to influenza vaccination using an assay for granzyme B activity. *J Immunol Meth* **190**, 11–20.

Plebanski, M. & Burtles, S.S. (1994) *In vitro* primary response of human T cells to soluble protein antigens. *J Immunol Meth* **170**, 15–25.

Polak, J.M. & van Noorden, S. (1997) *An Introduction to Immunocytochemistry: Current Techniques and Problems,* 2nd edn. BIOS, Blackwell Science, Oxford.

Rowland-Jones, S.L. & McMichael, A. (eds) (2000) *Lymphocytes: A Practical Approach.* Oxford University Press, Oxford.

Sewell, W.A., North, M.E., Webster, A.D. & Farrant, J. (1997) Determination of intracellular cytokines by flow cytometry following whole blood culture. *J Immunol Meth* **209**, 67–74.

Studzinski, G.P. (ed.) (1999) *Apoptosis: A Practical Approach.* Oxford University Press, Oxford.

Vermes, I., Haanen, C., Steffens-Nakken, H. & Reutelingsperger, C. (1995) A novel assay for apoptosis. Flow cytometric detection of phosphatidylseribe expression on early apoptotic cells using fluorescein labelled Annexin V. *J Immunol Meth* **184**, 39–51.

Weir, R.E., Morgan, A.R., Britton, W.J., Butlin, C.R. & Dockrell, H.M. (1994) Development of a whole blood assay to measure T cell responses to leprosy: a new tool for immuno-epidemiological field studies of leprosy immunity. *J Immunol Meth* **176**, 93–101.

Young, J.L., Daser, A. & Beverley, P.C.L. (1995) *In vitro* proliferative responses to human peripheral blood mononuclear cells to nonrecall antigens. *J Immunol Meth* **182**, 177–184.

Zhi-Jun, Y., Sriranganathan, N., Vaught, T., Arasti, S.K. & Ahmed, S.A. (1997) A dye-based lymphocyte proliferation assay that permits multiple immunological analyses: mRNA, cytogenetic, apoptosis and immunophenotyping studies. *J Immunol Meth* **210**, 25–39.

10

The cytokines

10.1 Bioassays for cytokines

A vast array of published information is available on the immunoregulatory molecules known as cytokines that are secreted by cells and thus modulate the behaviour, function or differentiation state of other cells.

With the original nomenclature, a cytokine produced by lymphocytes was called a lymphokine, and a cytokine produced by the monocyte lineage of cells, a monokine. However, such terms are restrictive and misleading; for example, the so-called lymphokine, interleukin 6, is produced by more than one cell type in addition to leucocytes: fibroblasts, epithelial cells, keratinocytes, monocytes, microglial cells, endothelial cells and uterine stromal cells.

Many cytokines that are intimately involved in the regulation of specific and non-specific immune function (e.g. as illustrated for IL-1 and IL-2 in Fig. 10.1) probably pre-date adaptive immunity in evolution and have retained important (more important?) roles outside the immune system. The cytokines so far identified have been shown to interact with their target cell via a specific receptor, though the route(s) of signal transduction to the nucleus remain to be defined.

Recombinant DNA technology, protein sequence analysis, the use of monoclonal antibodies and the development of a variety of bioassays has enabled many of the properties of these cytokines to be demonstrated. The precise physiological role of a cytokine is often difficult to determine; many have been shown to have several activities *in vitro* and so it is difficult to predict which activity might have *in vivo* relevance. Several cytokines have been shown to have

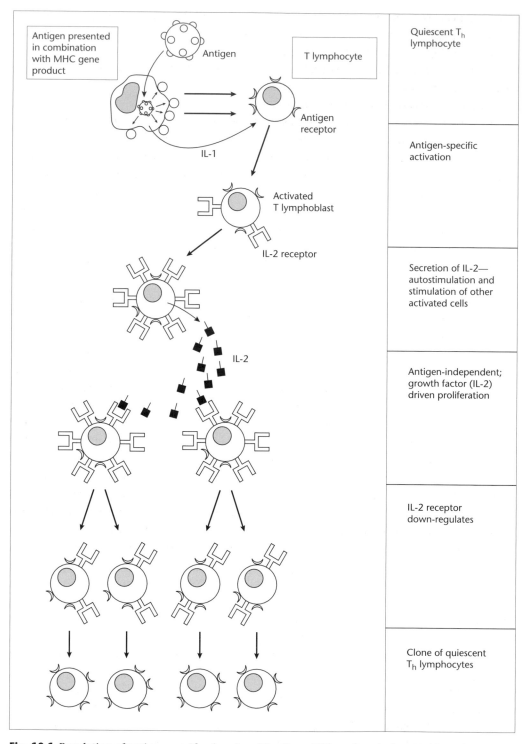

Antigen presented in combination with MHC gene product

Antigen

T lymphocyte

Antigen receptor

IL-1

Activated T lymphoblast

IL-2 receptor

IL-2

Quiescent T$_h$ lymphocyte

Antigen-specific activation

Secretion of IL-2— autostimulation and stimulation of other activated cells

Antigen-independent; growth factor (IL-2) driven proliferation

IL-2 receptor down-regulates

Clone of quiescent T$_h$ lymphocytes

Fig. 10.1 Regulation of antigen-specific clonal proliferation of T lymphocytes by cytokines. Antigen bridging between the antigen-presenting cell (APC) and T lymphocyte results in secretion of IL-1 by the APC. Interleukin 1 and antigen activate the T lymphocyte to express its preprogrammed effector function, in this case secretion of IL-2. At the same time, however, the T lymphocyte also up-regulates its high-affinity IL-2 receptors and so can respond to extracellular IL-2, including its own. Whereas the initial activation phase is antigen driven, the later proliferative phase is largely in response to IL-2. Feedback control is achieved in turn by the down-regulation of the IL-2 receptor by IL-2 in the presence of diminishing antigen concentration.

convergent effects in the immune system, e.g. both IL-2 and IL-4 maintain the proliferation of activated T cells. Although the molecules are structurally different, a response to a cytokine is elicited following cytokine binding to the specific receptor. The nature of the response is dependent on the type of cell being stimulated. When deciding on a method to measure cytokines there are two key assay systems:

1 bioassay that measures biological activity, and
2 immunoassay, such as an ELISA, that measures the concentration of the cytokine within the body fluid/cell lysate of interest, but does not determine whether it has any activity.

It seems likely that synergy or inhibition of activity between cytokines may occur, thus providing opportunities for highly discriminatory fine-tuning of the immune system. Nomenclature of the cytokines is confusing as many cytokines have been isolated independently in a number of different laboratories throughout the world. Thus similar or identical molecules are known by a variety of names. It is possible to standardize assays via a growing collection of international and national standard cytokine preparations obtainable from the National Cancer Institute (Bethesda, USA), or the National Institute for Biological Standards and Control (South Mimms, UK).

The majority of the cytokines described here are available as recombinant proteins, derived from *in vitro* expression in prokaryotic or eukaryotic systems. Although most recombinant molecules have a comparable activity they are not identical to the native cytokine, especially if derived by prokaryotic expression. In particular, glycosylation patterns may vary quite considerably.

Most cytokines occur in similar or equivalent forms throughout the mammals. However, although nucleotide and amino acid sequence analysis shows considerable homology between the species for some cytokines, the cross-reactivity between species is low or unidirectional. For example, human IL-2 will stimulate lymphocytes from the rat and the mouse, but rodent IL-2 cannot stimulate human lymphocytes (see the useful Table prepared by Horst Ibelgaufts, University of Munich, at the aptly named website: http://www.copewithcytokines.de/cope.cgi?001174).

To ensure that a functionally active cytokine is present in an unknown sample, a bioassay is required. Monoclonal antibodies have been developed into commercially available enzyme-linked immunosorbent assay (ELISA) and radioimmunoassay (RIA) kits. Dot blotting or northern analysis with DNA probes can also be used to define whether a cell is capable of cytokine production, though this is not as sensitive as a bioassay and not quantitative to any degree of accuracy.

Calculation of results

National/international standards for some cytokines are available. Here are some recommendations for when considering undertaking cytokines assay studies.

1 Calibrate your own laboratory standard which can then be used as a reference for all further assays.
2 Make a bulk preparation of the cytokine of interest, aliquot into convenient samples for storage at –70°C and do three or four repeat assays on aliquots of this stored material.
3 The standard preparation should give reproducible results (albeit some variation due to heterogeneity in the responder-cell population), and a mean of the dose–response curves will enable you to identify the dilution of standard which gives 50% stimulation of activity, cell killing, etc. Assign an arbitrary number of units to this and use as a positive control in all future experiments.

4 The cross-reactivity between species is variable, so care must be taken when attempting to determine cytokine activity on cells from different species.

Cytokines are molecules with a defined structure and with potent effector functions on cells. For simplicity, immunoassays, either radio- or enzymic, should be ideal for estimating cytokines. Antibodies provide very precise recognition of molecular structure, especially in two-site assays where two monoclonal antibodies recognize distinct epitopes on the cytokine, but such assays frequently fail to give correct information on the activity of the cytokine. With good standards they should give reliable information on mass.

Failure of correlation between recombinant cytokine mass and activity can be due to a number of causes. Glycosylation to produce the mature protein can be an important characteristic that has a functional role in a specific cytokine. However, if that cytokine is produced as a recombinant protein, e.g. in yeast, mammalian oligosaccharides will not be added and this can affect the biological activity. Even cytokines produced by cultured mammalian cells will often have altered glycosylation unless extreme care is taken to maintain nutrients and culture conditions in an optimal steady state. *In vivo* soluble cytokine receptors are often produced, frequently in greater quantity than the cytokine, and these may inhibit function while the cytokine is still detected in an immunoassay. For the above reasons bioassays are generally preferred when studies are being made that relate to cytokine function.

Problems with bioassays

Specificity is a key issue; cytokines are usually assayed *in vitro* on populations of cells and most cells have receptors for more than one cytokine so that care must be taken to ensure that the correct cytokine is being detected. To overcome this it may be advisable to combine bioassay with the specificity of antibody. If a neutralizing anticytokine antibody is available, the assay may be performed both with and without the antibody, the difference in activity being due to the cytokine in question, and it is essential to be aware that this still cannot prevent errors caused by cytokines yet to be discovered which may well be present in the test samples.

Cytokines may be assayed in whole animals, cells isolated from animals or on cell lines or clones. Obviously whole animal experiments are only ethical where no other method is available and their use is generally restricted to the later stages of drug development, for instance for testing the *in vivo* anticancer effects of a cytokine. An alternative to using a live animal would be to take cells from particular organs, such as spleen cells or thymocytes, and examine the effects of cytokines on these particular mixtures. This gives a good idea of how the cytokine relates to the *in vivo* mix of cells, but is highly complex for simply assaying cytokine activity. Sometimes, however, it is difficult to get hold of the correct cell line and we show below how to use animal-derived cell preparations and give recommendations for individual cell lines. If a large number of assays are to be performed over a period of time cell lines should be used as this will cut down on the requirement to use animals and will provide greater consistency than using cells from different animals each time.

Sample collection

Cytokines are frequently measured in blood samples and great care is needed to avoid artefacts. Lithium heparin, in certain collection tubes, is contaminated with endotoxin which will have potent effects on cytokine production by the cells within the blood sample. TNF-α (tumour necrosis factor α) has been detected after 2 hours and IL-1 and IL-6 after 3 hours of contact of the blood sample with the contaminated heparin. It is salutary to reflect that some of the confusions in the cytokine literature may be due to endotoxin.

10.2 Interleukin 1 (IL-1)

IL-1 is known as endogenous pyrogen, catabolin and haematopoietin 1. Almost every nucleated cell type can be induced to produce IL-1 but it is produced in greatest amount by activated monocytes and macrophages. IL-1 has stimulatory and regulatory effects in terms of growth and differentiation of numerous cell types, has profound effects on the immune system, regulating both T and B cells, and is a mediator of inflammatory responses.

Two distinct genes have been identified (*IL-1α* and *IL-1β*) whose gene products produce IL-1 activity that is essentially identical and which both bind to the IL-1 receptor. The IL-1 precursors have a MW_r of around 33 000, but when proteolytically cleaved produce mature proteins with a MW_r of around 17 000. The Il-1α precursor protein is biologically active, but the IL-1β must be processed in order to exert any activity. Yet most of the biological activity in the circulation is exerted by IL-1β.

10.2.1 Thymocyte costimulator assay

Thymocytes from young (6–10-week-old) mice are cultured in the presence of a submitogenic concentration of phytohaemagglutinin (PHA) that is potentiated by IL-1.

MATERIALS AND EQUIPMENT
Mouse thymocytes
Tissue culture medium
Fetal bovine serum (FBS)
Phytohaemagglutinin (PHA)
^{3}H-thymidine
96-well microtitre plates (round-bottomed wells)
Automated cell harvester
Beta spectrometer

METHOD

1   Remove the thymus from a freshly killed mouse and prepare a single-cell suspension, using aseptic technique.

2   Wash the cells twice by centrifugation and resuspend in medium at 1.5×10^7/ml.

3   Dispense 100 μl aliquots into individual wells of a 96-well microtitre plate.

4   Add 50 μl of PHA (diluted 1 : 250 in tissue culture medium containing 10% FBS) to each culture. The final dilution of 1 : 1000 should be submitogenic, i.e. it should not give a significant proliferative response in the absence of IL-1. If it does induce a mitogenic response, check

Continued on p. 306

---

that the dilution has been made correctly, then, if you are really sure, dilute the PHA further until it just becomes submitogenic.

5   Add the IL-1 samples under test at a range of dilutions, using 50 µl aliquots of each, to triplicate wells.

6   Appropriate controls are:

cells + medium alone

cells + PHA alone

cells + IL-1 alone

in each case in a final volume of 200 µl.

7   Incubate the plates at 37°C for 48–72 h and pulse with 18.5×10^3 Bq of ^{3}H-thymidine (74×10^{10} Bq/mol) for 4–6 h prior to harvesting.

8   Harvest the plates using an automated cell harvester and process the samples for β scintillation counting (see Section 9.5.1).

Assessment of results

A standard IL-1 preparation is available from the National Institute for Biological Standards and Controls, UK. Then a standard curve can be plotted of proliferation (^{3}H-thymidine uptake) against IL-1 concentration and units of activity shown by the unknown samples read off the curve. Alternatively, you may wish to assign an arbitrary number of units to the dilution giving 50% of maximal stimulation.

10.2.2 Calcium ionophore costimulation

Interleukin 1 plus calcium ionophore can stimulate certain IL-1-sensitive cell lines to produce IL-2 (see Section 10.3). The IL-2 produced is then measured using an IL-2-dependent T-cell line.

MATERIALS AND EQUIPMENT

EL4.6.1 cell line (IL-1 sensitive, IL-2 producer)

IL-2-dependent T-cell line, e.g. CT-6, CTLL-D, DIOS

Tissue culture medium

Fetal bovine serum (FBS)

Calcium ionophore, e.g. ionomycin or A6137

Dimethyl sulphoxide (DMSO)

96-well microtitre plates

^{3}H-thymidine (74×10^{10} Bq/mol)

Recombinant IL-2

Beta scintillation counter

Preparation in advance

1   Make a stock solution of calcium ionophore at 1×10^{-3} M in DMSO and store at –20°C.

2   Prepare subcultures of the two cell lines to be used 24–48 h in advance of the assay, to ensure that they are in their log phase of growth.

1 Add 100 µl aliquots of IL-1 samples, at a range of dilutions and in triplicate, to 96-well microtitre plates.

2 Add 50 µl of calcium ionophore diluted to 1×10^{-6} M in complete medium to each well.

3 Harvest EL4 cells from an actively growing culture, wash twice by centrifugation and resuspend at 4×10^6/ml.

4 Add 50 µl of the cell suspension to each well and incubate overnight at 37°C in a humidified atmosphere containing 5% CO_2 in air.

Controls should include calcium ionophore plus cells alone, the highest concentration of IL-1 plus cells alone and cells alone.

5 Remove 100 µl of medium from each well and transfer to the corresponding well of a second microtitre plate.

6 Harvest the CTLL-D (or equivalent) cells from an actively growing culture, wash three times to remove IL-2 from the growth medium and resuspend the cells at 1×10^5/ml.

7 Add a 100 µl aliquot of cell suspension to each microtitre well containing the transferred supernatants.

Be sure to include cultures containing CTLL-D cells with doubling dilutions of recombinant IL-2, for the construction of a standard curve.

8 Incubate the plates overnight at 37°C in a humidified atmosphere of 5% CO_2 in air.

9 Add 18.5×10^3 Bq of ^{3}H-thymidine to each well 4–6 h before harvesting the plates with an automated cell harvester.

10 Process the samples for liquid scintillation counting.

TECHNICAL NOTES

- The colorimetric MTT assay using the tetrazolium salt, 3-(4,5 dimethylthiazol-2-yl)-2,5-diphenyl tetrazolium bromide (see Section 9.5.2) can also be used to assay for cell proliferation.
- The DIOS murine helper T-cell line may also be used to measure IL-2 in a proliferative assay.

10.3 Interleukin 2 (IL-2)

Interleukin 2 was originally known as T-cell growth factor (TCGF). It is produced by activated T cells and is involved in stimulation of T cells in the cell cycle from the G1 to the S phase. IL-2 acts as both an autocrine and a paracrine T-cell growth factor. For experimental work native IL-2 is usually generated from mitogen-stimulated spleen or lymph-node cells or from an IL-2-producing T-cell line, e.g. Jurkat (human IL-2), EL4 (murine IL-2). IL-2 is important for the maintenance and proliferation of a number of cell types in the immune system, including T cells, B cells and NK (natural killer) cells, enhancing their cytolytic activity.

IL-2 can induce the secretion of other cytokines such as interferon γ (IFN-γ) and B-cell growth factor (BCGF).

Assays for IL-2 are based on the maintenance of the proliferation of activated T cells *in vitro* and can use the IL-2-dependent T-cell lines: CTLL-2 and HT-2.

Alternatively, phytohaemagglutinin (PHA)- or concanavalin A (Con A)-activated T-cell blasts, after extensive washing to remove residual mitogen, can be used as IL-2-dependent cells. The proliferative response to IL-2 is measured by a colorimetric assay or ^{3}H-thymidine uptake.

10.3.1 ^{3}H-thymidine uptake assay

This is similar to the colorimetric assay (see Section 9.5.2) but with the following modifications.

1 Use 2×10^4 cells/well in 100 μl complete tissue culture medium.
2 Add 100 μl aliquots of sample under test.
3 Add 18.5×10^3 Bq of ^{3}H-thymidine in 10 μl medium 4–6 h before the end of the assay.
4 Process the samples for counting in a β spectrometer.

The concentration of IL-2 in the sample can be determined as described above for the colorimetric assay.

TECHNICAL NOTE
It is possible to shorten the incubation time to 24 h; although the signal to noise ratio is less favourable the discrimination should still be sufficient for reproducible results.

10.4 Interleukin 3 (IL-3)

Interleukin 3 is also known as multilineage colony-stimulating factor (multi-CSF) and is predominantly a product of CD4$^+$ T cells that stimulates very immature bone marrow progenitor cells to differentiate into the mature cell types.

For experimental purposes it can be derived from the human bladder carcinoma cell line 5637 and also from the myelomonocytic cell line WEHI-3b.

IL-3 can be detected by its ability to promote the growth and differentiation of cells of monocytic and polymorphonuclear origin in colony-forming assays. It also supports the growth and proliferation of various IL-3-dependent lines, e.g. the cloned mast-cell line MC/9 or MO7e cells which can be assayed by ^{3}H-thymidine uptake or colorimetrically using the MTT assay, as described in Sections 9.5.2 and 10.3.

10.4.1 Proliferation assay

MATERIALS AND EQUIPMENT
Mast-cell line, e.g. MC/9
96-well microtitre plates
3-(4,5-dimethylthiazol-2-yl)-2,5-diphenyl tetrazolium bromide (MTT); stock solution at 5 mg/ml in phosphate-buffered saline (PBS) (stored in the dark)
Tissue culture medium, with and without phenol red
Fetal bovine serum (FBS)
2-mercaptoethanol (2-ME)
ELISA reader

Essentially the same as the colorimetric assay for IL-2, Section 9.5.2.

1 Dispense 100 µl aliquots of MC/9 cells (1×10^5/ml in tissue culture medium containing 4% FBS and 5×10^{-5} M 2-ME) into individual wells of a microculture plate.

2 Add test supernatants as 100 µl aliquots in a range of dilutions.

3 Incubate at 37°C for 20 h in a humidified atmosphere of 5% CO_2 in air.

4 Centrifuge the plates at 90 g for 10 min, flick off the medium by inverting the plate rapidly, add 100 µl of MTT in indicator-free medium and incubate for a further 3–4 h.

5 Centrifuge the plate as described above, flick off the medium and add 100 µl of isopropyl alcohol to each well.

6 Read the plates on an ELISA reader using a test wavelength of 570 nm, a reference wavelength of 630 nm and a calibration setting of 1.99.

Assessment of results

Plot a curve of concentration versus optical density (equivalent to cell proliferation) for the standard preparation of IL-3 and use this to determine your unknown samples by interpolation. If a standard preparation of IL-3 is not available, arbitrary units should be assigned to the dilution of IL-3 which gives 50% maximal stimulation.

10.5 Interleukin 4 (IL-4)

Interleukin 4 is also known as B-cell stimulating factor 1 (BSF-1), B-cell growth factor 1 (BCGF-1) and B-cell differentiation factor γ (BCDF-γ). Originally described in terms of its action on B cells, it induces an IgM to IgE class switch and increases immunoglobulin levels in B cells activated, for example, by treatment with anti-immunoglobulin antibodies.

IL-4 is a growth factor for mast cells and synergistic with IL-3 for stimulating their proliferation. It is antagonistic to interferon γ and inhibits macrophage activation but has been shown to enhance the proliferation of T cells and the generation of cytotoxic T lymphocytes. IL-4 promotes adhesion molecule expression, e.g. VCAM-1, and is found in local high concentration in areas of inflammation where there is eosinophil and monocyte involvement.

Il-4 may be measured by its effect on the proliferation of B cells in a costimulator assay.

10.5.1 B-cell costimulator assay

Anti-IgM-pre-activated IgM-bearing B cells and IL-4 supplementation are used, then cell proliferation is assessed by ^{3}H-thymidine incorporation.

MATERIALS AND EQUIPMENT
Purified murine splenic B cells
Anti-murine IgM antibody (conveniently added bound to polyacrylamide beads)
Tissue culture medium
Fetal bovine serum (FBS)
96-well microtitre plates

³H-thymidine
Automated cell harvester
Beta spectrometer

METHOD

1 Resuspend the B cells in tissue culture medium containing 10% FBS and dispense into microtitre trays at a concentration of 1×10^5 cells per well.

2 Add anti-IgM antibody at a range of dilutions to determine the stimulatory concentration (this can be replaced by a single dilution in subsequent assays).

3 Dilute the supernatants under test to obtain a range of concentrations and add to triplicate wells to give a final volume of 200 µl. Controls should include:

   cells + medium alone

   cells + anti-IgM antibody

   cells + IL-4 standard

   cells + anti-IgM antibody + IL-4 standard.

4 Incubate the plates at 37°C in a humidified atmosphere of 5% CO_2 in air for 72 h.

5 Add 18.5×10^3 Bq of ^{3}H-thymidine during the last 6 h of culture.

6 Harvest the plates using an automated cell harvester and process the samples for β scintillation counting.

Assessment of results

Plot ^{3}H-thymidine uptake (equivalent to proliferative response) against concentration for the IL-4 standard, and determine the units of activity in the unknown samples by interpolation.

TECHNICAL NOTE

Interleukin 4 acts on resting B cells and induces them to proliferate, as demonstrated above by enhanced ^{3}H-thymidine uptake. Incubation of resting B cells with IL-4 also causes marked enhancement of expression of class II major histocompatibility complex (MHC) molecules on the cell surface. This is detectable within 6 h and, by 24 h, can show a sixfold or greater increase in antigen density. This has been used to assay for active IL-4. It should be borne in mind, however, that other cytokines, notably IFN-γ, also enhance class II antigen expression.

10.6 Interleukin 5 (IL-5)

Interleukin 5 is also known as TRF (T-cell replacing factor) or EDF (eosinophil differentiation factor). It has B-cell growth factor activity and induces IgM secretion. It can be derived from some T-cell lines and from the T-cell hybridomas B151 and NIMP-TH1 after induction with PMA (phorbol myristate acetate).

10.6.1 Reverse plaque-forming cell assay

IgM secretion by B-cell lymphoma (BCL)1 cells is measured using a reverse plaque-forming cell assay for IgM total immunoglobulin.

MATERIALS AND EQUIPMENT

BCL$_1$ cells growing in a BALB/c mouse

Tissue culture medium

Fetal bovine serum (FBS)

96-well microtitre plates

Protein A-coupled sheep erythrocytes (SRBC)

Rabbit anti-IgM antibody

Other reagents for IgM plaque assay

METHOD

1. Prepare BCL$_1$ cells from the spleens of tumour-bearing BALB/c mice.
2. Deplete the spleen cells of T cells by treatment with anti-Thy-1 monoclonal antibody plus complement (see Section 7.8).
3. Dispense 1.5×10^5 BCL$_1$ cells into 96-well microtitre plates in 100 μl aliquots in tissue culture medium.
4. Add a range of dilutions of the samples under test, in 100 μl aliquots.
5. Incubate at 37°C in a humidified atmosphere of 5% CO$_2$ in air for 48 h.
6. Assay the cells for IgM production using a reverse plaque-forming cell assay with protein A-coupled SRBC and anti-IgM antibody (see Section 9.1.1).

Assessment of results

Plot plaque number versus concentration of sample. A unit of IL-5 activity is usually represented as that required to induce a half maximal response.

10.6.2 **Proliferation assay**

MATERIALS AND EQUIPMENT

BCL$_1$ cells prepared as described above, or, T-cell-depleted normal mouse spleen cells (from C57BL/6xDBA/2 F$_1$ mice)

Tissue culture medium

Fetal bovine serum (FBS)

^{3}H-thymidine

96-well microtitre plates

Automated cell harvester

Beta spectrometer

METHOD

1. Resuspend the B cells at 1×10^6/ml (normal mouse B cells) or 5×10^5/ml (BCL$_1$ cells) and add 100 μl aliquots to individual wells of a 96-well microtitre plate.
2. Add 100 μl aliquots of a range of dilutions of the supernatant under test to triplicate wells.
3. Incubate at 37°C in a humidified atmosphere of 5% CO$_2$ in air for 72 h.
4. Add 18.5×10^3 Bq of ^{3}H-thymidine and incubate for a further 6 h.
5. Harvest using an automated cell harvester and process the samples for liquid scintillation counting.

Assessment of results

Plot ^{3}H-thymidine uptake (equivalent to proliferative response) against concentration for the IL-5 standard, and determine the units of activity in the unknown samples by interpolation. If a standard preparation of IL-5 is not available, assign an arbitrary number of units to the concentration giving half maximal stimulation.

10.7 Interleukin 6 (IL-6)

Interleukin 6 is also known as B-cell differentiation factor 2 (BCDF-2) or interferon β2 (IFN-β2) and can be detected in the circulation following Gram-negative bacterial infections. It has several demonstrable activities *in vitro*; for example, when assayed for its ability to induce B-cell differentiation, it increases surface IgM expression and secretion of μ chains.

Il-6 enhances cytotoxic T lymphocytes and is a potent growth factor for myeloid cells. It also stimulates hepatocytes to produce acute-phase reactant proteins and therefore has a role in inflammation; it is also said to have nerve growth factor-like activity.

IL-6 can be produced *in vitro* by stimulating human fibroblasts with polyribonucleotides or cyclohexamide plus actinomycin D and is constitutively produced by the leukaemia virus-transformed human T-cell line TCL-Na1. IL-6 can also stimulate hybridoma cells used in monoclonal antibody production (see also Chapter 2).

10.7.1 ELISA assay for immunoglobulin secretion by an IL-6-responsive cell line

MATERIALS AND EQUIPMENT
IL-6-responsive cell line, e.g. SKW6-CL4 or CESS
Tissue culture medium
Fetal bovine serum (FBS)
96-well microtitre plates
Reagents for anti-IgM (using SKW6-CL4) or anti-IgG (CESS) ELISA (see Section 5.4.3)
ELISA reader

Preparation in advance

Subculture the indicator cell of choice 24–48 h before the assay to ensure that it is in log-phase growth.

METHOD

1 Harvest the indicator cells, wash twice by centrifugation and resuspend in tissue culture medium containing 10% FBS. Adjust the cell concentration to 4×10^4/ml (SKW6-CL4) or 6×10^4/ml (CESS).

2 Dispense 100 μl aliquots of either cell line into each well of a microtitre plate.

3 Prepare a range of dilutions of the supernatant under test and add 100 μl aliquots to wells in triplicate.

Continued

4 Incubate the plates in a humidified atmosphere of 5% CO_2 in air at 37°C for 72 h.

5 Transfer 100 µl aliquots of culture supernatant from each well to the corresponding well in a second microtitre plate.

6 Assay these supernatants using an anti-IgM or anti-IgG ELISA as appropriate for the cell line used (see Section 5.4.3).

Assessment of results

The amount of immunoglobulin secreted is proportional to the IL-6 concentration in the sample under test. A plot of concentration of the standard IL-6 versus optical density (OD) (immunoglobulin secretion) can be used to determine the activity of the sample. If a standard preparation is not available, assign arbitrary units to the concentration that gives half maximal stimulation.

10.7.2 Reverse plaque-forming cell techniques

Instead of determining the amount of immunoglobulin (IgM or IgG) secreted by CESS or SKW6-CL4 cells by an ELISA assay, one can assay activation by determining the number of IgM or IgG plaque-forming cells in a reverse plaque assay.

Reverse plaque-forming cell assay

MATERIALS AND EQUIPMENT
As for Section 10.7.1 but with reagents for reverse plaque assay.

METHOD

As for Section 10.7.1, but with the following modifications:

1 Incubate the cells for 48 h in a humidified atmosphere of 5% CO_2 in air.

2 Enumerate the antibody-forming cells in a reverse plaque assay, remembering to assay for IgM plaques for SKW6-CL4 cells and IgG plaques for CESS cells.

Assessment of results

The number of plaques is proportional to the IL-6 concentration in the sample under test. A plot of concentration of the standard IL-6 versus the number of plaque-forming cells can be used to determine the activity of the sample. If a standard preparation is not available, assign arbitrary units to the concentration which gives half maximal plaque numbers.

Assay for IL-6 by hybridoma proliferation

A highly sensitive assay for IL-6 utilizes hybridoma B9 cells (Aarden *et al.* 1987). In each microtitre plate well 5×10^3 cells are cultured in 200 µl Iscove's modified Dulbecco's medium supplemented with 50 µM 2-mercaptoethanol, 5% v/v fetal bovine serum, plus streptomycin and penicillin. Following addition of IL-6, and culture for 44 h, 7.4 kBq (0.2 µCi) ^{3}H-thymidine is added and 4 h later the thymidine incorporation is determined following cell harvesting and β-scintillation counting (see Section 9.1).

10.8 Interleukin 7 (IL-7)

Assay for IL-7 by proliferation

Interleukin 7 has potent proliferative effects on B- and T-cell progenitors, and can stimulate mature peripheral T-cells. It is assayed by measuring the stimulatory effects on B-cell progenitors or, more standardly, using a cell line 2bx(1xN/2b) which has been derived from these cells (Park *et al.* 1990). These cells are dependent on IL-7 for growth. Aliquots (50 µl) of cells (1.2×10^5/ml) in Iscove's modified Dulbecco's medium supplemented with 50 µM 2-mercaptoethanol, 2 mM L-glutamine, 50 µg/ml streptomycin and 50 U/ml penicillin are incubated with test samples for 44 h in 7.5% CO_2, 5% O_2. and then pulsed with 74 kBq per cell of ^{3}H-thymidine for 4 h. Cells are then harvested and counted as per standard proliferation assay procedures.

10.9 Interleukin 8 (IL-8)

Interleukin 8 is an inflammatory cytokine that exerts chemoattractant activity for neutrophils. It has activating properties and can be assayed by measuring either neutrophil chemotaxis or activation.

Chemotaxis assay is classically performed in Boyden chambers in which isolated cells to be tested are placed on one side of a chamber (Fig. 10.2) and separated by a membrane from medium containing the chemotactic stimulus. After incubation the membrane is stained and examined microscopically to determine how far the cells have migrated towards the stimulus. Multiwell forms of the chambers are now available for examining several samples. Cellulose ester filters, 150 µm thick, with 3–5-µm pores are suitable for neutrophils.

It is an assay requiring no special apparatus: cells are placed in small wells cut in agarose gels and allowed to migrate under the agarose towards a chemotactic signal placed in an adjacent well.

10.9.1 Agarose migration assay for human neutrophil chemotaxis

MATERIALS AND EQUIPMENT
Neutrophils (see Chapter 7)
IL-8 or other chemotactic test sample

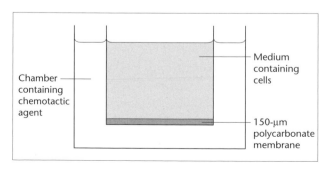

Chamber containing chemotactic agent

Medium containing cells

150-µm polycarbonate membrane

Fig. 10.2 Chamber for testing neutrophil or monocyte chemotaxis.

Plastic tissue culture dishes, 6-cm diameter

Agarose

Tissue culture medium, 10 × concentrated Eagle's MEM with HEPES buffer

Stainless steel punch 3 mm internal diameter with inside bevel

Glutaraldehyde 2.5% w/w in phosphate-buffered saline (PBS)

May–Grünwald and Giemsa stains

METHOD

Preparation of agarose plate

1 Dissolve 0.2 g agarose in 10 ml distilled water by careful boiling, e.g. in a water bath or microwave oven and cool to 56°C.

2 Warm double-strength medium, 10 ml containing 2 ml 10 × concentrated Eagle's MEM, 2 ml heat-inactivated fetal bovine serum (FBS) and 6 ml distilled water, to 56°C.

3 Mix the two solutions together.

4 Pour 6 ml portions of agarose/medium solution into plastic culture dishes on a level surface and allow to cool.

5 When set transfer to a refrigerator for 15–30 min to allow the gel to harden.

6 Cut the pattern (Fig. 10.3) with the steel punch.

7 Remove agarose plugs with a Pasteur pipette attached to a vacuum pump.

TECHNICAL NOTES

- Heat-inactivated FBS is included to cut down on absorption of cytokine to the agarose and to improve the gel handling properties. It must be tested to check that is does not have chemotactic activity as this would increase the random migration of the neutrophils. It is necessary to inactivate the serum as agarose will activate the alternative complement pathway in fresh serum.

- Care must be taken not to scratch the plate when punching the wells.

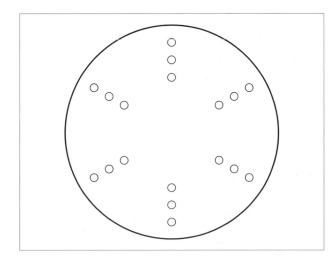

Fig. 10.3 Pattern for cell migration under agar.

- Do not worry at slight lifting of gel when removing plugs as this will aid the neutrophils in moving under the gel.
- It is advisable to prepare a template corresponding to the pattern in Fig. 10.3. If this is constructed in Perspex, about 3 mm thick, mounted on side supports, this will guide the punch to produce vertical wells.
- Any liquid that collects in the wells after punching should be carefully removed with a Pasteur pipette.

Chemotaxis assay

1 Fill the middle well of each set of three with 10 μl neutrophils, 5×10^7/ml.
2 Add 10 μl of control solution, e.g. medium, to inner well of three.
3 Add 10 μl of test solution or standard IL-8 solution to outer well of three.
4 Incubate plate in humidified chamber at 37°C for 2 h.
5 Terminate migration by flooding plates with 2.5% glutaraldehyde for 1 h at room temperature or overnight at 4°C.
6 Carefully remove the agarose with a small spatula taking care not to rotate the gel.
7 Stain cells with May–Grünwald and Giemsa solutions.
8 Determine migration by either: (i) counting the number of cells which have migrated out of the well; or (ii) measuring the distance migrated by the cells.

TECHNICAL NOTES
- A positive control for migration may be obtained by using agarose-activated fresh serum. Simply place fresh human serum in a well 1 h before rest of samples.
- Longer incubation times may be used but all materials will need to be prepared and used under sterile conditions.

Calculation of results

The migration distance for the positive samples must be corrected for random migration. This is accomplished by subtracting the distance moved towards the control well. The result may be expressed as corrected distance moved or as a stimulation index (SI):

$$SI = \frac{\text{Corrected distance moved}}{\text{Random distance moved}}$$

10.10 Interleukin 9 (IL-9)

Interleukin 9 supports the growth of some helper T-cell clones and enhances proliferation of mast-cell lines in the presence of IL-3.

Il-9 is assayed on MO7e cells, a human megakaryoblastic cell line (Yang *et al.* 1989). The MO7e cells are cultured in modified Eagle's medium supplemented with 20% v/v heat inactivated fetal bovine serum (FBS) and either 10 U/ml IL-3 or 4 ng/ml (40 IU/ml) granulocyte–macrophage colony-stimulating factor (GM-CSF). After washing the cells are resuspended to 10^5 cells/ml and 10 000 cells are placed in each of the wells of a microtitre plate together with 0.1 ml of test sample in medium. Cells are allowed to grow for 72 h and then pulsed for 4 h with 0.5 µCi ^{3}H-thymidine.

Then cells are harvested and radioactivity determined by scintillation counting.

TECHNICAL NOTE

IL-9 stimulates on its own but the assay is made more sensitive by the inclusion of the stem-cell factor.

10.11 Interleukin 10 (IL-10)

IL-10 has multiple activities on B, T and mast cells. On its own it has little effect on mast cells but if added with either IL-3 or IL-4 it potentially enhances proliferation.

The mast-cell line MC/9 provides a convenient source of mast cells for assay (Thompson-Snipes *et al.* 1991).

1   5×10^3 MC/9 cells in 1 ml RPMI 1640 medium containing 10% v/v fetal bovine serum and 50 mM 2-mercaptoethanol are placed in each well of a flat-bottomed 24-well plate.

2   IL-4 is added at 200 U/ml and IL-10 in the range of 1–100 ng/ml.

3   After 3 days in culture cells are counted to assess proliferation.

10.12 Interleukin 11 (IL-11)

Interleukin 11 has comparable activities to IL-6 and can be assayed in a similar way to IL-6, but it is necessary to remove IL-6 activity from test samples in order to determine the effect due to IL-11.

IL-6 is depleted from samples by addition of monoclonal antibody to IL-6. The B9 hybridoma cells used in IL-6 assay are not particularly sensitive to IL-11 but subclones, which are IL-11 responsive, may be produced by cloning B9 cells in the presence of IL-11 and selecting positively growing cells. The subclone B9–11 (Lu *et al.* 1994) is very effective for the assay of IL-11 in the same system as that described for IL-6 above.

10.13 Interleukin 12 (IL-12)

IL-12 is a key cytokine with multiple activities.

When produced by antigen-presenting cells it induces proliferation of T-helper cell clones. It induces the production of interferon γ by T cells and NK cells and has stimulatory effects on NK and antibody-dependent cell-mediated cytotoxicity (ADCC) activity. IL-12 is frequently assayed using its ability to maintain the proliferation of mitogen-activated T cells. As described above for the assay of IL-2, PHA-activated lymphoblasts may be used to determine the levels of IL-12, in the presence of monoclonal antibody to IL-2.

10.14 Interleukin 13 (IL-13)

Interleukin 13 has a range of activities including inhibitory effects on monocyte cytokine release and stimulatory effects on B lymphocytes. Labit-Le Bouteiller *et al.* (1995) cultured B-hybridoma cells in the presence of IL-13 to produce an IL-13-dependent subclone of B9 cells. The B9-1-3 subclone may be used in the same experimental format as for the B9 assay for IL-6 but with the addition of monoclonal antibody to neutralize IL-6.

10.15 Interleukin 14 (IL-14)

Interleukin 14 is a potent enhancer of the proliferation of activated B cells but inhibits immunoglobulin synthesis. The bioassay is accomplished by activating B cells with *Staphylococcus aureus* (Cowan I strain) and measuring the proliferation induced by IL-14.

MATERIALS AND EQUIPMENT

Human B cells (see Chapter 6)

Tissue culture medium RPMI 1640 containing 5% v/v fetal bovine serum (FBS)

Staphylococcus aureus (Cowan I strain (SAC); immunoprecipitin, Bethesda Research Laboratories, Gaithersburg, MD)

IL-14 standard

^{3}H-thymidine

Cell harvesting equipment

Beta spectrometer

METHOD

1 Incubate 2×10^5 cells/ml of B cells in RPMI 1640 containing 10% v/v FBS and a 1 : 25 000 dilution of *Staphylococcus aureus* (Cowan I strain).

2 Remove dead cells by Ficoll–Hypaque methods (see Chapter 6).

3 Wash the B cells with phosphate-buffered saline (PBS) and resuspend the cells at a concentration of 10^6 cells/ml in RPMI containing 5% v/v FBS.

4 Place 100 µl of B-cell suspension in each well of a 96-microtitre plate.

5 Add 100 µl of test samples in tissue culture medium to wells.

6 Incubate at 37°C in a CO_2 incubator for 54 h.

7 Add 37 kBq ^{3}H-thymidine to each well and culture for a further 18 h.

8 Harvest the cells from each well onto filter mats and count in a liquid scintillation counter or other appropriate equipment.

10.16 Interleukin 15 (IL-15)

Interleukin 15 has similar activity to IL-2 and interacts with part of the IL-2 receptor (Giri *et al.* 1994). It can be assayed on an IL-2-dependent cell line such as CTLL-2 as shown above, but with the addition of monoclonal antibody to block IL-2.

10.17 The interferons

These cytokines were first described on the basis of their antiviral activity, even though they are not directly toxic to viruses but instead induce the various host cells to exhibit antiviral activity.

Interferon α (IFN-α) is a leucocyte-derived interferon that induces antiviral activity and enhances NK cell and mixed-lymphocyte reaction. It stimulates the increased expression of HLA on lymphocytes and inhibits the growth of human lymphoblastoid cell lines. IFN-α can be prepared from activated lymphocytes (helper T cells, B cells and macrophages) and from Namalva cells.

Interferon β (IFN-β) is a fibroblast-derived interferon that enhances NK-cell activity, induces antiviral activity and inhibits the growth of fibroblasts. It can be prepared from poly IC (polymer of inosine and cytosine)-induced fibroblasts, human foreskin cells, fetal muscle cells, epithelial cells, myeloblasts and lymphoblasts.

Interferon γ (IFN-γ) is an immune cell-derived interferon that stimulates macrophage activation, up-regulates class II antigen expression, activates cytotoxic T lymphocytes and induces antiviral activity (but poorly compared with IFN-α and -β). IFN-γ can be prepared from activated lymphocytes and T-cell lines.

Interferons can be assayed using commercially available ELISA or RIA kits that are based on specific antibody. However, antiviral assays are used to give assessments of units of activity.

10.17.1 Interferon assays

Described below are two assays for determining the antiviral activity of interferon.

Inhibition of viral nucleic acid synthesis

MATERIALS AND EQUIPMENT
Indicator cell line, e.g. L929
Plastic or glass scintillation vials (5 × 1.3 cm)
Semliki forest virus (SFV) at 1×10^7 PFU/ml
Actinomycin D
^{3}H-uridine
Trichloroacetic acid (TCA)
Soluene–toluene 1 : 2 mix
Tissue culture medium
Fetal bovine serum (FBS)
Beta spectrometer

Preparation in advance

Plate the indicator cells into a 150-cm^2 growth area tissue culture flask and allow to grow to confluence.

METHOD

1 Harvest the indicator cell line by trypsin treatment, wash twice and resuspend in 200 ml of tissue culture medium containing 10% FBS.
2 Dispense 1 ml aliquots of cell suspension into the individual vials.
3 Incubate for 24 h at 37°C in a humidified atmosphere of 5% CO_2 in air.
4 Remove the tissue culture supernatant by aspiration and add 200 µl aliquots (in triplicate) of a range of dilutions of the samples under test, made up in medium containing 2% serum.
5 Incubate overnight under conditions as described in step 3.
6 Add 200 µl of SFV at 1×10^7 PFU/ml in medium containing 2% FBS and 3 µg/ml actinomycin D.
7 Incubate for 3 h.
8 Add 100 µl medium containing 2% FBS and 1 µg/ml actinomycin D and 37×10^4 Bq/ml ^{3}H-uridine.
9 Incubate for a further 3 h.
10 Aspirate the medium and wash the cell monolayer twice with 1 ml of 5% ice-cold TCA and once with 1 ml ethanol.
11 Aspirate the residual ethanol and dry the vials at 60°C for 15 min.
12 Add 500 µl soluene–toluene and 2 ml scintillant. Count the vials in a β spectrometer.

Assessment of results

Plot the mean c.p.m. for replicate cultures against $\log_{10}$ IFN dilution. The inhibition of virus proliferation, measured as inhibition of ^{3}H-uridine uptake into untreated control cells, is proportional to IFN concentration.

Cytopathic effect reduction

MATERIALS AND EQUIPMENT
Indicator cell line, usually Hep/2c
Murine encephalomyocarditis virus (EMCV), 1×10^7 PFU/ml
96-well microtitre plates
Gentian violet stain and filter
Tissue culture medium
Fetal bovine serum (FBS)

Preparation in advance

1 Prepare a stock solution of the gentian violet stain at 1% w/v in 20% ethanol in phosphate-buffered saline, warm to 60°C and filter to remove insoluble material.
2 Subculture the indicator cell line 24–48 h before use to ensure it is in log-phase growth.

1. Harvest the indicator cells from a culture in log-phase growth and wash twice by centrifugation. Resuspend in tissue culture medium at 5×10^5/ml.
2. Dispense 100 μl aliquots of cell suspension into individual wells of a microtitre plate.
3. Incubate at 37°C in a humidified atmosphere of 5% CO_2 in air for 5 h.
4. Aspirate the medium and add the samples under test to triplicate wells, at a range of dilutions, in medium containing 15% serum.
5. Incubate at 37°C overnight.
6. Aspirate the medium, add 100 μl formal saline to each well and leave on the bench for 5 min.
7. Aspirate the formal saline and add 3 drops per well of gentian violet stain and leave on the bench for 10 min.
8. Wash gently with running tap water for 3 min.
9. Read the cytopathic effect by counting the number of plaques.

In practice, the results of the experiment can usually be determined by scanning the plate directly by eye to give an end point. Counting plaques will give a more accurate result for determining the titre of the samples. Alternatively the plate can be read by solubilizing the stain with 100 μl of 50% ethanol and reading with an ELISA reader at a wavelength of 700 nm.

Assessment of results

Interferon gives a concentration-dependent reduction in virus plaque number compared with untreated virus-infected cells. This may be used to construct a standard curve for the determination of IFN concentration in unknown samples.

If standard preparation of interferon is not available, assign an arbitrary number of units to the dilution giving 50% reduction in plaque number compared with controls.

10.18 **Tumour necrosis factors**

Tumour necrosis factors α (TNF-α) and β (TNF-β—sometimes referred to as lymphotoxin) are distinct and separate gene products but have similar functions and activities *in vitro*, and appear to bind to the same receptor.

TNF-α was originally described as a monocyte/macrophage product derived from certain macrophage-like cell lines, but also produced by T cells. It has cytostatic and cytocidal effects on transformed cells; it stimulates bone resorption and inhibits bone reformation; and it inhibits lipoprotein lipase activity in adipocytes.

TNF-β is produced by T lymphocytes and has properties similar to TNF-α. The only effective means of distinguishing between the two molecules at present is by the use of appropriate neutralizing antibodies. Identical assays can be used for both TNF-α and TNF-β.

10.18.1 L929 cell-killing assay

MATERIALS AND EQUIPMENT

L929 tumour cells

Tissue culture medium

Fetal bovine serum (FBS)

Actinomycin D

96-well microtitre plates

Phosphate-buffered saline (PBS)

Crystal violet, 1% w/v aqueous solution

ELISA reader

Preparation in advance

1 Actinomycin D sensitizes cells for lysis by TNF. L929 cells can vary in their susceptibility to TNF. It is advisable to work with cell cultures maintained and subcultured for relatively short periods. If TNF assays are to be done on a regular basis, it is recommended that a large number of cells with proven sensitivity to TNF be cryopreserved. Frozen vials can then be used to start up fresh cultures at regular intervals.

2 Subculture the cell line 24 h prior to use to ensure that the cultures are subconfluent.

METHOD

1 Prepare a suspension of L929 cells, by trypsin treatment of a subconfluent culture, and wash twice by centrifugation.

2 Resuspend the cells at 4×10^5/ml in medium containing 5% serum.

3 Dispense 100 μl aliquots of cells into individual wells of microtitre plates.

4 Incubate for 4 h at 37°C in a humidified atmosphere of 5% CO_2 in air to allow the cells to adhere.

5 Remove the medium by inverting the plate with a rapid flicking motion.

6 Add 100 μl aliquots of a range of dilutions of the samples under test, in medium containing 2% serum and actinomycin D (2 μg/ml initial concentration).

7 Incubate the plates overnight at 37°C in a humidified atmosphere of 5% CO_2 in air.

8 Remove the medium as described and wash the wells once with PBS.

9 Remove the PBS by flicking the plate as described and add 100 μl methanol to each well to fix the cells.

10 Remove excess methanol and dry the plates briefly in air.

11 Add 100 μl of aqueous crystal violet and incubate at room temperature for 5 min.

12 Wash the wells thoroughly with tap water; finally empty the wells by flicking the plate.

13 Solubilize the contents of the wells with 100 μl of 33% acetic acid (in water) and read the plates on an ELISA reader at a test wavelength of 570 nm and a reference wavelength of 420 nm.

Assessment of results

Reduced OD relative to controls without TNF indicates cell killing. Plot OD against sample dilution to determine the dilution of the unknown sample that gives 50% target-cell death.

10.18.2 WEHI-164 killing assay

The recently derived subclone 13 of the WEHI-164 murine fibrosarcoma has provided a highly sensitive assay for TNF/LT (lymphotoxin) activity; it is similar in principle to the standard L929 but has the following modifications.

1 Actinomycin D is not required in the medium.
2 The cells are plated at 2×10^4/ml in the presence of the test samples.
3 The culture plates are incubated at 37°C for 20 h. Viability can then be assessed using crystal violet staining (see Section 10.19.1) or the MTT assay (Section 9.5.2).

Assessment of results

Reduced OD relative to controls without TNF indicates cell killing. Plot OD against sample dilution to determine the dilution of the unknown sample that gives 50% target-cell death.

10.19 ELISPOT assay for the evaluation of cytokines

Estimation of cytokines in serum can only give an average view of cytokine production. It is informative to look at cells within particular tissues. The expression of cytokine mRNA can give useful information although it does not always correlate with the production of cytokine.

The ELISPOT assay may be adapted to quantify cytokine-producing cells using solid-phase anticytokine antibody to capture cytokines produced by individual cells.

Earlier versions of the assay used nitrocellulose supports but conventional ELISA plates have been found to give greater sensitivity and specificity (Rönnelid & Klareskog 1997).

TECHNIQUE
1 Microtitre plates are coated with anticytokine antibody and cells, with or without stimulation, are placed in the wells and allowed to layer on the plate bottom.
2 Secreted cytokines are captured by the solid-phase antibody and revealed, after washing away the cells, by adding labelled anticytokine antibody.

10.19.1 ELISPOT assay for single-cell production of cytokine

MATERIALS
96-well flat-bottomed microtitre plates, e.g. Immunon II (Dynatech) or Maxisorb (Nunc)
Anti-cytokine antibody, e.g. monoclonal anti-IFN-γ
Phosphate-buffered saline (PBS)
Cells, e.g. peripheral blood mononuclear cells (PBMC) prepared on Ficoll–Hypaque
Tissue culture medium RPMI 1640 with 10% fetal bovine serum (FBS), penicillin, streptomycin, glutamine and HEPES buffer
Mitogen, e.g. PHA
CO_2 incubator
Biotinylated anticytokine antibody
Avidin–alkaline phosphatase conjugate

Substrate 5-bromo-4-chloro-3-indoyl-phosphate (BCIP) solution, made up as per manufacturer's instructions, e.g. Sigma-Aldrich.

Low-power microscope

METHOD

1 Coat the wells of a microtitre plate with 50 μl anticytokine antibody, 15 μg/ml, at 4°C overnight.

2 Wash four times with sterile PBS.

3 Add 100 μl cell suspension 10^6 cells/ml in RPMI 1640 with FBS.

4 Add mitogen if required, e.g. PHA, to 5 μg/ml.

5 Incubate at 37°C in a humidified incubator with 5% CO_2 for 0–72 h to examine kinetics.

6 Flick out cells and wash four times with PBS.

7 Add 50 μl biotinylated anticytokine antibody, 1 μg/ml, and incubate overnight at 4°C.

8 Wash three times with PBS.

9 Add 50 μl avidin–alkaline phosphatase conjugate, 1 μg/ml, and incubate at room temperature for 2 h.

10 Wash three times with PBS.

11 Add 50 μl BCIP–phosphatase substrate solution and incubate at room temperature for 1–5 h.

12 Wash with water and dry.

13 Count spots using × 20 magnification.

TECHNICAL NOTES

• Pilot experiments will be necessary to ensure that optimum numbers of cytokine-producing cells are placed in the wells. With too many positive cells the 'spots' merge and become difficult to count.

• The kinetics vary for different cytokines and will need to be examined experimentally.

• The FBS must be checked to ensure that it does not stimulate cytokine production itself but that it does have good cytokine-producing support properties.

10.20 **Further reading**

Aarden, L.A., De Groof, E.R., Schaap, O.L. & Lansdorp, P.M. (1987) Production of hybridoma growth factor by human monocytes. *Eur J Immunol* **17**, 1411–1416.

Ambrus, Jr, J.L., Chesky, L., Stephany, D., McFarland, P., Mostowski, H. & Fauci, A.S. (1990) Functional studies examining the subpopulations of human B lymphocytes responding to high molecular weight B cell growth factor. *J Immunol* **145**, 3949–3955.

Balkwill, F. (ed.) (2000) *Cytokine Cell Biology: A Practical Approach*. Oxford University Press, Oxford.

Balkwill, F. (ed.) (2000) *Cytokine Molecular Biology: A Practical Approach*, 3rd edn. Oxford University Press, Oxford.

Chianelli, M., Signore, A., Hicks, R., Testi, R., Negri, M. & Beverley, P.C.L. (1993) A simple method for evaluation of receptor binding capacity of modified cytokines. *J Immunol Meth* **166**, 177–182.

Collins, D.P. (2000) Cytokine and cytokine receptor expression as a biological indicator of immune activation, important considerations in the development of *in vitro* model systems. *J Immunol Meth* **243**(1–2), 125–145.

Evans, T.J. (2000) *Septic Shock: Methods and Protocols*. Blackwell Science, Oxford.

Frussin, C. & Metcalfe, D.D. (1995) Detection of intracytoplasmic cytokine using flow cytometry and directly conjugated anticytokine antibodies. *J Immunol Meth* **188**, 117–128.

Giri, J.G., Ahdieh, M., Eisenman, J. *et al.* (1994) Utilization of the β and γ chains of the IL-2 receptor by the novel cytokine IL-15. *EMBO J* **13**, 2822–2830.

Kopp, W., Reynolds, C. & Ruscetti, F. (1999) The immunoassay of cytokines and growth factors in biological fluids. *Dev Biol Stand* **97**, 29–37.

Labit-Le Bouteiller, C., Astruc, R., Minty, A., Ferrara, P. & Lupker, J.H. (1995) Isolation of an IL-13 dependent subclone of the B9 cell line useful for the estimation of human IL-13 bioactivity. *J Immunol Meth* **181**, 29–36.

Lakew, M., Nordstrom, I., Czerkinsky, C. & Quiding-Jarbrink, M. (1997) Combined immunomagnetic cell sorting and ELISPOT assay for the phenotypic characterization of specific antibody-forming cells. *J Immunol Meth* **203**, 193–8.

Lalani, A.S., Barrett, J.W. & McFadden, G. (2000) Modulating chemokines: more lessons from viruses [Review]. *Immunol Today* **21** (2), 100–106.

Lu, Z.-Y., Zhang, X.-G., Gu, Z.-J. *et al.* (1994) A highly sensitive quantitative bioassay for human interleukin-11. *J Immunol Meth* **173**, 19–26.

Mire-Sluis, A.R., Gaines-Das, R. & Thorpe, R. (1995) Immunoassays for detecting cytokines: What are they really measuring? *J Immunol Meth* **186**, 157–160.

Mire-Sluis, A.R., Page, L. & Thorpe, R. (1995) Quantitative cell line based bioassays for human cytokines. *J Immunol Meth* **187**, 191–199.

Nelson, R.D. & Herron, M.J. (1988) Agarose method for human neutrophil chemotaxis. *Methods Enzymol* **162**, 50–59.

O'Connor, E., Roberts, E.M. & Davis, J.D. (1999) Amplification of cytokine-specific ELISAs increases the sensitivity of detection to 5–20 picogrammes per millilitre. *J Immunol Meth* **229**, 155–160.

Ozenci, V., Kouwenhoven, M., Press, R., Link, H. & Huang, Y.M. (2000) IL-12 ELISPOT assays to detect and enumerate IL-12-secreting cells. *Cytokine* **12**, 1218–1224.

Park, L.S., Friend, D.J., Schmeirer, A.E., Dower, S.K. & Namen, A.E. (1990) Murine interleukin-7 (IL-7) receptor: characterization on an IL-7 dependent cell line. *J Exp Med* **171**, 1073–1079.

Pashenkov, M., Kouwenhoven, M.C., Ozenci, V. & Huang, Ymn. (2000) Phenotypes and cytokine profiles of enriched blood dendritic cells in healthy individuals. *Eur Cytokine Netw* **11**(3), 456–463.

Riches, P., Gooding, R., Millar, B.C. & Rowbottom, A.W. (1992) Influence of collection and separation of blood samples on plasma IL-1, IL-6 and TNF-α concentrations. *J Immunol Meth* **153**, 125–131.

Rönnelid, J. & Klareskog, L. (1997) A comparison between ELISPOT methods for the detection of cytokine producing cells: greater sensitivity and specificity using ELISA plates as compared to nitrocellulose membranes. *J Immunol Meth* **200**, 17–26.

Sander, B., Höidén, F., Andersson, U., Möller, E. & Abrams, J.S. (1993) Similar frequencies and kinetics of cytokine producing cells in murine peripheral blood and spleen. Cytokine detection by immunoassay and intracellular immunostaining. *J Immunol Meth* **166**, 201–214.

Thompson-Snipes, L., Dhar, V., Bond, M.W., Mosmann, T.R., Moore, K.W. & Rennick, D.M. (1991) Interleukin 10: a novel stimulatory factor for mast cells and their progenitors. *J Exp Med* **173**, 507–510.

Thomson, A. (ed.) (1998) *The Cytokine Handbook.* Academic Press Inc., New York.

Wadhwa, M. & Thorpe, R. (1998) Cytokine immunoassays: recommendations for standardization, calibration and validation. *J Immunol Meth* **219**, 1–5.

Yang, Y.C., Ricciardi, S., Ciarletta, A., Calvetti, J., Kelleher, K. & Clark, S.C. (1989) Expression cloning of a cDNA encoding a novel human haematopoietic growth factor: human homologue of murine T-cell growth factor P40. *Blood* **74**, 1880–1884.

11 Immunological manipulations *in vivo*

Much immunological experimentation is carried out *in vitro,* but sometimes it is necessary, particularly to raise antisera, to work *in vivo.*

For obvious ethical reasons, serious consideration should always be given to finding alternatives to living animals. If the human immune system is being studied, it is often possible to work on volunteers, by careful choice of acceptable antigens that have been approved by the local ethical committee. Only where there is no acceptable alternative to non-human animals should animal experiments be considered. It is mandatory to conform to the legal requirements of the country in which one is working, and to take care to minimize the suffering to the animals. Detailed procedures for handling animals are beyond the scope of this book, but a list of helpful references is included at the end of the chapter.

11.1 Production of polyclonal antisera

Although monoclonal antibodies offer distinct advantages, the potential diversity of epitopes recognized by polyclonal antisera, even against a single molecular species of antigen, can yield enormous benefits in immunoassays.

Every laboratory has its own methods for raising antisera. Those we describe below are known to work and are rapid. There is considerable variation in the route and frequency of immunization as well as the choice of adjuvant depending on the species being immunized. Surprisingly, there is little variation in the amount of antigen: both mice and goats can be immunized effectively with 100–200 μg of foreign protein.

Inflammation can be intense and supporters of Polly Matzinger's danger/damage hypothesis might regard this as an important part of the adjuvant effect (Matzinger 1994; see also her website http://cmmg.biosci.wayne.edu/asg/polly.html).

A useful guide to polyclonal antibody production (theory and practice) is provided by Hanley *et al.* (1995).

11.1.1 Adjuvants

Antigens are more immunogenic when presented in an insoluble form or with an adjuvant; the most commonly used adjuvant is Freund's complete adjuvant. The mode of adjuvant action is unclear, but it is probable that the slow release of the antigen from the emulsion 'depot' acts as a prolonged series of small injections. A proportion of the subsequent antibody production occurs within the granuloma induced by the *Mycobacterium tuberculosis* in the adjuvant.

Freund's complete adjuvant is a mixture of oil (Bayol F) and detergent (mannide mono-oleate) containing *M. tuberculosis*. Freund's incomplete adjuvant is a mixture of oil and detergent alone. The complete and incomplete adjuvant may be purchased commercially. However, please note that Freund's adjuvant is not clinically acceptable for human use; care should be taken to avoid personal contamination during its experimental use. Substitutes for Freund's adjuvant have replaced whole mycobacteria with muramyl dipeptide, a synthetic dipeptide originally identified in the cell wall of *Corynebacterium parvum*. This is available as a synthetic derivative in a water-in-oil emulsion from Chiron Corporation, Emeryville, California, USA, as Syntex Adjuvant Formulation.

A related adjuvant, N-acetylglucosaminyl-N-acetyl-L-alanyl-D-isoglutamine with dimethyl-dioctadecylammonium chloride and zinc-L-proline complex (Gerbu adjuvant; Gerbu Biotechnik GmbH, Gaiberg, Germany) is reported to be an effective adjuvant without side-effects (Grubhofer 1995).

Saponin is a safer immunostimulating agent and used in a variety of veterinary vaccines. It consists of a mixture of water-soluble triterpene glycosides extracted from the bark of a South American tree *Quillaia saponaria*, and when purified is known as Quill A. Saponin is highly surface active and forms stable complexes with proteins released from the viral envelopes of viruses, such as para-influenza, influenza, measles and rabies. The complexes are about 30 nm in diameter and are referred to as ISCOMs—immunostimulating complexes (Morein *et al.* 1993).

Other adjuvants include aluminium hydroxide (one of the few adjuvants approved for human use) which precipitates in the presence of antigen and is absorbed onto nascent particles. The incorporation of *Bordetella pertussis* organisms can make this a highly effective adjuvant (Hay & Torrigiani 1973).

Frequently the investigator ends up with an antigen as a band on a nitrocellulose blot. The band may be cut out, dissolved in dimethyl sulphoxide (DMSO) and reprecipitated as micro-particles of nitrocellulose suitable for immunization (Forrest & Ross 1993).

Methods described in the next few sections are applicable for polyclonal antisera against any protein or glycoprotein antigen.

Freund's complete adjuvant

MATERIALS AND EQUIPMENT

Mouse γ-globulin
Freund's complete adjuvant
Glass syringe with Luer lock
Large rabbits

Please refer to your local animal research facility to obtain guidelines for injecting animals—such procedures should only be performed by experienced personnel.

METHOD

1 Dissolve 500 μg of mouse γ-globulin in 1 ml saline.
2 Add protein dropwise to 1 ml of Freund's complete adjuvant. Homogenize with a syringe and needle to a white cream after each addition.
3 Continue homogenizing until a stable water-in-oil emulsion is obtained. Check this by gently placing 1 drop from the syringe onto saline. If the emulsion is stable the first or second drop will not disperse.
4 Inject approximately 250 μl of the emulsion intramuscularly into each hindquarter of the rabbit. (Many investigators favour a foot-pad injection regime. Theoretically this is advantageous as there is good lymphatic drainage to the local nodes. In practice, however, it is not advisable, especially if the rabbits are housed over wire grilles.)
5 Two weeks later repeat the injections in incomplete Freund's adjuvant (omitting the *M. tuberculosis*).
6 After 2 further weeks take a 5-ml sample bleed from the central ear artery. This technique must be performed by experienced personnel only, and under the strict guidelines of your local animal research facility.
7 Transfer the blood to a glass tube and allow it to clot at room temperature for 1 h. Loosen the clot from the sides of the tube to aid retraction.
8 Leave at 4°C until serum is expressed, and harvest as in Section 11.3.1.
9 Test the antiserum in an interfacial ring test (see Section 11.4).

Alum precipitation of proteins

MATERIALS AND EQUIPMENT

Protein antigen
1 M sodium bicarbonate
0.2 M aluminium potassium sulphate
Phosphate-buffered saline (PBS)

METHOD

1 For each 10 ml of protein solution add 4.5 ml of 1 M sodium bicarbonate.
2 Add 10 ml of 0.2 M aluminium potassium sulphate while stirring. Add slowly to minimize frothing.
3 Leave for 15 min.
4 Spin off precipitate (300 g for 15 min) and wash three times with PBS by centrifugation.
5 Resuspend the insoluble protein to the required concentration.

TECHNICAL NOTES

• Addition of 2×10^9 *Bordetella pertussis* organisms per animal with alum–antigen mixture has pronounced immunostimulating properties.
• Experience shows that the older the solution of aluminium hydroxide, the better the adjuvant effects. This may be due to physical changes or simply to increased endotoxin content.

Suggested routes of immunization

Subcutaneous (s.c.)

For protein antigen emulsified in Freund's complete adjuvant/incomplete Freund's adjuvant water-in oil emulsion, e.g. in mice for hybridoma generation and rabbits for polyclonal antibody production. Multiple sites may be used, and reasonably large volumes (mice 100 μl, rabbits 400 μl). There is lymphatic drainage into local lymph nodes.

Intramuscular (i.m.)

As above for protein antigens, e.g. useful in hindquarters of rabbit. It enables slow release of antigen into local lymph nodes. It is also useful for DNA preparations, e.g. plasmids.

Intradermal (i.d.)

Used for the slow release of antigen in larger animals, e.g. rabbits.

Intraperitoneal (i.p.)

Used for delivering particulate or soluble antigen in saline, e.g. for boosting mice. It is a particularly effective route for generating antibodies to cells.

Intrasplenic (i.s.)

Applicable when there is minimal antigenic material available, e.g. neural crest cells.

Intravenous (i.v.)

Used for directing antigen to organs such as the spleen. It is applicable for final boosting prior to fusing and hybridoma generation.

11.2 Immunization schedules

Common sense and experience provide the best guide to effective immunization. For example, if immunization is being used to obtain antibody-secreting plasma cells or an antiserum, the interval between immunization and use will be much shorter than if the intention is to generate memory B lymphocytes.

Serum should be obtained from the animal(s) prior to immunization. If the animal is large (rabbit, goat, etc.) a blood sample of 50 ml or more will yield a useful quantity of normal or pre-immunization serum. If the animal is small (mouse, guinea pig, etc.) it is not usually feasible to prebleed the individual intended for immunization. In this case a pool of serum is a practical alternative, derived from non-immunized animals of the same strain and the same colony (i.e. same environmental antigens) and of approximately the same age.

Important: do *NOT* take more than 15% of the total blood volume from normal laboratory species over any 4-week period. Blood volume averages about 65 ml/kg. Therefore one can take up to a maximum of 1.5 ml from a mouse over 4 weeks, with each bleed of around 300 µl (5 bleeds including Day 0). A typical single bleed from a rat can be about 2.5 ml, a hamster 0.5 ml, a guinea-pig 5 ml and a rabbit 30 ml.

11.2.1 **Rabbits**

1 Use between 50 and 500 µg foreign protein antigen, in Freund's complete adjuvant, injected subcutaneously into areas of loose skin, up to 0.1 ml at each of the two sites.
2 Repeat the inoculation after 2 weeks using Freund's incomplete adjuvant, being careful to inject into different sites from those previously used.
3 If a good precipitating antiserum is not obtained 2 weeks after the second inoculation of antigen, continue boosting with 300 µg of alum-absorbed antigen given subcutaneously.

Sample bleed

It is relatively easy to obtain a 10–30 ml blood sample (under aseptic conditions) by bleeding from the central ear artery using a hypodermic syringe and needle. When required, exsanguination can be accomplished by cardiac puncture under phenobarbital anaesthesia. A 2.5-kg rabbit should yield 100–120 ml blood, equivalent to 70–80 ml serum, when killed.

11.2.2 **Rats and mice**

Good B-cell responses in mice can be obtained by intraperitoneal immunization with 0.1 ml alum-precipitated protein (400 µg) mixed with standard 'whooping cough' vaccine (equivalent to 2×10^9 killed *Bordetella pertussis* organisms).

IgG and IgM plaque-forming cells can be detected in the spleen after 8 days and the serum antibody levels are maximal by 10–14 days (with slight variations, depending on the antigen used). If memory B cells are required then at least 2–3 months should be allowed to elapse after the last immunization. If T-cell priming is required, immunization in Freund's complete adjuvant is advised. Use 10–100 µg of antigen in 100 µl Freund's complete adjuvant and inject the emulsion subcutaneously near the nape of the neck.

Immunization of mice against membrane antigens is particularly effective when saponin (Quill A purified extract) is used as an adjuvant. Mix 15–20 µg of saponin with 10–100 µg of antigen in phosphate-buffered saline and inject the mixture subcutaneously near the nape of the neck. The adjuvant effects of saponin are highly dose dependent—20 µg is about the maximum subtoxic dose that can be given to a mouse.

Mice can be selectively immunized for an IgE response by immunization with the antigen of choice and infection with the nematode *Nippostrongylus brasiliensis*. Animals are primed with alum-precipitated antigen, followed 2–3 weeks later with infection with 300–500 *N. brasiliensis* larvae. On further boosting with antigen, pronounced IgE responses are induced.

Exsanguinate mice either by cardiac puncture or by severing the underarm vessels (see Fig. 6.2) under ether anaesthesia.

Rats may be immunized by subcutaneous or intramuscular injection of 10–100 µg antigen in 500 µl Freund's complete adjuvant, distributed at three sites. Exsanguinate by cardiac puncture under general anaesthesia.

11.2.3 Goats, sheep and pigs

These large animals can be immunized easily and provide relatively large volumes of serum (up to 1.5 l) even when done commercially as a customer request. They are immunized by subcutaneous injection with up to 1 mg of foreign protein antigen in Freund's complete adjuvant to a maximum of 0.25 ml at each of the four sites, and boosted for repeated bleeding. Test bleeds can be taken from the jugular vein and exsanguination accomplished by insertion of an arterial shunt.

The size of these animals puts the inexperienced immunizer at a considerable disadvantage. It is wise to seek expert help or a commercial supplier.

11.3 Serum and plasma

Serum is to be preferred to plasma for any immunoassay due to the tendency of the clotting factors in plasma to form spontaneous clots and so mimic or mask antigen–antibody reactions.

11.3.1 Collection of serum

MATERIALS AND EQUIPMENT
Blood without anticoagulant
Glass containers (test tubes or conical flasks)
Low-speed centrifuge

METHOD

1. Collect the blood into a glass container and allow it to clot at room temperature for 1 h.
2. Once the clot has formed, loosen it from the walls of the container to aid retraction.
3. Transfer to 4°C and leave overnight if necessary.
4. Collect the expressed serum and centrifuge at 150 g for 5 min (to sediment the erythrocytes) and then at 350 g for 15 min.
5. Transfer the serum (straw-coloured supernatant) to containers suitable for long-term storage and heat at 56°C for 30 min to destroy the heat-labile components of complement.

TECHNICAL NOTES
- Blood clots better in glass than in plastic containers.
- Although heating to destroy the complement components is largely of historical interest, it is still good practice as the unrecognized activation of complement in an antiserum can have far-reaching consequences in some immunoassays.
- Serum may be frozen at –20°C for long-term storage but repeated freezing and thawing should be avoided. Protein denaturation at room temperature is minimal if serum is sterilized by filtration (0.22-μm pore size). For filter sterilization of volumes of serum greater than 20 ml use a combination of filters; 0.45-μm prefilter pad, 0.22-μm filter. A single 0.22-μm filter will block very rapidly. Alternatively, storage at 4°C is possible after the addition of merthiolate (0.01% w/v, final concentration) as a preservative. Preservation of non-sterile serum for

transport without refrigeration can be achieved by the addition of 50% v/v glycerol with no interference with its immune reactivity.

11.3.2 Serum preparation from plasma

Pooled plasma is frequently the only source of human serum for use as a tissue culture supplement or for the isolation of plasma proteins.

The action of the anticoagulant used to prevent clotting can be successfully reversed, but some plasma proteins are degraded during the preparation.

Citrate-dextrose anticoagulant

MATERIALS
Plasma with citrate anticoagulant
Thrombin solution
1 M calcium chloride solution

METHOD

1 Prepare thrombin solution for use by diluting to 100 IU/ml in calcium chloride solution.
2 Warm plasma to 37°C, add 1/100 volume of thrombin solution and mix vigorously to promote clot formation over 5–10 min.
3 Leave at room temperature for 60 min and collect supernatant.
4 Centrifuge at 20 000 g for 20 min at 4°C and collect the supernatant.
5 Filter sterilize (0.22 μm), if required, and heat inactivate at 56°C for 45 min.
6 Store at –20°C until used.

TECHNICAL NOTE
For filter sterilization of volumes of serum greater than 20 ml use a combination of filters; 0.45-μm prefilter pad, 0.22-μm filter. A single 0.22-μm filter will block very rapidly.

Heparin anticoagulant

MATERIALS
Plasma with heparin anticoagulant
Protamine sulphate
Thrombin solution
1 M calcium chloride solution

METHOD

1 Prepare thrombin solution for use by diluting to 100 IU/ml in calcium chloride solution and adding 5 mg/ml protamine sulphate.
2 Warm plasma to 37°C, add 1/100 volume of thrombin solution and mix vigorously to promote clot formation over 5–10 min.
3 Leave at room temperature for 60 min and collect supernatant.
4 Centrifuge at 20 000 g for 20 min at 4°C and collect the supernatant.
5 Filter sterilize (0.22 μm), if required, and heat inactivate at 56°C for 45 min.
6 Store at –20°C until used.

Additional protamine sulphate may be added if a clot does not form.

11.4 **Interfacial ring test**

A rapid check on the efficacy of immunization.

MATERIALS AND EQUIPMENT

Test serum

Durham tubes (glass), or other thin glass capillary-like vessels, e.g. drawn glass section of a Pasteur pipette

Antigen solution (10–20 mg/ml protein solution)

METHOD

1   Place 0.1 ml of serum into the small rimless (Durham) test tube.
2   Carefully layer over 0.1 ml of the solution of immunizing antigen.

If a visible interfacial precipitate is not formed within 1–2 min you must continue boosting the animal.

11.5 **Experimental mice**

In vivo experimental work, especially that which involves cell transfer, tissue or organ transplantation and the use of animal models of human disease, relies crucially on the availability of inbred animal strains.

Reproducibility and genetic homogeneity is guaranteed in these strains by brother–sister mating through many generations. Although a wide range of rat and mouse inbred strains are available, those of rabbit, guinea-pig and pig origin are more limited in genetic range and availability.

Common strains of inbred mice are widely available from commercial breeders.

Several strains of congenic mice have now been developed where each strain is identical to the next except for a single gene and short stretch of associated chromosome.

The B10 series was derived by the introduction of different H-2 loci onto a C57BL/10 genetic background (different strains representing more than 18 different loci are commercially available) and has been used extensively for the investigation of the linkage of various immunological phenomena to different regions of the H-2 gene complex.

Spontaneous mutations with immunological consequences have been identified in inbred mice or introduced into inbred mice by back-crossing and progeny selection. The best known example of this is the mutation which arose in about 1960 in an outbred stock of mice and was observed to result in both hairlessness and a congenital failure of thymus development. The mutated gene is referred to as *nu* and a homozygous *nu/nu* mouse is 'nude'. This mutation has now been introduced into the BALB/c, CBA/Ca and C57BL/10ScSn inbred lines and has virtually replaced the experimental counterpart of thymectomy, irradiation and bone marrow reconstitution.

1 Inbred strains have been developed as experimental models of human autoimmune and lymphoproliferative disease as described below.

2 Histocompatibility antigens were discovered as a result of the generation of inbred mouse strains. The most important set of these antigens is determined by closely linked genes in the so-called H-2 or major histocompatibility complex (MHC).

3 The term haplotype is used to indicate alternative forms of the entire H-2 complex which consist of several regions and subregions. This gene family is very complex (highly polymorphic) and so the number of loci in each subregion of the entire H-2 complex has yet to be determined.

Note: The H-2 complex is carried on chromosome 17.

Genetic defects of the immune system

C57BL/6-bg/bg. Beige mutant of previously black strain. Deficiencies in natural killer (NK)-cell activity and lysosomal function.

AKR. Over 90% of either sex develop spontaneous thymomas and leukaemias by 6–8 months.

SCID. Although these mice have a severe combined immunodeficiency (hence SCID) they can be kept alive in a clean, but not necessarily germ-free, environment. They are ideal recipients for cells from histocompatible strains of mice, for example in reconstitution experiments, and will also support the growth of xenogeneic human lymphoid and tumour cells. They augment the 'nude' mouse in studies on the function of the immune system.

Nude. Congenital thymic aplasia, T-cell deficiency, heightened NK cells and macrophage activities, and hairless.

Motheaten. Impaired humoral and cell-mediated responses. Granulocytic skin lesions.

W/Wv. Mast cell-deficient mice.

Models of autoimmune disease

EAMG. Experimental autoimmune myasthenia gravis.

EAE. Experimental autoimmune encephalitis.

EAT. Experimental autoimmune thyroiditis.

NZB. Autoimmune haemolytic anaemia with Coombs' test-positive erythrocytes (autoantibodies binding to, but not agglutinating, erythrocytes).

(NZBxNZW) F$_1$. Develops a lupus-like syndrome with glomerulonephritis and anti-DNA antibodies.

MRL/Mp-lpr/lpr. Model for human systemic lupus erythematosus and rheumatoid arthritis, with enlarged lymph nodes owing to generalized lymphoproliferation. This strain shows an early production of anti-DNA antibodies and rheumatoid factor (anti-immunoglobulin antibody), and has a mutation within the *Fas* gene.

MRL/Mp-+/+0. Develops chronic glomerulonephritis and anti-DNA antibodies late in life but no lymphadenopathy.

C57BL/KS-db/db. Obese mouse strain which develops severe diabetes owing to decreased insulin secretion at about 4 months.

NOD. Non-obese diabetic mouse strain. Its genetically based disease is thought to parallel human diabetes more closely than other murine models.

BXSB mice. Unusual male-associated lupus-like syndrome with Coombs' positive haemolytic anaemia, anti-DNA antibodies and immune complex-mediated glomerulonephritis.

BB rats. The diabetes-prone variant of BB rat also develops autoimmune thyroiditis.

OS chicken. Develops autoimmune thyroid disease similar to Hashimoto's thyroiditis.

11.6 Evaluation of cells

11.6.1 Morphology of thymus and blood leucocytes

Blood film

MATERIALS AND EQUIPMENT
Mouse or human blood
Microscope slides (clean overnight in acetone–ethanol 50 : 50 v/v)
95% methanol in water

METHOD

1 Grasp the mouse firmly by the nape of the neck using your thumb and forefinger. Hold the mouse's tail between your little and third fingers with its abdomen towards you; use your middle finger to flex its spine slightly so it cannot struggle. This is a general position for immobilizing a mouse for intraperitoneal injection or, as here, cutting the tip from its tail with a pair of scissors. Humans are usually more cooperative; in this case a finger prick with a sterile needle will draw sufficient blood.

2 Squeeze out 1 drop of blood and place it at one end of a clean glass slide.

3 Use a second, 'spreader' slide and touch the extreme edge of the drop of blood. Hold this slide at an angle of about 45 degrees.

4 Allow the blood to flow along the edge of the spreader slide and then push it away from the drop to obtain a film of cells (ideally in the shape of a bunsen flame).

5 Wave the slide in the air to dry it rapidly.

6 Fix in 95% methanol for 2 min.

With practice a serviceable, if not perfect, blood film can be produced. It is necessary to vary the size of the drop of blood and the amount taken up on the spreader slide to obtain an optimal distribution of cells.

11.6.2 Smears of single-cell suspensions

Blood plasma is viscous and so protects the cells in whole blood from damage as they are smeared. Smears are more difficult to obtain from single-cell suspensions taken from organs.

Using a cytocentrifuge it is possible to obtain excellent preparations by simply suspending the cells in neat serum and smearing them as in the previous section.

MATERIALS AND EQUIPMENT
Mouse
Phosphate-buffered saline (PBS)
Fetal bovine serum (FBS)
Microscope slides (clean overnight in acetone–ethanol 50 : 50 v/v)
95% methanol in water

METHOD

1 Kill the mouse by cervical dislocation and remove the thymus into a Petri dish containing PBS or tissue culture medium.
2 Prepare a single-cell suspension.
3 Place 1 drop of the cell suspension on a clean slide and smear with a second slide.
4 Dry the slide in the air and fix in 95% methanol for 2 min.
5 Wash the slide in running tap water for 30 min to remove the FBS.

11.6.3 Cytocentrifuge technique

MATERIALS AND EQUIPMENT
Mouse
Phosphate-buffered saline (PBS)
Fetal bovine serum (FBS)
Microscope slides (clean overnight in acetone–ethanol 50 : 50 v/v)
95% methanol in water
Cytocentrifuge

METHOD

1 Prepare a single-cell suspension from the mouse thymus as described in Section 6.3. After washing, finally resuspend in tissue culture medium with 10% FBS.
2 Load cytocentrifuge with glass slides and filter-paper strips.
3 Add 1 drop of cell suspension and 3 drops of tissue culture medium to each carrier block being used.
4 Centrifuge at 300 g for 10 min at room temperature.
5 Unload the glass slides, being careful to keep the slide and filter-paper strip together as you remove them from the carrier.
6 Remove the strip without smearing the cell preparation.
7 Dry the slide in the air and fix in 95% methanol for 2 min.
8 Wash the slides in running tap water for 30 min and then stain as required.

TECHNICAL NOTES

• The concentration of the cells in the suspension and the volume used should be varied to obtain the required cell density in the smear.
• Human lymphocytes tend to be more fragile and should be centrifuged at 250 g.

To examine the morphological details of the prepared cells, it is necessary to stain them. Pleasing results can be obtained with May–Grünwald/Giemsa staining.

11.7 May–Grünwald/Giemsa staining

MATERIALS AND EQUIPMENT
Smears of cells, fixed in methanol
Giemsa buffer
May–Grünwald stain
Giemsa stain
Staining racks and troughs
Neutral mounting medium (DePeX)

METHOD

1 Immerse the fixed cells in buffer for 5 min.
2 Transfer to May–Grünwald stain (freshly diluted 1 : 2 with buffer) for 5 min.
3 Rinse the slides in buffer and blot dry.
4 Stain in the Giemsa solution (freshly diluted with buffer) for 15 min.
5 Rinse in the buffer.
6 If the cells are over-stained (too blue) allow them to stand in the buffer.
7 Dry the slides in air and examine them under the microscope. If permanent preparations are required the cells may be mounted in a neutral mounting medium under a coverslip (use DePeX; Canada Balsam, although sold in a neutral form, eventually decolorizes the stained cells).

TECHNICAL NOTES

- These stains are based upon dyes dissolved in methanol which undergo a polychromasia upon dilution with water. For this reason stains must be prepared freshly for each staining session.
- A precipitate forms upon dilution of the stains: this is normal and will not affect the preparation as it is removed during washing of the slides. If you filter the precipitate from the stain you will also remove its staining properties.

Examination of cell smears

During smearing, white cells tend to move differentially to the red cells and are found at the edges and extreme end of the film. Figures 7.1 and 7.2 show the typical morphology of cells encountered in stained blood.

It is likely that you will rarely look at stained cells because, although lymphocytes in the blood are heterogeneous with regard to size and morphology (Fig. 7.2), there is no correlation with their function or antigen specificity.

Stained cells from the thymus are much more homogeneous than those of the blood; the majority have the morphological appearance typical of small lymphocytes (Fig. 7.2a).

11.8 Viable lymphocyte count

When handling living cells, maximum *in vitro* viability is usually maintained if the cells are kept at 0°C, i.e. in melting ice. Guinea-pig lymphocytes, however, are the exception to this rule; they should not be cooled below room temperature.

Cells used in an experiment must be freshly removed and the protocol completed, or the cells put into culture or transferred *in vivo* as quickly as possible.

In general, living cells will not remain functional if left overnight in a refrigerator.

The plasma membrane of a viable cell does not permit the entry of non-electrolyte dye substances. This phenomenon is used to distinguish dead from living lymphocytes. Many dyes are suitable for this purpose; for example, Trypan blue or eosin in dilute, physiological solution. However, we have found that nigrosin has invariably been the least toxic dye for estimation of cell viability.

11.9 Chicken thymus and bursa

Chicken thymus has up to nine pairs of lobes running up its neck alongside the carotid arteries and increases in cellularity with the onset of each moult, unlike the mammalian thymus that involutes at puberty and is a relatively small and acellular organ thereafter. The bursa of Fabricius is a large sac-like organ dorsal to the cloaca. Its internal surface is plicated and has a direct connection with the rectum. Cell suspensions from the thymus and bursa provide virtually pure T- and B-lymphocyte populations, respectively.

The cell suspensions from these organs have already been described (see Section 6.3). The technique for cell-surface immunofluorescence (see Section 8.2.1) is modified by the use of a rabbit anti-chicken, rather than mouse, immunoglobulin serum.

11.10 Cell counting

11.10.1 Cell counting with a haemocytometer

For counting lymphocyte suspensions, use $\times$ 40 objective lens and count in the central, triple-ruled area of the haemocytometer (this area is used for red-cell counting in haematology).

Count the cells in the large triple-ruled squares (improved Neubauer ruling, Fig. 11.1) until a minimum of 100 unstained (viable) lymphocytes have been counted (see Fig. 11.2).

Calculation of the number of viable cells

Number viable lymphocytes/ml $\times 10^4$

$$= \frac{\text{Number lymphocytes counted}}{\text{Number triple-ruled squares} \times \text{original dilution (if any)}} \times 25$$

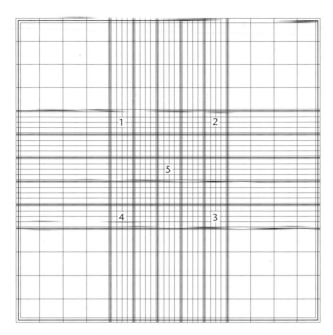

Fig. 11.1 The improved Neubauer ruling haemocytometer. For most applications in experimental immunology, the haemocytometer provides a cost-effective alternative to an electronic particle counter, unless you wish to use it for volume measurements. In principle, the number of cells in small volumes taken at random is counted to predetermined rules, and this value multiplied up to give an estimate of the total population. The figure shows the appearance of the central ruled area of the haemocytometer as it would appear under a low-power lens on the light microscope. There are nine squares, each of 1 mm^2; as the depth of the counting chamber is 0.1 mm, cells settling into one of these squares have come from a volume of 0.1 mm^3. If dealing with high-density cell populations, use a high-power lens ($\times$ 40) and count in the central triple-ruled areas (see Fig. 11.2); at low cell density count in one of the four peripheral, single-ruled areas. When counting lymphocyte suspensions, it is convenient to use a phase-contrast microscope and so distinguish viable (phase-bright) from dead (phase-dark) cells, as an adjunct to dye exclusion (see Section 11.10.2).

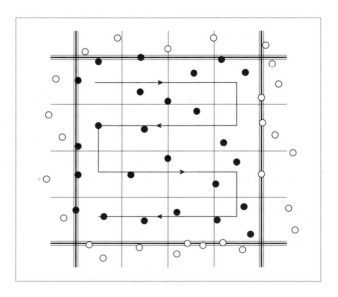

Fig. 11.2 Counting lymphocyte suspensions in a haemocytometer. The figure shows an enlarged view of square 1 from Fig. 11.1. Cells falling across the top and left border lines of a square are considered to be in that square, whereas cells on the bottom and right borders are excluded. The diagram shows 25 cells (filled circles) in an area of 1/25 mm^2, depth of chamber 0.1 mm. To gain an acceptable degree of accuracy in this technique, you should count cells in the triple-ruled squares in the order shown in Fig. 11.1 until at least 100 cells have been included in the sample.

11.10.2 Dye exclusion test

This test is an extension of the method used to estimate cell viability (see Section 11.10.1).

MATERIALS
Anti-lymphocyte serum (ALS)
Rabbit anti-mouse immunoglobulin
Guinea-pig serum (complement)
Nigrosin dye
Inbred mice, 4–6 weeks old

METHOD

1 Absorb the complement with mouse spleen and erythrocytes, approximately 0.1 ml packed cells/ml of serum, for 30 min at 4°C.
2 Centrifuge the absorbed complement. Use immediately or store at –20°C.
3 Prepare thymus and lymph-node suspensions from mouse donors. Estimate viability and adjust to 5×10^7 viable lymphocytes/ml.
4 Prepare cell and serum mixtures according to the following Protocol, and incubate at 37°C for 30 min.

Protocol.

	Tube number					
	1	2	3	4	5	6
Anti-lymphocyte or normal rabbit serum final dilution	1 : 20	1 : 40	1 : 80	1 : 160	1 : 320	1 : 640
Lymph-node cells (5×10^7/ml)	0.1 ml———————————————————→					
Absorbed guinea-pig serum (1 : 5 initial dilution)	0.1 ml———————————————————→					

Repeat this Protocol using thymus cells with the same dilution of ALS and normal rabbit serum (NRS).

Assay 1 (see Protocol above)
Cells: lymph node.
Antisera: ALS and preimmunization serum (NRS). Titrate NRS only to 1 : 40.

Assay 2 (see Protocol below)
Cells: lymph node.
Antisera: anti-immunoglobulin (if assays 1 and 2 are performed simultaneously a second NRS control is not required).
5 After incubation stand the tubes in ice to prevent further complement fixation and cell lysis.
6 Count the number of viable cells in each suspension.
   Calculate the number of viable cells/ml and from this the percentage lysis for each tube according to the following equation:
   % lysis = $C_N - C_A \times 100/C_O$

Continued

where C_N is number of live cells in NRS, C_A is number of live cells in ALS or anti-Ig, and C_O is original number of live cells.

Table 11.2 Protocol.

	Tube number				
	1	2	3	4	5
Anti-immunoglobulin dilution	1 : 10	1 : 20	1 : 40	1 : 80	1 : 160
Lymph-node cells (5×10^7/ml)	0.1 ml————————————————————————→				
Absorbed guinea-pig serum (1 : 5 initial dilution)	0.1 ml————————————————————————→				

Repeat this Protocol using thymus cells with the same dilutions of anti-immunoglobulin.

8 Plot a graph of percentage lysis against antiserum dilution for each tissue and antiserum.

Interpretation of results

- You should find that ALS kills all nucleated cells in the thymus and the lymph-node suspension to a high dilution of antiserum. This lack of T-cell specificity is, of course, to be expected as lymphocytes share many surface antigens.
- The percentage of cells killed by the anti-immunoglobulin serum should coincide with the expected percentage of B cells in the tissue used.
- If the killing of thymocytes by anti-immunoglobulin or NRS exceeds 5%, there are probably anti-species antibodies present, not related to the original immunizing procedure. In this case it is necessary to absorb all sera with liver membranes.

TECHNICAL NOTES
- The sensitivity of this assay depends upon a high initial cell viability. Frequently 20–30% dead cells are encountered in lymph-node suspensions. Dead cells may be removed as described in Section 6.4.
- The guinea-pig serum complement source must be absorbed with spleen and red cells before use as it is sometimes itself cytotoxic. It was discovered that an agarose absorption may also be used to remove anti-mouse antibodies. Use 100 mg of agarose/ml of serum; absorb for 60 min at 4°C.
- In this assay it is advisable to count the number of viable cells after lysis rather than the number of dead cells, especially if centrifugation steps are included after killing. Dead cells are often broken up and lost during centrifugation.

11.11 Lymphoid organs of the mouse

Figure 6.2 shows the major lymphoid organs of the mouse and their cellular composition. There is a continuous traffic of recirculating small lymphocytes from the blood into the other peripheral lymphoid organs such as the spleen, lymph nodes, etc. From here the cells enter the other tissues and finally return to the blood via the lymphatic vessels, e.g. the thoracic duct. The intact immune response involves great changes in the 'trafficking' pattern of recirculating antigen-reactive lymphocytes. When specific small lymphocytes are confronted with antigen they will leave this recirculating pool, congregate at the site of the greatest antigen concentration and migrate to the draining lymph node.

11.12 X-irradiation of mice

Mice may be immunosuppressed by 6.0–8.0 Gy whole body irradiation, the precise dose being dictated by the degree of immunosuppression required and the 'cleanliness' of the environment. Under these conditions there is only the occasional death by 7 days post irradiation without bone marrow therapy.

Early X-ray death is usually due to gut damage; accordingly, X-ray resistance may be increased by starving the mice 24 h before irradiation. If infection-associated deaths are noted after routine immunosuppression the following antibiotic regime may be used: in drinking water, ad libitum 1 g neomycin and 400 mg polymixin B to 10 l distilled water.

Again it must be emphasized that this technique must be performed by experienced personnel only, and under the strict guidelines of your local animal research facility.

Figure 11.3 shows the variation in numbers of peripheral blood mononuclear cells, neutrophils and platelets measured at various times after irradiation, in C57Bl mice given 6.0 Gy whole body irradiation. See below for details of a protocol for the dose–response curve of X-ray-induced immunosuppression.

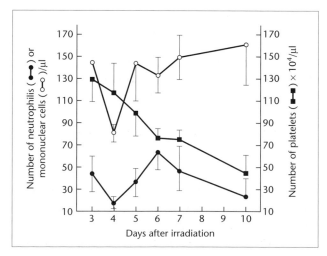

Fig. 11.3 Response of peripheral blood cells to whole body irradiation. Male C57B1 mice were given 6.0 Gy whole body irradiation and the numbers of peripheral blood cells determined at various days thereafter. Initial values of cells: neutrophils $1300 \pm 340/\mu l$; mononuclear cells $8900 \pm 1500/\mu l$; and platelets $1200 \pm 180 \times 10^{-3}/\mu l$. Each population showed marked variation in the response to irradiation. At 4–5 days maximum leucocyte suppression was seen, with only minimal depression of platelet numbers. Lower doses of irradiation produced much less dramatic effects on cell numbers; for example, the 4-day neutrophil count in response to 4.0 and 5.0 Gy was 170 ± 46 and $180 \pm 31/\mu l$, respectively. Whole body irradiation has no acute effects on the plasma levels of the complement components.

11.12.1 Suppression of the immune response by X-irradiation

The dose of X-rays required to kill most types of non-dividing cells is much greater than that required to kill actively dividing cells. One of its major effects is to induce chromosomal breaks so the cells are unable to complete mitosis. Lymphocytes, however, are unusual among mammalian cells in being susceptible to X-ray induced death in G0. They have a D_{37} of only 1.0 Gy. The dose-dependent immunosuppressive effect of X-irradiation may be demonstrated in a primary immune response against sheep erythrocytes. This experiment may also be designed to determine the lethal and immunosuppressive X-ray doses of recipient animals for other experiments (see Technical notes).

MATERIALS AND EQUIPMENT
Mice (preferably inbred)
Sheep erythrocytes (SRBC)
Irradiation source
Materials for haemolytic plaque assay (see Section 9.1)

METHOD

Irradiate and prime the mice according to the Protocol.

Protocol.

	Group (3–5 animals per group)							
	1	2	3	4	5	6	7	8
Irradiation dose (Gy)	0	0	2	4	6	8	8.5	9
Immunising antigen—SRBC intravenously	0.2×10^7							→

1 Challenge the animals with antigen immediately before or after X-irradiation.
2 Assay the anti-SRBC haemolytic plaque response 5 days after antigen challenge.
3 Calculate the total number of plaques per spleen for each animal and the geometric mean for each group.
4 Plot a graph of the X-ray dose against the log mean plaque response.

TECHNICAL NOTES
- See above for changes in blood leucocytes following whole body irradiation.
- For most laboratory strains of mice there should be very few deaths during the period of assay due to X-irradiation over the range indicated. For long-term survival, however, it is necessary to reconstitute the mice with bone marrow as X-irradiation suppresses not only lymphoproliferation, but also proliferation of the haemopoietic system.

11.12.2 Radioresistance

Experiments suggest that T and B cells show a differential radioresistance in the whole animal. Thus, if an animal is primed with sheep erythrocytes and X-irradiated 4 days later, functional T cells remain, whereas B-cell activity is suppressed.

Inbred mice

Sheep erythrocytes (SRBC)

Materials for haemolytic plaque assay (Section 9.1)

METHOD

1 Prime recipient mice with 2×10^7 sheep erythrocytes intravenously. X-irradiate (8–8.5 Gy) 4 days after priming.

2 Prepare spleen and thymocyte suspensions from normal donor mice.

3 Treat aliquots of the spleen suspension with anti-Thy-1 and complement or an irrelevant monoclonal and complement (see Section 7.8).

4 Reconstitute the X-irradiated mice according to the Protocol.

Protocol.

Group	Recipients per group	Previous treatment	Cells transferred	SRBC challenge
1	3–5	2×10^7 SRBC + 8 Gy*	None	2×10^7
2	3–5	2×10^7 SRBC + 8 Gy*	Thymocytes	2×10^7
3	3–5	2×10^7 SRBC + 8 Gy*	Spleen treated with anti-Thy-1 + complement	2×10^7
4	3–5	2×10^7 SRBC + 8 Gy*	Spleen treated with irrelevant monoclonal + complement	2×10^7

* 8.0 Gy 4 days after SRBC challenge.

5 Assay all mice for anti-SRBC haemolytic plaques 8 days after cell transfer.

6 Calculate the total plaque-forming cells per spleen for each individual and the geometric mean for each group.

Knowing the cell phenotype specificity of the anti-Thy-1 serum, you should be able to identify the radiosensitive and radioresistant lymphocyte populations. This is an extremely useful method by which to prepare helper cells.

TECHNICAL NOTES

- We have assayed at only one time point; both T and B cells have phases of relative radioresistance after antigen stimulation.
- Differential radioresistance is not shown by T and B cells *in vitro*.

11.13 **Further reading**

Allison, A.C. & Byars, N.E. (1991) Immunological adjuvants: Desirable properties and side-effects. *Mol Immunol* **28**, 297–284.

Amyx, H.L. (1987) Control of animal pain and distress in antibody production and infectious disease studies. *J Am Vet Med Assoc* **191**, 1287–1289.

Bennett, B., Check, I.J., Olsen, M.R. & Hunter, R.L. (1992) A comparison of commercially available adjuvants for use in research. *J Immunol Meth* **153**, 31–40.

BVA/FRAME/RSPCA/UFAW. (1993) Removal of blood from laboratory mammals and birds. First report of the BVA/FRAME/RSPCA/UFAW Joint Working Group on Refinement. *Lab Anim* **1**, 1–22.

Festing, M.F.W. (1987) International index of laboratory animals. Laboratory Animals Ltd, London.

Flecknell, P.A. (1996) Laboratory animal anaesthesia, 2nd edn. Academic Press, London.

Forrest, J.M. & Ross, H.A. (1993) Splenic implantation of nitrocellulose pellets as a means of raising antibodies to nanogram quantities of antigen. *J Immunol Meth* **159**, 275–276.

Freund, J. (1951) The effect of paraffin oil and mycobacteria on antibody formation and sensitization. *Am J Clin Pathol* **21**, 645–656.

Grubhofer, N. (1995) An adjuvant formulation based on N-acetylglucosaminyl-N-acetylmuramyl-L-alanyl-D-isoglutamine with dimethyldioctadecylammonium chloride and zinc-L-proline complex as synergists. *Immunol Lett* **44**(1), 19–24.

Hart, L.A. (1999) *Responsible Conduct with Animals in Research*. Oxford University Press, Oxford.

Hay, F.C. & Torrigiani, G. (1973) The effect of pertussis adjuvant on antibody production: the need for thymus dependent lymphocytes. *Eur J Immunol* **3**, 657–659.

Hanley, W.C., Artwohl, J.E. & Bennett, B.T. (1995) Review of polyclonal antibody production procedures in mammals and poultry. *ILAR J.* **37**, 93–118.

Howard, G.C., Bethell, D.R. & Vilsaint, F. (2000) *Basic Methods in Antibody Production and Characterization*. Cambridge University Press, Cambridge.

Hrapkiewicz, K., Medina, L. & Holmes, D.D. (1999) *Clinical Laboratory Animal Medicine: An Introduction*. Iowa State University Press, Iowa, USA.

Jackson, I.J., Smith, C.W.J. & Abbott, C. (2000) *Mouse Genetics and Transgenics: A Practical Approach*. Oxford University Press, Oxford.

Lembeck, F. (1990) *Scientific Alternatives to Animal Experiments*. Chapman & Hall, Andover.

Matzinger, P. (1994) Tolerance, danger, and the extended family. *Ann Rev Immunol* **12**, 991–1045.

Polly Matzinger's web site: The real function of the immune system, or Tolerance and the four Ds (danger, death, destruction and distress). http://cmmg.biosci.wayne.edu/asg/polly.html

Morein, B., Villacres-Erikson, M., Åkerblom, L. & Lövgren, K. (1993) Initiation of immune response with ISCOM. In: *New Generation Vaccines: The Role of Basic Immunology* (eds G. Gregoriadis, B. McCormack, A.C. Allison & G.C. Poste). Plenum Press, Dordrecht.

O'Hagan, T. (1998) Recent advances in vaccine adjuvants for systemic and mucosal administration *J Pharm Pharmacol* **50**, 1–10.

Orlans, F.B. (1996) *In the Name of Science: Issues in Responsible Animal Experimentation*. Oxford University Press, Oxford.

Parliamentary Office of Science and Technology (1992) *The Use of Animals in Research, Development and Testing*.

Parsons, M., Herzenberg, L.A., Stall, A.M. & Herzenberg, L.A. (1997) Mouse immunoglobulin allotypes. In: *Handbook of Experimental Immunology*. (eds L.A. Herzenberg, D.M. Weir, L.A. Herzenberg C. Blackwell). pp. 97.1–97.17. Blackwell Science, Oxford.

Poole, T.B. (1995) *The UFAW Handbook on the Care and Management of Laboratory Animals*, 6th edn. Longman Scientific and Technical, Harrow.

Poole, T. (1999) *The UFAW Handbook on the Care and Management of Laboratory Animals*, Vol. 1: Terrestrial Vertebrates; Vol. 2: Amphibious and Aquatic Vertebrates and Advanced Invertebrates. Blackwell Science, Oxford.

Schade, R. (2001) *Chicken Egg Yolk Antibodies, Production and Application*. IgY Technology (Springer Lab. Manual) Springer Verlag, New York.

Tuffery, A.A. (1995) *Laboratory Animals: an Introduction for New Experimenters*, 2nd edn. John Wiley & Sons.

United Kingdom Co-ordinating Committee on Cancer Research (1988) *UKCCCR Guidelines for the Welfare of Animals in Experimental Neoplasia*. UKCCR, 20 Park Crescent, London W1N 4AL, UK.

Vogel, F.R. (1998) Adjuvants in perspective. *Dev Biol Stand* **92**, 241–248.

APPENDIX A

Buffers and media

All solutions must be made up in distilled water which has been prepared by an endosmosis purification system or double-glass distillation.

Acetate–acetic acid buffer, pH 4.0, ionic strength 0.1

MATERIALS

0.6 M sodium acetate (49.2 g/l).
0.6 M acetic acid (34.4 ml glacial acetic acid in 1000 ml distilled water)

METHOD

1 Mix 435 ml 0.6 M acetic acid with 130 ml 0.6 M sodium acetate.
2 Adjust to 1000 ml with distilled water.

0.001 M acetate–acetic buffer, pH 4.4

MATERIALS

Sodium acetate (CH_3COONa) (8.20 g/l)
Acetic acid (6.0 g/l)

METHOD

1 Mix 1/3 sodium acetate solution with 2/3 acetic acid solution.
2 Dilute 1 : 1000 to give 1 mM.

Balanced salt solution (BSS)

MATERIALS

Calcium chloride (0.14 g/l)
Sodium chloride (8.00 g/l)
Potassium chloride (0.40 g/l)
0.8 mM magnesium sulphate ($MgSO_4 \cdot 7H_2O$) (0.20 g/l)
1.0 mM magnesium chloride ($MgCl_2 \cdot 6H_2O$) (0.20 g/l)
0.4 mM potassium dihydrogen phosphate (0.06 g/l)
1.4 mM disodium hydrogen phosphate ($Na_2HPO_4 \cdot 2H_2O$) (0.24 g/l)

METHOD

1 If required, 1 g/l of glucose may be added.
2 Dissolve all components in 1000 ml.
3 Membrane filter, if required to be sterile.

Barbitone buffer, pH 8.2, ionic strength 0.08

MATERIALS

Barbital sodium (5′5-diethyl barbituric acid, Na salt)
Barbital (5′5 diethylbarbituric acid)
5 M sodium hydroxide
Merthiolate

METHOD

1 Dissolve 12.00 g sodium barbital in 800 ml distilled water.
2 Dissolve 4.40 g barbital in 150 ml distilled water at 95°C.
3 Mix solutions 1 and 2 and adjust pH to 8.2 with concentrated sodium hydroxide.
4 Add 0.15 g merthiolate (preservative) and adjust final volume to 1000 ml.

TECHNICAL NOTE

For electrophoresis on cellulose acetate membranes use 0.05–0.07 M barbitone buffer, pH 8.6. The exact buffer composition and concentration can be adjusted according to requirements. At lower concentrations, the protein bands are wider and their mobility increased. A higher buffer concentration produces the reverse effect with crowding of the bands.

0.15 M barbitone-buffered saline, pH 7.6
(for complement fixation test)

MATERIALS

Sodium chloride
Barbital (5′5 diethylbarbituric acid)
Barbital sodium (5′5 diethylbarbituric acid, Na salt)
Magnesium chloride
1.0 M calcium chloride (111.1 g/l)

STOCK SOLUTIONS

A: 85.0 g sodium chloride + 2.75 g sodium diethylbarbiturate in 1400 ml of distilled water

B: 5.75 g diethylbarbituric acid in 500 ml hot
  distilled water

C: 20.3 g $MgCl_2 \cdot 6H_2O$ (2.0 M) dissolved in 50 ml
  distilled water + 30 ml 1.0 M calcium chloride
  solution. Adjust to 100 ml with distilled water.
  Final concentrations 1.0 M $MgCl_2$, 0.3 M $CaCl_2$

METHOD

1 Mix solutions A and B and cool to room
  temperature.
2 Add 5 ml of C.
3 Adjust final volume to 2 l with distilled water
  and store at 4°C.

TECHNICAL NOTE

This buffer is five times the concentration used
in the text. Dilute just before use.

0.1 M borate buffer, pH 7.4

MATERIALS

Disodium tetraborate ($Na_2B_4O_7 \cdot 10H_2O$) (9.54 g
  in 250 ml distilled water)
Boric acid (24.73 g in 4 l distilled water)

METHOD

Add approximately 115 ml borate solution to
4 l boric acid solution until pH reaches 7.4.

Borate–saline buffer, pH 8.3–8.5, ionic strength 0.1

MATERIALS

Boric acid (6.18 g/l)
Sodium tetraborate (borax) (9.54 g/l)
Sodium chloride (4.38 g/l)

Make up to 1000 ml with distilled water.

0.15 M borate–succinate buffer, pH 7.5
(for tanning erythrocytes)

MATERIALS

Solution A: 0.05 M sodium tetraborate
  ($Na_2B_4O_7 \cdot 10H_2O$) (19.0 g/l)
Solution B: 0.05 M succinic acid (5.9 g/l)
Sodium chloride
Horse serum

METHOD

1 Take 1000 ml of A and add B until pH is 7.5.
2 Add sodium chloride to 0.14 M final
  concentration and 1% (v/v) horse serum (final
  concentration) previously heat inactivated
  (56°C for 45 min).

0.28 M cacodylate buffer, pH 6.9

MATERIALS

Sodium cacodylate
3 M hydrochloric acid

METHOD

1 Dissolve sodium cacodylate (60 g/l) in distilled
  water.
2 Titrate to pH 6.9 with 3 M HCl.
3 Adjust to 1000 ml with distilled water.

Carbonate–bicarbonate buffer

Stock solution A: 0.2 M solution of anhydrous
  sodium carbonate (21.2 g in 1000 ml)
Stock solution B: 0.2 M solution of sodium
  hydrogen carbonate (16.8 g in 1000 ml)

For use: x ml of A + y ml of B, diluted to a total of
200 ml will yield the approximate pH shown. If an
accurate final pH is required, titrate the two
solutions on a pH meter using the volumes given
below as a guide.

Table A1.1

x	y	pH
5.0	45.0	9.2
7.5	42.5	9.3
9.5	40.5	9.4
13.0	37.0	9.5
16.0	34.0	9.6
19.5	30.5	9.7
22.0	28.0	9.8
25.0	25.0	9.9
27.5	22.5	10.0
30.0	20.0	10.1
33.0	17.0	10.2
35.5	14.5	10.3
38.5	11.5	10.4
40.5	9.5	10.5
42.5	7.5	10.6
45.0	5.0	10.7

Adjust volume to achieve the required molarity
using distilled water.

0.1 M citrate buffer, pH 3.0–7.0

MATERIALS

0.1 M citric acid ($C_6H_8O_7·H_2O$) (21.01 g/l)
0.1 M disodium hydrogen phosphate
($Na_2HPO_4·2H_2O$) (17.80 g/l)

METHOD

1 pH 5.0: approximately a 50 : 50 mixture of citric to phosphate.
2 Below pH 5.0: titrate pH of citric acid with phosphate.
3 Above pH 5.0: titrate pH of phosphate with citric acid.

C1q buffers

Buffer 1

MATERIALS

Ethylene glycol-bis-(b-amino-ethyl ether)-N, N′-tetra-acetic acid (EGTA) (19.76 g)
11 M sodium hydroxide solution

METHOD

1 Add 1500 ml distilled water to the EGTA.
2 Slowly add strong NaOH (about 8 ml of 11 M NaOH) to both dissolve the EGTA and adjust to pH 7.5.
3 Add distilled water to a total volume of 2 l.

Buffer 2

MATERIALS

0.02 M sodium acetate (1.64 g in 1000 ml distilled water)
Acetic acid 0.02 M, 1.14 ml glacial acetic acid in 1000 ml distilled water
Ethylene diamine tetra-acetic acid (EDTA), disodium salt (1.79 g)
Sodium chloride (21.91 g)

METHOD

1 Add the EDTA and sodium chloride to 300 ml of the acetic acid.
2 When dissolved, add further acetic acid and sodium acetate solution to attain pH 5.0 and a volume of 500 ml.

Buffer 3

MATERIALS

Ethylene diamine tetra-acetic acid (EDTA), disodium salt (86 g)
Concentrated HCl

METHOD

1 Dissolve EDTA in 3.5 l of water.
2 Adjust to pH 5.0 with HCl and add distilled water to 4 l, final volume.

Buffer 4

MATERIALS

Potassium dihydrogen phosphate (0.34 g in 500 ml distilled water)
Sodium chloride (21.91 g)
Ethylene diamine tetra-acetic acid (EDTA), disodium salt (1.79 g)

METHOD

1 Dissolve the sodium chloride and EDTA in about 200 ml of the disodium hydrogen phosphate solution.
2 Add further disodium hydrogen phosphate and potassium dihydrogen phosphate solution to pH 7.5 and a volume of 500 ml.

Buffer 5

MATERIALS

Ethylene diamine tetra-acetic acid (EDTA), trisodium salt (50.15 g)
Concentrated HCl

METHOD

1 Dissolve the EDTA in 3.5 l distilled water.
2 Titrate to pH 7.5 with concentrated HCl.
3 Make up the volume to 4 l with distilled water.

Buffer 6

MATERIALS

As for Buffer 2

METHOD

1 Dissolve EDTA and the sodium chloride in 300 ml sodium acetate solution.
2 Adjust to pH 7.5 and a volume of 500 ml with further sodium acetate and acetic acid solutions.

Diamino ethane–acetic acid buffer, pH 7.0, ionic strength 0.1

MATERIALS

Diamino ethane
1 M acetic acid (57.3 ml glacial acetic acid in 1000 ml distilled water)

METHOD

1 Mix 2.88 g diamino ethane with 73.0 ml 1 M acetic acid.
2 Adjust to 1000 ml with distilled water.

0.05 M diethylamine–HCl buffer, pH 11.5

MATERIALS
  Diethylamine
  1.0 M HCl

METHOD
1 Dissolve 365.5 mg diethylamine in 50 ml distilled water.
2 Titrate to pH 11.5 with 1.0 M HCl.
3 Adjust to 100 ml final volume with distilled water.

ELISA conjugate buffer

To 9 ml of phosphate-buffered saline (as below) add:
  100 µl sheep serum
  10 mg casein
  10 µl Tween 20
  5 µl antibody–enzyme conjugate.
Make up to a final volume of 10 ml.

Giemsa buffer
(for May–Grünwald/Giemsa staining)

MATERIALS
  0.1 M citric acid (21.01 g/l)
  0.2 M disodium hydrogen phosphate (Na_2HPO_4) (28.39 g/l)

METHOD
1 Mix 85 ml 0.1 M citric acid with 115 ml 0.2 M disodium hydrogen phosphate and adjust pH to 5.75.
2 Make up to 1000 ml.

0.1 M glycine–HCl buffer, pH 2.5 or 2.8
(for acid elution of antibodies from immunoadsorbents)

MATERIALS
  0.2 M glycine (15.01 g/l)
  0.2 M HCl

METHOD
1 Titrate 500 ml of 0.2 M glycine to pH 2.5–2.8 as required, with 0.2 M HCl.
2 Make up to 1000 ml with distilled water.

0.5 M glycine–saline buffer, pH 8.6
(for immunofluorescence mountant and latex agglutination)

MATERIALS
  Glycine (14.00 g)
  Sodium hydroxide, solid (0.7 g)

Sodium chloride (17 g)
  Sodium azide (preservative) (1 g)

METHOD
1 Dissolve components in 500 ml of distilled water and adjust to pH 8.6 with alkali, as required.
2 Make up to 1000 ml with distilled water.

Mounting medium made as follows: 30 ml above buffer plus 70 ml glycerol.

Hank's saline

There are other formulations for this medium.

MATERIALS
  Sodium chloride (8.00 g/l)
  Calcium chloride (0.20 g/l)
  Magnesium sulphate (0.20 g/l)
  Potassium chloride (0.40 g/l)
  Potassium dihydrogen phosphate (0.10 g/l)
  Sodium bicarbonate (1.27 g/l)
  Glucose (2.00 g/l)

METHOD
1 Dissolve in 1000 ml of distilled water.
2 Sterilize by membrane filtration.

(Concentrated Hank's saline is sold commercially, but often has phenol red added as a pH indicator. This makes visualization of haemolytic plaques difficult.)

Jacalin storage buffer

MATERIALS
  10 mM HEPES
  150 mM sodium chloride
  100 mM calcium chloride
  20 mM galactose
  0.08% sodium azide as preservative

METHOD
Mix together
  4.38 g NaCl
  5.55 g $CaCl_2$
  1.80 g galactose
  1.19 g HEPES
  0.4 g sodium azide
and adjust to 500 ml with water.

0.5 M phosphate buffers

MATERIALS
  Sodium dihydrogen phosphate 1 hydrate ($NaH_2PO \cdot 4H_2O$) (69.0 g/l)

Disodium hydrogen phosphate, anhydrous
(Na$_2$HPO$_4$) (71.0 g/l)

METHOD

Prepare stock solutions of each salt in water and add 1 drop of chloroform as a preservative. Store at room temperature. Mix the two solutions to obtain the required pH using a pH meter and then adjust to the desired molarity. Take care not to add too much chloroform, especially if the buffer is to be used with plastic chromatography columns.

0.15 M phosphate-buffered saline (PBS), pH 7.2

MATERIALS

Sodium chloride (8.00 g/l)
Potassium chloride (0.20 g/l)
0.008 M disodium hydrogen phosphate
(Na$_2$HPO$_4$) (1.15 g/l)
Potassium dihydrogen phosphate (0.20 g/l)

METHOD

Dissolve in 1000 ml of distilled water.

TECHNICAL NOTES

- It is convenient to make up a × 10 solution for storage and dilute as required.
- Sterilize by autoclaving or add 20 mM (final concentration) sodium azide as a preservative.
- Remember that azide is not compatible with many experimental systems (not only cell culture)—it will inactivate lactoperoxidase, bind to ion exchangers, etc.

0.20 M phosphate–saline buffer, pH 7.2
(for tanning erythrocytes)

MATERIALS

0.02 M potassium dihydrogen phosphate
(KH$_2$PO$_4$) (12.2 g)
0.06 M disodium hydrogen phosphate
(Na$_2$HPO$_4$) (40.4 g)
0.12 M sodium chloride (36.0 g)

METHOD

Dissolve in 5 l of distilled water.

Polyacrylamide running buffer

Stock solution

Tris–glycine buffer × 10:
144 g glycine in 1000 ml water, pH 8.3
30 g Tris (tris(hydroxymethyl)-aminomethane)
Dilute stock solution × 10 then add 3 ml 20% SDS to 600 ml of diluted stock solution.

Polyacrylamide sample buffer

MATERIALS

20% sodium dodecyl sulphate (SDS) (in water)
(6.0 ml)
Glycerol (3.0 ml)
1 M tris(hydroxymethyl)-aminomethane
(Tris)–HCl, pH 6.8 (2.4 ml)
Distilled water (15.6 ml)
Bromophenol blue, few grains

METHOD

Mix the above quantities together to prepare the final sample buffer.

TECHNICAL NOTES

- Prepare Tris solution on each occasion; the others may be kept as stock solutions.
- Glycerol is added to increase the density of the solution and so aid loading of the polyacrylamide gel. It can be replaced by a 60% w/v sucrose solution.
- Bromophenol blue dye is used as a marker to monitor the progress of the protein front during electrophoresis.
- Prepare 2 M dithiothreitol as a stock solution and store at –20°. Add to sample dissolved in sample buffer just before boiling, if the separation is to be performed under reducing conditions.

0.14 M saline physiological or 'normal' saline

Sodium chloride (8.5 g/l). Store at a × 10 concentration and dilute as required. Sterilize by autoclaving.

Scintillation fluid

MATERIALS

2,5-diphenyloxazole (PPO) (6 g)
2,2'-p-phenylene-bis (5-phenyloxazole)
(POPOP) (0.05 g)
Toluene (1000 ml)

METHOD

Dissolve the PPO and POPOP in toluene in a fume cupboard.

TECHNICAL NOTE

Many institutions require the use of aqueous scintillation fluid, available ready prepared, although efficiency must be checked in individual systems.

Tissue culture media
(see also information on general *in vitro* culture techniques in Appendix B)

Many different culture media are available, each usually in an 'old' and 'new' or 'improved' formulation. For general use we suggest Eagle's minimal essential medium (EMEM) and Dulbecco's modification of Eagle's minimal essential medium (DMEM) or RPMI 1640 for culture under more demanding conditions.

Tris–ammonium chloride
(for erythrocyte lysis)

MATERIALS
0.17 M tris(hydroxymethyl)-aminomethane (Tris) (20.60 g/l)
0.16 M ammonium chloride (8.30 g/l)

METHOD
Add 10 ml of 0.17 M Tris to 90 ml of 0.16 M ammonium chloride and adjust to pH 7.2.

This buffer induces red-cell lysis without reducing lymphocyte viability, unlike 1.0% acetic acid which is also used to lyse erythrocytes during white cell counts.

Tris–HCl buffers

MATERIALS
Tris(hydroxymethyl)-aminomethane (Tris) (12.1 g)
1 M HCl

METHOD
1 Dissolve Tris in 100 ml distilled water to prepare a 1.0 M stock solution.
2 Titrate to desired pH with HCl, then dilute to the required molarity.

TECHNICAL NOTE
To measure and adjust the pH of a Tris solution, it is necessary to purchase a special Calomel Tris electrode—the electrochemistry of the normal electrode does not apply to Tris.

3.0 M Tris–HCl, pH 8.7

Dissolve 181.65 g Tris in 450 ml distilled water, titrate to pH 8.7 with 1 M HCl, finally adjust to 500 ml with distilled water.

0.1 M Tris-buffered saline, pH 8.0
(for IgM preparation)

MATERIALS
Tris(hydroxymethyl)-aminomethane (12.1 g)
Sodium chloride (29.22 g)
Glycine (0.75 g)
Sodium azide (0.2 g)
1 M HCl

METHOD
1 Dissolve ingredients in 800 ml distilled water and adjust to pH 8.0 with HCl.
2 Make volume up to 1000 ml with distilled water.

Tris–glycine buffer, pH 8.3; 0.25 M Tris, 1.92 M glycine

MATERIALS
Tris(hydroxymethyl)-aminomethane (30.3 g)
Glycine (134.6 g)
Sodium dodecyl sulphate (10 g)

METHOD
Dissolve materials in water and make up to 1000 ml.

Veronal-buffered saline
(for PEG precipitation)

MATERIALS
Sodium chloride (85.0 g)
Sodium barbitone (3.75 g)
Barbitone (5.75 g)

METHOD
Dissolve and make up to 2 l with distilled water.

This buffer is 5 times the concentration used in the text, as it is more stable as a concentrated stock solution. Dilute just before use.

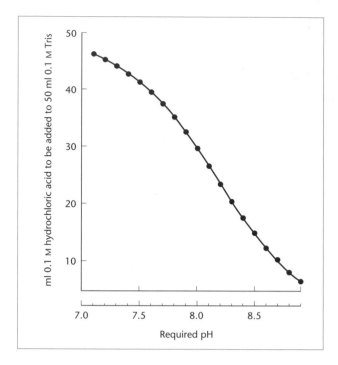

Fig. A.1 Tris buffer. Variation in pH of Tris buffer obtained by adding 0.1 M hydrochloric acid to 50 ml 0.1 M Tris base. Dilute the resulting mixture to the required molarity.

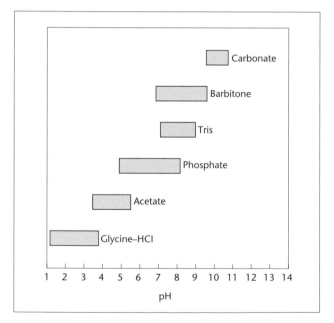

Fig. A.2 Working ranges for useful buffers.

APPENDIX B

Basic techniques and useful data

B.1 **Basic column technique**

Figure B.1 shows a suitable basic arrangement of equipment for gel filtration.

B.1.1 **Equipment**

Columns. Many different types of column are available, each with their own advantages and disadvantages. Many manufacturers supply a wide range of apparatus, from simple manual columns to fully integrated systems.

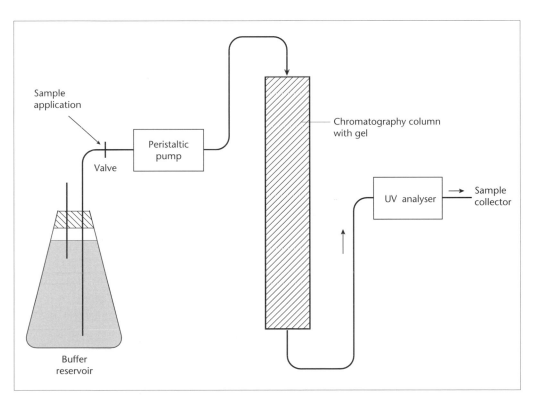

Fig. B.1 Equipment for column chromatography. The equipment shown allows efficient chromatographic separation of protein mixtures. It is an advantage to have an insulating jacket around the column to protect it from draughts and temperature changes. If the column is equipped with flow adaptors at either end, this will allow the column to be inverted and run in the opposite direction, or to be run with the buffer flow in the ascending direction which will lessen the chances of the column packing down.

Pumps. Peristaltic pumps provide an even flow rate with little solvent turbulence. Alternatively, a simple reservoir such as a Marriotte flask can be used. It is important to maintain a constant pressure on the column.

Monitoring and collection of fractions. A fraction collector and flow-through UV analyser connected to a chart recorder are necessary.

B.1.2 Fractionation of serum on Sephacryl S-200

Sephacryl S-200 is a preswollen gel that excludes proteins of over 250 000 molecular weight and so is extremely useful for the isolation of IgM. The same principles apply to the use of other gels fractionating in different size ranges.

MATERIALS AND EQUIPMENT

Sephacryl S-200

Phosphate-buffered saline (PBS)

Column chromatography equipment (Fig. B.1)

Serum

METHOD

1 De-gas the gel under a vacuum. Air bubbles in the gel will distort the protein bands during the run.

2 Pour the gel into the column along a glass rod to avoid air bubbles. Take great care that the column is vertical. All the gel must be poured into the column at one time. Use an extension tube or reservoir. Leave the column outlet open during packing. A column of 100×2.5 cm generally takes about 5 h to settle.

3 Once the gel has settled fit the flow adaptor.

4 Pack the column by running through at least 2 column volumes of buffer. The flow rate should be about 20 ml/h (faster flow rates are possible with Sephacryl). After packing lower the flow adaptor if necessary.

   If the column tends to pack down after several runs you are probably running the column too fast. If a flow adaptor is used, packing after extended use may be avoided by using descending and ascending flow chromatography alternatively.

5 When the column is not in use add thiomersal to a concentration of 0.005% to stop microbial growth. This must be completely flushed out of the column before adding a sample as it absorbs at the same wavelength as protein. Alternatively, columns may be run with buffer containing sodium azide 0.01 M. Azide gives less absorption at 280 nm.

Sample application

Gel surface must not be disturbed during sample application as this would cause distortion of the bands.

Feed the sample through the pump and then through the flow adaptor, but note, this will cause some mixing and dilution of the sample in the dead space of the pump tubing. If an adaptor is not available place a nylon net or a layer of G-25 Sephadex (about 5 mm) on top of the gel to protect the surface.

Add a little sucrose to the sample to increase its density and layer it gently onto the gel surface below the free buffer with a long Pasteur pipette or a syringe with capillary tubing.

1 Apply a sample volume of up to 8 ml of serum.
2 Run the column at 20 ml/h.
3 Collect samples of 2–5 ml.

Distribution of serum proteins in eluted volume

Three major peaks should be eluted on fractionation of mouse serum.

Peak 1

The first peak contains the macroglobulins, IgM and α_2-macroglobulin, plus some lipoproteins. Also, on some occasions, large haemoglobin–haptoglobin complexes are present. These are easily distinguishable by their reddish-brown colour. Some IgA may be found towards the end of the elution of this peak.

Peak 2

Most of the IgG is in this peak, together with IgA in the first fractions.

Peak 3

This contains mainly albumin and other small globulins.

Occasionally the first two peaks are not resolved satisfactorily. This is due to weak non-covalent interactions between the IgG molecules causing them to aggregate and so contaminate the first peak. In these cases, run the column in 0.1 M acetate buffer, pH 5.0. Lowering the pH increases the positive charges on the IgG molecules increasing the repulsive forces between them, so preventing aggregation.

Examination of fractions

After concentrating the fractions, examine either with reference to their molecular weight, by SDS polyacrylamide gel electrophoresis (see below), or immunologically by immunoelectrophoresis (see Chapter 3).

B.1.3 High-pressure liquid chromatography (HPLC)

Columns have been developed which have increased the HPLC molecular weight fractionation range sufficiently to deal with immunoglobulins. They are useful for analysing the products of enzymic digestion and for monitoring the purity of fractions from gel exclusion columns (e.g. they are capable of resolving F(ab')$_2$ from whole IgG) and they are very fast, taking typically 30 min instead of the hours needed on a conventional gel column.

Such columns are generally small with sensitive detection systems capable of detecting 1–5 µg of protein, making them more suitable for analytical than preparative purposes.

B.1.4 Buffer exchange and desalting of protein solutions

Dialysis is often used to remove small molecular contaminants or to change the buffering conditions of a macromolecular solution. The same effect can be achieved rapidly by the use of a Sephadex G-25 column. Small molecules, e.g. free dinitrophenol, ions of the original buffer, are retarded by the Sephadex while protein molecules are excluded from the gel and can be collected in the effluent, already equilibrated in the column buffer.

Rapid dialysis is often important when the protein is under harsh conditions, where conventional dialysis would be too slow and would allow irreversible denaturation. The technique described is a similar principle to size fractionation of proteins by molecular sieving. But a word of caution: since the required molecules are excluded from the gel, they cannot be size fractionated, so filtration through the gel is faster and the whole procedure is less critical.

B.1.5 Preparation of exchange column

MATERIALS AND EQUIPMENT
Sephadex G-25, fine
Chromatography column
Blue dextran, 1% w/v in water
Peristaltic pump for column

Determination of column void volume

1   Pour the Sephadex into a chromatography column and pack under pressure.
2   Ensure that the surface of the gel is level, open the flow-control valve and allow the water to completely enter the column. (With Sephadex G-25, the gel bead size is sufficient to support the column of water inside the gel by surface tension; consequently, liquid flow stops as the meniscus comes into contact with the top of the gel. With fine grades of Sephadex this does not happen. The column may dry out and crack if left to flow unattended.) Close the column outflow.
3   Add 1 ml of blue dextran solution to the surface of the gel. Allow this to enter the gel completely while collecting the effluent into a graduated cylinder. Close the column.
4   Add water to the surface of the gel and continue collecting the effluent until the blue dye just appears. The liquid collected represents the void volume of the column.

Repeat the void volume determination for different heights of the gel. Plot a graph of void volume against column height. If you use the same diameter column each time then the void volume may be read off from the graph using the column height.

Molecules in the excluded fraction of Sephadex G-25, for example proteins, leave the gel just after the void volume, and their volume is expanded to approximately 1.5 times the original sample volume.

B.1.6 Use of column for buffer exchange

MATERIALS AND EQUIPMENT
Sephadex G-25 column
1% w/v blue dextran solution

Peristaltic pump
Protein solution to be dialysed

METHOD

1 Determine void volume of the column.
2 Equilibrate the gel with buffer; equivalent to 3 times the void volume of the column.
3 Apply the sample in a volume not greater than half the void volume.
4 Allow the void volume of buffer to leave the column and collect up to 1.5 times the original sample volume.

If you are using small sample volumes and mini-columns, for example during radioiodination of protein, it is advisable to determine the volume of the final sample more precisely by using a test volume of blue dextran equal to the original sample volume. This avoids unnecessary dilution.

After one run, the column may be re-equilibrated with 3 times the void volume of buffer, provided the retained material has not irreversibly bound to the column, e.g. as occurs with fluorescein isothiocyanate, or has not altered the gel chemically.

B.2 Estimating molecular weight by polyacrylamide gel electrophoresis

B.2.1 Sodium dodecyl sulphate polyacrylamide gel electrophoresis (SDS-PAGE)

Electrophoresis involves the migration of proteins and is dependent upon the charge, size and shape of the molecules. With SDS-PAGE, proteins bind the SDS and become negatively charged, so have similar charge : weight ratios. When SDS-coated proteins are placed in an electric field, their spatial separation will depend only upon their size and shape. By varying the concentration of the polyacrylamide gel used as the medium for the electrophoretic separation, different resolution ranges of molecular weights may be obtained. Proteins may be fractionated in the native state, but better resolution is usually obtained if the disulphide bonds are first reduced, allowing separation of the individual peptide chains.

Briefly, the technique involves the protein solution being heated to 100°C in the presence of reducing agents and SDS; the proteins unfold and bind about 1.4 g SDS/g protein. The strong negative charge on the proteins means that their electrophoretic mobility is inversely proportional to the logarithm of their molecular weight. There are some exceptions to this behaviour and they include:

(a) heavily glycosylated proteins, which bind less SDS than unglycosylated molecules of similar molecular weight; and

(b) some proteins, e.g. immunoglobulin J chains, which do not unfold completely and retain some of their native configuration.

A stacking gel is cast on top of the separating gel with a lower percentage polyacrylamide concentration (typically between 3 and 5%) and is prepared using a buffer with a slightly different composition. The different mobilities of chloride and glycine and the slow rate of entry into the separating gel relative to the rate of progression through the stacking gel concentrate the proteins in a narrow band at the interface between the stacking and separating gels. This allows the loading of variable volumes of sample. Improved resolution can be obtained by running a two-dimensional gel in which the proteins are separated:

1st direction: isoelectric focusing in the absence of reducing agents; and

2nd direction: at right angles to the first, under reducing conditions.

This technique allows the determination of the molecular weight of a protein in its multichain structure and also the composition and weight of its individual chains.

MATERIALS AND EQUIPMENT

Vertical slab gel system

Acrylamide

N,N′-methylene bis acrylamide

3.0 M tris(hydroxymethyl)-aminomethane (Tris)–HCl buffer, pH 8.7

1.0 M Tris–HCl buffer, pH 6.8

Ethylene diamine tetra-acetic acid (EDTA)

Sodium dodecyl sulphate (SDS)

N,N,N′,N′-tetramethylethylene diamine (TEMED)

Water-saturated butan-3-ol

Ammonium persulphate

Bromophenol blue

Sucrose

Solutions	Separating gels				Stacking gel 5%
	15%	10%	7.5%	6%	
40% acrylamide	11.25	7.5	5.6	4.5	1.25
1% bis acrylamide	7.8	7.8	7.8	7.8	1.3
3 M Tris–HCl, pH 8.7	3.75	3.75	3.75	3.75	1.25
10% ammonium persulphate	0.2	0.2	0.2	0.2	0.1
Distilled H_2O	6.84	10.35	12.25	13.35	5.0
20% SDS	0.15	0.15	0.15	0.15	0.05
TEMED	0.02	0.02	0.02	0.02	0.01
100 mM EDTA	–	–	–	–	1.0
Molecular weight range	8000–50 000	20 000–100 000	40 000–150 000	55 000–175 000	

* Use 1 M Tris–HCl buffer for the stacking gel.

Casting the gel

1 Wash thoroughly plates, spacers, etc., rinse in distilled water and air dry. Rinse in 70% ethanol and dry.

2 Assemble the slab gel mould, check it is vertical.

3   Mix the solutions for the separating gel according to the table above, but omit the SDS and TEMED at this stage. The precise final volume of reagents needed depends on the type of equipment being used, but the table gives a guide to the proportions required to produce gels for separation in various molecular weight ranges.

4   De-gas the solution under vacuum.

5   Add the SDS and TEMED and run the solution between the plates, within 4 cm of the top of the plates. Take care to avoid air bubbles.

6   Overlay the top of the separation gel with aqueous isobutanol (butan-3-ol saturated with distilled water). This reduces surface tension and ensures that the polymerized gel will have a flat surface.

7   Leave to polymerize for about 30–60 min and then wash off the butanol with three changes of distilled water and dry the surface carefully with filter paper. Alternatively, prepare an excess of stacking gel solution and use this to rinse away all traces of the isobutanol.

8   Mix the stacking gel and de-gas under vacuum prior to the addition of TEMED and SDS, pour into the mould over the separating gel and insert the plastic comb to form the sample wells. Leave the stacking gel to polymerize for 30 min.

Sample preparation

MATERIALS
Polyacrylamide sample buffer
Dithiothreitol
Bromophenol blue
Molecular weight standards, e.g. rainbow markers

METHOD

1   If the sample to be analysed is in a strong buffer, dialyse it against sample buffer, otherwise proceed to step 2.

2   Add 40 μl sample (containing 2–20 μg protein) to 20 μl of sample buffer (containing 31 mg/ml dithiothreitol) and 3 μl bromophenol blue (1 mg/ml in water). For unreduced samples omit the dithiothreitol.

3   Prepare the molecular weight standards in the same way.

4   Heat for 3 min in a boiling water bath.

Running the gel

MATERIALS AND EQUIPMENT
Power supply
Gas-tight glass syringe (50 μl)
Plastic capillary tubing
Polyacrylamide running buffer: tris(hydroxymethyl)-aminomethane (Tris)–glycine, pH 8.3, containing 3 ml 20% sodium dodecyl sulphate (SDS) per 600 ml buffer

1 Carefully remove the comb from the polymerized gel, clean wells of any unpolymerized acrylamide with running buffer, mount the gel plate in the electrophoresis apparatus and fill with running buffer.

2 Add samples to wells using a 50-µl syringe with plastic capillary tubing or a fine pipette. Do not forget the molecular weight standards.

3 Connect to power supply with anode at the bottom. Run at constant current: 20 mA while the sample is in the stacking gel and 40 mA after it enters the separating gel. The precise power requirements will vary according to the length and thickness of gel and whether the apparatus has a cooling pattern.

4 Once the bromophenol blue marker dye is approximately 1 cm from the bottom of the gel, turn off the power and remove the gel for either fixation and staining or electrophoretic transfer to nitrocellulose (see Chapter 4).

TECHNICAL NOTES

• Although this is a relatively robust technique, it is prone to artefacts from various sources. If too much current is applied to speed separation, then heating effects can distort the separation pattern and are seen as a horizontal wave pattern after protein staining. Either use cooling or reduce the current across the gel. Individual tracks are sometimes seen to give vertical streaks; this is due to a high salt content in the initial sample allowing a local increase in the current. This may be corrected by sample dialysis against the running buffer.

• Samples in the outside tracks may show an upward curve in their polypeptide bands due to greater electrical resistance at the edge of the gel. This is usually only a problem if the gel is being run to analyse and compare complex protein mixtures. This may be eliminated by running a sample of an irrelevant protein, such as bovine serum albumin, in the outside tracks.

• It is possible to prepare an 'in-house' mixture of molecular weight standards by buying pure proteins from one of the chemical suppliers. In addition, these can be radiolabelled using ^{14}C-formaldehyde. However, commercial mixtures are now available which contain intensely dyed proteins. It is therefore possible to monitor the progress of polypeptide bands across the whole gel during electrophoresis.

B.2.2 Staining and molecular weight estimation

To locate and recover a particular polypeptide band, e.g. for use in T-lymphocyte stimulation assays, we recommend the use of Aurodye rather than the methods described below. This procedure is said to be as sensitive as silver staining and yet does not affect mitogenesis assays.

Proteins (minimum detection limit 1 µg)

MATERIALS
Methanol
Acetic acid
Coomassie blue

1   Fix the gel in a mixture of 40% methanol, 10% acetic acid for 4 h.
2   Stain in 0.1% w/v Coomassie blue in methanol–acetic acid for 5 h.
3   Destain in 30% methanol, 10% acetic acid for 2 h.
4   Complete the destaining in 10% methanol, 10% acetic acid.
5   Reswell and store in 7% acetic acid.

Carbohydrates (minimum detection limit 5 µg)

MATERIALS
Methanol
Acetic acid
Periodic acid
Schiff's reagent
Sodium metabisulphite

1   Fix gel in 40% methanol, 20% acetic acid for 4 h.
2   Reswell in 7% acetic acid.
3   Oxidize in a mixture of 1% periodic acid in 7% acetic acid for 1 h in the dark.
4   Wash in 7% acetic acid for 24 h, changing the wash several times.
5   Stain with Schiff's reagent at 4°C for 1 h in the dark.
6   Differentiate in 1% w/v sodium metabisulphite in 0.1 M hydrochloric acid.

The apparent relative molecular weight (app. MW_r) of unknown polypeptide or glycopeptide bands may be determined by reference to the set of internal standards which should be run in each gel.

1   Identify each polypeptide band in the track of molecular weight standards and measure its migration distance from the interface between the stacking and separating gels.
2   Plot a graph of log molecular weight against distance travelled and use this to read back from the distance travelled by the unknown band to its log molecular weight.

TECHNICAL NOTES

• The molecular mass estimate determined by this technique is an apparent relative molecular weight as it is obtained by comparison with the set of molecular weight marker proteins run in the same gel. The value thus obtained should be expressed as a simple number, without units.

• Size determination by this technique can produce surprising and dramatic deviations from reality, due to artefacts produced by unexpected behaviour or unrecognized peculiarities of the unknown protein, for example:

   (a) Unfolding of a protein mixture to random coils may occur to different degrees.

   (b) Inactivation of proteinases from cell-based assays may be incomplete, thus permitting protein degradation during sample preparation. Some proteinases are poorly inactivated by boiling and SDS treatment; consequently, the unfolded proteins are likely to be even more susceptible to proteolytic cleavage than in their native state.

(c) The unknown proteins might be heavily glycosylated or phosphorylated and so not show the full charge for weight gain expected after SDS treatment. When some glycophospho-proteins have been compared as native proteins and *in vitro* translation products by this technique, the latter show increased app. MW_r, even though the molecular mass of the unglycosylated and unphosphorylated *in vitro*-derived protein is smaller.

- A reducing agent, dithiothreitol or 2-mercaptoethanol, is included to reduce both inter- and intrachain disulphide bonds. Remember to include unreduced samples when analysing unknown proteins by this technique.

B.2.3 Gradient gels

Homogeneous polyacrylamide gels are widely used, partly because of the ease of pouring these gels, but gradient gels give increased resolution. Gradients of varying ranges may be prepared, e.g. from 4 to 30%. Proteins continue to move within the gel until they effectively reach their pore size in the sieving gradient.

B.2.4 Two-dimensional SDS-PAGE

Increased information may be obtained about a protein by running a two-dimensional electrophoresis.

A conventional SDS-PAGE may be run in one direction in non-reducing conditions, then fol-lowing incubation of the gel with reducing agent, the proteins may be run into a second reducing SDS-PAGE. From this analysis the molecular weight of the native protein may be calculated and also, if the protein is made up of several polypeptide chains, this will be revealed in the second dimension.

Alternatively: the first dimension may be run as an isoelectric focusing gel, to give information on the isoelectric point, and the second dimension can be run as an SDS-PAGE to reveal the molecular weight.

B.3 Detergent solubilization of cells

Ionic detergents such as sodium dodecyl sulphate (SDS, anionic detergent) or acetyltrimethyl ammonium bromide (cationic detergent) are very efficient at solubilizing cells but, except at low concentrations (for SDS < 0.1%) tend to disrupt proteins by destroying their secondary, ter-tiary or quaternary structure. Non-ionic detergents, such as Nonidet P-40, Triton X-100 or Renex 30, tend to be less efficient solubilizers but do preserve protein structure and protein–protein interaction.

Many multichain cell-surface macromolecules have their non-covalent interchain binding preserved when cells are solubilized in detergent excess and lipids and membrane proteins trans-fer from the membrane into the detergent micelles. The configuration of most of the protein molecules and the external orientation of many is sufficiently preserved that antibodies are still able to react with antigens from solubilized cells for radioimmunoassay, immunoprecipitation, etc.

Non-ionic detergents are able to solubilize the surface membranes of cells but leave the nuclear membrane intact; the intact nuclei are removed by centrifugation. Consequently, it is possible to solubilize cells without the viscosity changes due to released DNA. For most purposes, the aliphatic polyoxyethylene isoalcohol Renex 30 is preferable to either Nonidet P-40 or Triton X-100 (aromatic detergents of the polyoxyethylene p-t-octyl phenol series) as it does not absorb at 280 nm (and so may be used for application where UV monitoring of protein content is required), does not interfere with the Lowry estimation of protein and is not labelled during the iodination procedures described above.

MATERIALS AND EQUIPMENT

Radiolabelled viable cells (10^7 lymphocytes, use pro rata and adjust for significant variations in cell surface area)

Phosphate-buffered saline (PBS), containing 5×10^{-7} M potassium iodide

Renex 30, 1% v/v in PBS

Protease inhibitors

High-speed centrifuge, Sorval

METHOD

1   Wash the cells three times in PBS by centrifugation (150 g for 10 min at 4°C) and resuspend the dry pellet by vortexing.

2   Add 100 µl of Renex solution and mix by vigorous vortexing while adding the protease inhibitors.

3   Leave solubilized cells for 20 min on ice, vortex and then centrifuge at 250 g for 10 min at 4°C to remove the intact nuclei (and unsolubilized cell membranes, if the detergent was not in excess).

4   Clarify the solubilized membranes by centrifugation at 100 000 g for 20 min at 4°C.

5   Determine the fraction of total radioactivity associated with protein and also the specific activity, if required.

6   Store at −80°C until use. The low temperature is preferable to retard proteolytic degradation.

TECHNICAL NOTES

- During cell-surface iodination, up to 10% of the apparent coupling of ^{125}I is through non-covalent interaction with membrane lipids. A significant proportion of this unwanted label can be exchanged back into the medium during the 20-min incubation on ice.

- If a gel forms during solubilization the nuclei have been disrupted, usually because one of the solutions is not isotonic. Ideally start again. However, if the cells are very valuable vortex very violently to try to reduce the viscosity by shearing the DNA and then add 40 µg/ml DNAse II and 20 µg/ml phosphodiesterase (both final concentrations) per 10^7 cells and incubate at room temperature for 30 min. Some proteolytic degradation is inevitable as most nucleases are contaminated with proteinases.

- Some cells, particularly exotic protozoan parasites, tend to contain membrane-partitioned proteolytic enzymes which can significantly degrade proteins from solubilized cells. In the case of *Trypanosoma cruzi* epimastigotes, the released proteinases can produce a Cleveland peptide map without the need to add V8 proteinase. Consequently, it is advisable to use a good range of proteinase inhibitors, add them with the aid of an assistant while vortexing the cell–detergent mixture, keep everything cold and generally complete the whole procedure as rapidly as possible, prior to storage at −80°C.

- The final protein concentration may be measured by the Lowry technique as Renex 30, unlike Nonidet P-40 and Triton X-100, does not induce precipitation with the Folin–phenol reagent.

- Incorporated radioactivity may be measured; however, lipids, which still might be carrying unexchanged ^{125}I, are precipitated by treatment with trichloroacetic acid (TCA). It is good practice at the beginning of a series of labelling experiments to determine the amount of residual, lipid-bound radioactivity by soaking an additional TCA/ethanol-treated filter in 2 ml of a 2 : 1 mixture of chloroform–methanol for 10 min at room temperature prior to drying.

- Significant losses can occur during washing of the cell pellet. If the cells are destined for immunoprecipitation (see Section 3.13), it is acceptable to reduce the number of washes because of the rigorous washing procedure after the adsorption of the immune complex on to the immunoabsorbent. Even so, the protein-associated radioactivity should be > 60% for iodinated cells and > 85% for metabolically labelled cells.

- Renex 30 is often semisolid at room temperature; if so, warm in a 60°C water bath prior to use.

B.4 Inhibitors of proteolytic degradation

There are four classes of proteolytic enzymes:
serine proteinases
cysteine proteinases
aspartic proteinases
metalloproteinases.

Unless you have detailed knowledge of the range of proteinases present in the cells lysed with detergent, or are attempting to work within a system which relies on one of the classes of protease for its action (e.g. blood clotting or complement activation), it is usual to choose a cocktail made up of a range of non-specific inhibitors with activity against each of the above classes of enzymes. The information below will help you to choose a useful combination of inhibitors.

Serine proteinases

Aprotinin (Trasylol) inhibits plasmin, kallikreins, trypsin and chymotrypsin with high activity; it does not inhibit thrombin or Factor Xa. Phenylmethane sulphonylfluoride (PMSF) inactivates a wide variety of enzymes including chymases, tryptases, elastases and serine proteinases of the plasma; for example, the blood coagulation proteinases. The sulphonyl–enzyme derivative is stable at neutral pH but may hydrolyse at non-neutral pH. The reaction of PMSF with enzyme can be slow, and the PMSF can itself undergo spontaneous hydrolysis. Other inhibitors of trypsin-like enzymes are (N_α-p-tosyl-L-lysine chloromethyl ketone) TLCK, an irreversible chloromethyl ketone inhibitor, and soya bean trypsin inhibitor.

Cysteine proteinases

p-Chloromercuriphenyl sulphonic acid (CMPS) is more soluble than p-chloromercuribenzoate (PCMB), but both inhibit sulphydryl-dependent enzymes. N-ethylmaleimide and sodium tetrathionate are less commonly used inhibitors.

Aspartyl proteinases

Pepstatin is usually employed in inhibitor cocktails to nullify the effects of aspartyl proteinases such as pepsin and cathepsin D. Lysosomal cathepsin D can be a problem in cell homogenates especially if buffers with a pH < 7.0 are used.

Metalloproteinases

Ethylene diamine tetra-acetic acid (EDTA) tends to be rather non-selective in cation binding and will chelate Ca, Mg, Cu, Fe, Mo, Zn, etc. Ethylene glycol-bis [β-aminoethyl ether] N, N, N',N'-tetra-acetic acid (ECTA) is more selective than EDTA for Ca. Consequently EGTA can be used to inhibit Ca-dependent enzymes in the presence of Mg-dependent ones; for example, treating serum with EGTA while supplementing the Mg^{2+} levels will inhibit the classical pathway of complement activation but leave the alternative pathway intact. O-phenanthroline shows selectivity towards the chelation of Zn, Fe and to a lesser extent other cations, but does not chelate Ca. Therefore a cocktail with both phenanthroline and EGTA would be more selective than EDTA, and would be Mg sparing.

B.5 Estimation of protein concentration

B.5.1 Absorption of UV light

Proteins containing tryptophan, tyrosine or phenylalanine residues absorb UV light at 280 nm in a concentration-dependent manner. Consequently, a spectrophotometer may be used to determine the increased absorption obtained when a protein is dissolved in a buffer (the buffer alone is used to 'zero' the spectrophotometer, so this 'difference' is obtained directly) and this value used: (i) to calculate the concentration of a pure solution using a published extinction coefficient ($E^{1\%}_{1\ cm}$—the absorbance at 280 nm due to a 10 mg/ml solution measured in a quartz cuvette with a 1-cm light path; values for commonly used proteins are given in Table B.1); or (ii) if the solution contains more than one protein, to estimate their total concentration.

MATERIALS AND EQUIPMENT
Protein solution, of unknown concentration
Buffer solution, used for dissolving the protein
Spectrophotometer, capable of operating at UV wavelengths
Quartz cuvettes, typically with 1.0- or 0.5-cm light path

METHOD

1 Turn on the spectrophotometer and allow it to stabilize for 15 min at 280 nm, in the absorbance rather than transmission mode.
2 Add buffer to the cuvette and use it to adjust the absorbance to zero.
3 Replace the buffer with protein solution (or use another cuvette if you have a matched set) and read the absorbance.
4 Using its extinction coefficient calculate the concentration of protein, remembering to allow for any dilutions made, and standardize for a 1-cm cuvette.

Table B.1 Molecular weights and spectral properties of immunoglobulins and antigens of immunological interest

Protein	Molecular weight	$E_{1\,cm}^{1\,\%}$	Wavelength (nm)	Solvent
IgG	160 000	14.3	280	0.2 M NaCl pH 7.5
IgA	170 000	10.6	280	
IgM	900 000	11.85	280	0.2 M NaCl pH 7.5
IgD	184 000			
IgE	188 000			
μ chain	73 814			
α chain	59 582	10.6	280	5 M guanidine HCl
γ chain	50 179	13.7	280	0.01 N HCl
light chain	25 170	11.8	280	0.01 N HCl
Fab$_\gamma$	50 000	15.3	278	PBS
F(ab$_\gamma$)$_2$	104 000	14.8	280	PBS
Fc$_\gamma$	50 000	12.2	278	PBS
pFc$'_\gamma$	26 000	13.8	280	PBS
Ovalbumin	43 500	7.35	280	PBS
Human serum albumin	68 460	5.3	279	PBS
Bovine serum albumin	67 000	6.67	279	Water
Fowl γ-globulin		13.5	280	–
Keyhole limpet haemocyanin	3 000 000 (*Megathura crenulata*)			
Squid haemocyanin	611 800 (*Ommatostrephes sloani pacificus*)			
Murex haemocyanin		18.1	278	Water
Limulus haemocyanin		11.2	278	Water
2,4-dinitrophenyl (DNP)	184	14 900 ($E_M^{1\,cm}$)	358	0.5 M phosphate pH 7.4
4-hydroxy-3-nitro-5-iodo phenacetyl azide (NIP azide)	348	–	–	–
Fluorescein	389	53 000 ($E_M^{1\,cm}$)	490	0.15 M NaCl, p.02 M K phosphate pH 7.4

TECHNICAL NOTES

- To ensure that the relationship between concentration and UV absorption is linear, the absorbance should be below 2.0, and ideally between 0.1 and 1.5 absorbance units.
- If the extinction coefficient of the protein is not known, or if the solution is a mixture of several proteins, total protein concentration may be calculated according to the following equation:

Protein concentration, mg/ml = $1.55 \times A_{280} - 0.77 \times A_{260}$

where A_{280} is absorbance value at 280 nm and A_{260} is absorbance value at 260 nm.

- Protein solutions frequently show much greater absorbance at wavelengths below 280 nm; however, so do many other materials. The ratio of the A_{280} and A_{260} readings should be below 0.6 for protein solutions; higher ratios usually indicate contaminants such as nucleic acids, peptides, detergents and preservatives such as sodium azide. If you know this to be a problem, use a colorimetric method.
- The technique is reasonably accurate for protein solutions at concentrations greater than 0.1 mg/ml.

B.5.2 Lowry technique

The estimation of protein concentration by UV absorption may be altered by the presence of certain detergents and buffers that absorb light strongly in these wavelengths. This problem is overcome by selecting chemicals with low UV absorption, e.g. substitution of the non-ionic detergent Renex 30 for Nonidet P-40. More often, however, it is necessary to use a different principle for estimation of protein content; for example, the colorimetric method developed by Lowry.

The Lowry technique involves the construction of a standard curve of colour versus protein concentration by reacting different concentrations of a known protein with Folin and Ciocalteu's phenol reagent (bovine serum albumin as a ubiquitous standard). The blue colour generated by the unknown protein solution can then be converted into concentration units by reference to the standard curve. Accuracy is enhanced if the known and unknown proteins are structurally related.

Preparation in advance

MATERIALS AND EQUIPMENT
As Section B.5.2, but in addition:
Protein for use as standard
Phosphate-buffered saline (PBS)

METHOD

1   Dissolve the standard protein in PBS to 1 mg/ml.
2   Centrifuge or filter to remove any undissolved material.
3   Determine the 280 nm absorbance of the protein solution and calculate its precise concentration using the extinction coefficient.
4   Dispense in small aliquots and store at –20°C for use.

Estimation of unknown protein solution

MATERIALS AND EQUIPMENT
Standard and unknown protein solutions
Sodium carbonate, 2.0% w/v in 0.1 M sodium hydroxide
Cupric sulphate, 1.0% w/v in distilled water
Sodium potassium tartrate, 2.0% w/v in distilled water
Folin and Ciocalteu's reagent
Spectrophotometer, visible light

METHOD

1   Prepare a dilution series of the standard protein solution in five steps between 0 and 500 μg/ml in 100 μl (final volume).
2   Prepare a series of dilutions of the unknown protein solution so that at least one tube falls within the range of the standard series. (As a first approximation, prepare a 1 : 5 dilution series through three steps and use 100 μl of each.) Include also a tube containing only the buffer used to dissolve the unknown protein, if this differs from that used to dissolve the protein standard.

Continued on p. 368

3   Mix an equal volume of copper sulphate and sodium potassium tartrate solutions, remove 1 ml and mix with 50 ml sodium carbonate solution (this mixture must be freshly prepared for each assay). Add 1 ml of this final mixture to each of the tubes containing standard or unknown protein solutions.

4   Add 100 µl of Folin and Ciocalteu's reagent to each tube and mix vigorously.

5   Incubate the tubes at room temperature for 15 min and quantify the colour reaction in a spectrophotometer at 650 nm.

6   Plot absorbance against protein concentration for the standard solution (the curve deviates slightly from linearity) and from this determine the protein concentration equivalent to the colour reaction of the unknown.

TECHNICAL NOTES

- As a guide, a protein solution of 250 µg/ml initial concentration yields a colour reaction with an absorbance of approximately 0.4. The lower limits of detection are about 5 µg/ml.
- If the buffer used to prepare the unknown solution gives a colour reaction in the absence of protein, this value should be subtracted from the absorbance of the unknown solution. In addition, it is not uncommon to find that buffer molecules or non-ionic detergents react with the phenol reagent to form a precipitate, without affecting the validity of the colour reaction in the supernatant.
- If a blue reaction is seen in the tube containing only the buffer used to prepare the standard curve, this indicates protein contamination, usually of the phenol reagent.
- The cupric sulphate and sodium potassium tartrate should be dissolved independently before mixing, to avoid precipitation.

B.5.3 BCA protocol for protein estimation

This is a colorimetric method for measurement of total protein in aqueous solution. It utilizes bicinchroninic acid (BCA) and the reduction of copper ions ($Cu^{2+} \rightarrow Cu^+$) in the presence of protein to produce a colour change which is read at an absorbance of 562 nm.

- BCA reagent is commercially prepared by and available from Pierce & Warriner Ltd.

B.5.4 Bradford method for total protein estimations

This is a colorimetric assay, but uses Coomassie brilliant blue G-250. When this reagent binds to proteins at an acidic pH there is an absorbance shift, and the colour change is read spectrophotometrically at 595 nm. As above, a commercially prepared reagent is available from Pierce & Warriner Ltd.

B.6 Tissue culture techniques

Tissue culture should be carried out in a sterile environment (usually a lamina flow hood where the air is filtered to remove airborne bacteria and fungi) using aseptic technique.

- If cells being cultured constitute a potential biohazard, e.g. human clinical specimens or virus-infected cell lines, then a class II hood should be used so that both operator and culture are protected.

Tissue culture media

Many different culture media are available, each usually in an 'old', 'new' and 'improved' formulation. For general use, we suggest a simple medium such as Eagle's minimal essential medium (EMEM) for growth of 'robust' cell lines. Cell growth under more demanding conditions, e.g. during cell cloning or for the growth of more fastidious lines, requires a more complex medium, such as Dulbecco's modification of Eagle's medium (DMEM) or RPMI 1640.

Buffers for culture media

Sodium bicarbonate (26 mM) is buffered by CO_2 in air, as this is at least physiological under closed-culture conditions (5% CO_2 in air in a gassed incubator). Although its buffering capacity is low, it is relatively cheap and has a low toxicity. Double-buffering systems have been used to good effect, e.g. RPMI 1640 containing bicarbonate, 24 mM and HEPES, 50 mM (N-2-hydroxyethylpiperazine N-2-ethanesulphonic acid). (In general, the HEPES concentration must be double that of the bicarbonate for good buffering.) In this case, under low CO_2 tension, the pH is maintained by the interaction of the bicarbonate with the HEPES; and in the culture, under high CO_2 tension (5%), the bicarbonate also acts as a buffer, as described above. Although 20 mM HEPES alone can control the pH of the culture medium within physiological limits, cells grow better in the presence of CO_2 and HCO_3^-. Oxygen tension is also important for the growth of cells—in static culture the depth of medium should not be greater than about 5 mm. However, to avoid the expense of large volumes of relatively expensive media, cells may be prepared from the animal in PBS and washed into medium immediately before culture. For *in vitro* handling of lymphocytes, not involving culture, we have used DMEM containing HEPES, 20 mM, adjusting to pH 7.4 with 1 M sodium hydroxide. Most cells grow well at pH 7.4. At this pH the most commonly used indicator, phenol red, is red, becoming blue-red at pH 7.6 and purple at pH 7.8; on the acidic side it is orange at pH 7.0 and yellow at pH 6.5.

Antibiotics for culture media

Researchers may have their own recipe. We suggest penicillin 200 U/ml and streptomycin 100 µg/ml or gentamycin 30 µg/ml. Where there is persistent yeast contamination, add Fungizone (amphotericin B) at up to 10 µg/ml (final concentration); cell lines vary in their sensitivity, so start at 2 µg/ml.

Serum supplements

Autologous serum may be collected at the same time as the cells for use in assays and or cell culture. Serum may be heat-inactivated at 56°C for 30 min without losing its growth-enhancing properties. Moreover, serum previously collected from the same donor that has been stored at –70°C may also be used.

Pooled human serum may be collected and prescreened for efficacy in the assay or culture system. Serum may be obtained from the National Blood Service; however, to avoid cross-reactivity with blood-group antibodies, it is advisable to use human AB serum.

For murine cells use 10% fetal bovine serum (FBS). It is necessary to select a 'good' batch of serum, i.e. giving acceptable cell survival, without a high background of incorporation of the DNA analogue due to mitogenic stimulation by the FBS. The proportion of FBS required may be reduced by adding 2-mercaptoethanol. The medium listed below was developed for murine mixed-lymphocyte cultures, but it may be used for the maintenance of mouse cell lines (including hybridoma lines).

Dulbecco's modification of EMEM containing:

arginine (200 mg/l)

folic acid (12 mg/l)

asparagine (36 mg/l)

2-mercaptoethanol (5×10^{-5} mol/l)

HEPES (1×10^{-2} mol/l)

FBS 5% v/v.

Horse or calf serum can be used as a cheaper alternative to fetal bovine serum for the maintenance of some cell lines, e.g. the hybridoma parent lines X-63. However, a period of 'adaptation' (probably resulting in cell selection) is required, during which the concentration of one supplement is decreased while the other is increased.

Serum-free media are available that are advantageous if secreted products, such as antibodies or cytokines, are to be purified from the culture supernatant. However, in general these media still contain high concentrations of added proteins and are relatively expensive.

Complete DMEM-5, -10 and -20 medium supplemented (adapted from Cerottini *et al.* 1974)

Note: The final concentration of each of the individual supplements is critical. Therefore where the commercially prepared DMEM has already been supplemented, e.g. with sodium pyruvate, then the concentration must be adjusted accordingly.

4.5 g/l DMEM (high-glucose formulation)

5%–20% v/v heat-inactivated fetal bovine serum

10 mM MOPS (3-(*N*-morpholino)propanesulphonic acid)

0.05 mM 2-mercaptoethanol

100 µg/ml streptomycin

100 U/ml penicillin

216 mg/l L-glutamine (final concentration 1.5 mM)

116 mg/l L-arginine (final concentration 0.7 mM)

36 mg/l L-asparagine (final concentration 0.3 mM)

2 g/l sodium bicarbonate (final concentration 25 mM)

110 mg/l sodium pyruvate (final concentration 1 mM)

6 mg/l folic acid (final concentration 14 µM)

Subculture of cell lines

The growth curve of a typical line is shown in Fig. B.2. This curve should be determined for every cell type in long-term culture, as it yields essential information on the growth characteristics and requirements of the line. Most cultures have an optimum lower cell density at initiation and tend to die at plateau densities, when nutrients or toxic waste become limiting. To maintain high viability, cells should be 'fed' by changing the medium once the indicator dye turns orange-yellow and the cell density should be reduced by dilution of the culture before the plateau phase is reached.

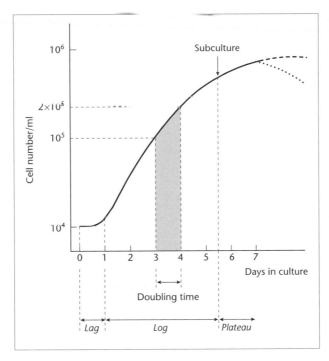

Fig. B.2 Typical growth curve of a continuous cell line. The data shown were obtained from a cell line growing in suspension culture. Growth of adherent cells follows the same curve but cell density values are approximately 10-fold lower. There are three distinct phases to cell growth *in vitro*: lag, log and plateau. In the lag phase, there is little increase in cell numbers as this is a period of recovery and adaptation; for example, the cell may need to resynthesize elements of its glycocalyx after trypsinization. This process is often cell-density dependent; if cells are subcultured at too low an initial density they may never escape into log phase. Log phase is the optimum time for cell use as the population is phenotypically at its most homogeneous and has high viability. As cell numbers increase exponentially the time taken for the cell number to increase twofold is equal to the cell doubling time. This should not be confused with the cell cycle time, which is a measure of the time taken for a population of synchronized cells to traverse the cell cycle and return to the starting point. Cells growing in log phase are not normally synchronous but instead are uniformly distributed throughout the stages of the cell cycle (G1→S→G2→M→return to G1, etc.). The plateau phase occurs towards the end of log phase and is evidenced by a rapid reduction in growth rate. Growth eventually ceases, after one or two divisions, to terminate in the G1 phase of the cell cycle. Normal cells, for example fibroblasts, stop growing at high density and remain viable for several weeks (dashed line). Cultures of transformed cells and cell lines deteriorate rapidly (dotted line) and so should be subcultured as described in the text.

Subculture of non-adherent cells

Shake the culture vessel gently to bring all the cells into suspension and count the cell number using a haemocytometer. Then either remove and discard a fraction of the suspension before adding fresh medium, or transfer an aliquot of suspension to a fresh flask containing medium. In each case the intention is to reduce the cells back to their optimum inoculation density (Fig. B2).

Subculture of adherent cells

MATERIALS AND EQUIPMENT
Phosphate-buffered saline (PBS)
Trypsin 0.25% in PBS, with or without 1 mM ethylene diamine tetra-acetic acid (EDTA)
Tissue culture medium containing a serum supplement

METHOD

1 Pour the spent medium off the culture and wash with PBS to remove all traces of serum (this would inhibit the action of the trypsin).
2 Add 3.0 ml of trypsin solution per 25 cm² growth area of cells, tip the flask to cover the culture and leave for 30 s at room temperature.
3 Pour off the trypsin solution and incubate the culture at 37°C until the cells are seen to detach, usually 5–15 min.
4 Add tissue culture medium containing serum (this inhibits the residual trypsin so there is no need to wash the cells), disperse the cells by gentle aspiration with a pipette and count using a haemocytometer.
5 Withdraw an aliquot containing an appropriate seeding number of cells and transfer to a fresh flask containing medium.

TECHNICAL NOTES

- EDTA should only be used if treatment with trypsin alone fails to release the adherent cells.
- Cross-contamination between cell lines can lead to overgrowth by the fastest grower. Never use the same pipette for different cell lines and work out a routine in which only one line at a time is subbed in the lamina flow hood.

B.7 **Cryopreservation of cells**

Cells may be stored for an indefinite period in a frozen state under liquid nitrogen. To optimize freeze viability, use actively growing cells whenever possible; they are your insurance against accidental loss.

MATERIALS
Cryoprotective solution; by volume:
    fetal bovine serum (FBS), 50%
    dimethyl sulphoxide (DMSO), 20%
    tissue culture medium, 30%

METHOD

1 Harvest the cells by centrifugation (150 g for 10 min at 4°C), count and adjust to 1×10^7/ml.
2 Add cell suspension dropwise to an equal volume of cryoprotective solution.
3 Dispense convenient volumes into ampoules suitable for storage in liquid nitrogen.
4 Freeze slowly (at about 10/min) down to at least –50°C and then immerse in liquid nitrogen.

TECHNICAL NOTES

- DMSO (or alternatively, glycerol) allows water to go from a liquid to a solid state without the formation of ice crystals.
- Use a fresh bottle of DMSO every 2–3 months to avoid the accumulation of toxic peroxides. Alternatively, redistil with care.

- DMSO must be handled with care: it can penetrate the skin and carry with it any harmful substance in regular use; for example, carcinogens.

Thawing

Cells may be recovered from liquid nitrogen storage by thawing rapidly to 37°C (in a water bath) and washing three times in tissue culture medium by centrifugation (150 g for 10 min at room temperature).

B.8 Cell lines

Most of the cell lines described in this book are generally available in laboratories throughout the world, from which they may be begged, borrowed but hopefully not stolen. In addition many are available from commercial suppliers; for example, the American Type Culture Collection (ATCC), or the European Collection of Animal Cell Cultures (ECACC) (see Appendix C). If all else fails the originator of the cell line will often respond positively to a polite request for a starter culture.

When importing a cell line it is advisable to screen for *Mycoplasma* infection. Mycoplasma do not necessarily slow down cell growth, but can play havoc with the results of *in vitro* bioassays. If a culture is contaminated, discard it and start again. It is possible to have cell lines 'cured' of the infection, but this is rarely complete. We have indicated availability through the ECACC or ATCC as the first point of contact; otherwise, original references are quoted.

B151	Takatsu *et al.* (1980) *J Immunol* **125**, 2646.
BCL$_1$	ATCC. Slavin and Strober (1977) *Nature* **272**, 62.
BW-5147	ATCC.
CESS	Muraguchi *et al.* (1981) *J Immunol* **127**, 412.
CT-6	Ho *et al.* (1987) *J Immunol Meth* **98**, 99.
CTLL-D	Gearing *et al.* (1987) *J Immunol Meth* **99**, 7.
Daudi	ATCC.
EL4.6.1	ATCC. Luscher *et al.* (1985) *J Immunol* **135**, 3951.
FS6-14.13	Kappler *et al.* (1981) *J Exp Med* **153**, 1198.
Hep/2c	ECACC and ATCC.
Human bladder carcinoma cell line 5637	ATCC.
HT-2	Ho *et al.* (1987) *J Immunol Meth* **98**, 99.
Jurkat	ECACC and ATCC. Gillis and Watson (1980) *J Exp Med* **152**, 1709.
K-562	ATCC.
L929	ATCC and ECACC.
MC/9	ATCC. Nabel *et al.* (1981) *Nature* **291**, 332.
Me-180	ATCC.
MLA-144	ATCC. Rabin *et al.* (1981) *J Immunol* **127**, 1852.

Gibbon cell line with constitutive production of a mixture of growth factors, including IL-2. Like all primate lines, assume that it contains xenotropic viruses and handle accordingly.

MOLT-4	ECACC and ATCC.
MOPC 21	ATCC.
Namalwa	ATCC.

NIMP-TH1	Warren and Sanderson (1985) *Immunology* **54**, 615.
NS1-Ag4-1	ECACC and ATCC.
P-815	ATCC.
P3/X63-Ag8	ECACC and ATCC.
SKW6-CL4	ATCC. Saiki and Ralph (1981) *Eur J Immunol* **13**, 31.
Sp2/O-Agl4	ECACC and ATCC.
T-24	ATCC.
TCl-Nal	Shimizu *et al.* (1985) *J Immunol* **134**, 1728.
WEHI-3	ATCC and ECACC. Luqer *et al.* (1985) *J Immunol* **134**, 915.
WEHI-164	ATCC. Clone 13 Espevik and Nissen-Meyer (1986) *J Immunol Meth* **95**, 99–105.

B.9 Defibrination of blood

MATERIALS AND EQUIPMENT

100-ml bottles

Glass balls

Blood without anticoagulant

1 M HCl

Preparation in advance

1　Wash the glass balls overnight in 1 M HCl then wash three times with a free rinsing detergent, e.g. Deconex.

2　Wash the balls thoroughly with distilled water and dry them in an oven.

3　Add 3 g of the glass balls to each 100 ml bottle and autoclave at 138 kPa for 20 min.
　　A 100-ml bottle, prepared as above, can be used to defibrinate 50 ml of blood.

METHOD

1　Add blood to bottles and mix by inverting until the clot has completely formed (10–20 min). Do not allow the blood to clot without mixing.

2　Allow the clotted blood to stand for 30 min and remove the serum which will contain free cells.

Virtually pure lymphocytes may be prepared from this cell suspension using density gradient centrifugation. Overall yield of lymphocytes is approximately $0.25–0.5 \times 10^6$/ml of original blood.

B.10 Siliconizing plastic and glassware

MATERIALS AND EQUIPMENT

Items for siliconizing

Dichlorodimethylsilane

Large glass desiccator

All items of glassware should be baked at 180°C for 2 h before use, and all plastic ware should be rinsed five times with distilled water.

Useful data

- Serum concentration of human immunoglobulins and distribution of subclasses.
- Molecular weights and spectral properties of immunoglobulins and antigens of immunological interest.
- Common acids.
- Immunoelectrophoresis of human serum in agar, sodium–barbitone buffer, pH 8.2. The main immunoglobulin classes are shown together with several other major proteins.
- Immunoelectrophoresis of normal BALB/c serum in agar, sodium–barbitone buffer, pH 8.6. Proteins are visualized with a rabbit antiserum to mouse immunoglobulin. Such antisera invariably contain antibodies to α_2-macroglobulin.

Further reading

Affinity Chromatography—Principles and Methods. Available from Amersham Biotech Limited.

Bailon, P., Ehrlich, G.K., Fung, W.-J. & Wolfgang Berthold, B. (eds) (2000) *Affinity Chromatography: Methods and Protocols.* Humana Press, New Jersey.

Ballance, P.E. (1992) *Phosphorus-32: Practical Radiation Protection.* H and H Scientific Consultants Ltd., Leeds.

Cerrotini, J.C., Engers, H.D., MacDonald, H.R. & Brunner, T. (1974) Generation of cytotoxic T lymphocytes *in vitro*. I. Response of normal and immune mouse spleen cells in mixed lymphocyte cultures. *J Exp Med* **140** (3), 703–717.

Davis, J.M. (1995) *Basic Cell Culture Techniques: A Practical Approach.* Oxford University Press, Oxford.

Deutscher, M.P., Simon, M.I. & Abelson, J.N. (eds) (1997) *Guide to Protein Purification: Methods in Enzymology, Vol. 182.* Academic Press, London.

Harrison, M.A. & Rae, I.F. (1997) *General Techniques of Cell Culture.* Cambridge University Press, Cambridge.

HMSO (1999) *The Ionizing Radiations Regulations.* The Stationery Office, London.

HMSO (2000) *Ionizing Radiations: Medical Exposure Regulations.* The Stationery Office, London.

ICRP (1997) *General Principles for the Radiation Protection of Workers*, Publication 75, Vol. 27/1. International Commission on Radiological Protection.

ICRP (1998) *Individual Monitoring for Internal Exposure of Workers*, Publication 78, Vol. 27/3–4. International Commission on Radiological Protection.

Kompala, D.S. & Todd, P. (eds) (1999) *Cell Separation Science and Technology*. Oxford University Press, Oxford.

Mayer, V.R. & Meyer, V.R. (1994) *Practical High-Performance Liquid Chromatography*. J. Wiley & Sons, Chichester.

Websites that provide comprehensive details on radioisotope health and safety procedures as well as useful information regarding detection and half-life include:

http://www.practicingsafescience.org

http://www.hse.gov.uk

Useful websites

1 Practical Immunology updates: http://www.sghms.ac.uk/depts/immunology/frankhay

2 Useful list of CD antigens: http://www.grt.kyushu-u.ac.jp/~hidehiro/public_old/cd_table.html

3 Brilliant site that produces individual buffer recipes based on the book: Beynon, R.J. & Easterby, J.S. (1996) *Buffer Solutions: The basics*. IRL Press at Oxford University Press, Oxford: http://www.bi.umist.ac.uk/buffers.html

4 Technical information on two-dimensional PAGE and many other techniques: http://expasy.org

5 Mike Clark's Home Page—a wealth of information on immunoglobulins and immunology in general: http://www.path.cam.ac.uk/~mrc7/mikeimages.html

6 IMGT, the international *ImMunoGeneTics* database, is an integrated database specializing in immunoglobulins (Ig), T-cell receptors (TcR) and major histocompatibility complex (MHC) molecules of all species. IMGT includes two databases: LIGM-DB (for Ig and TcR) and MHC/HLA-DB (in development). An IMGT tool, DNAPLOT, will allow Ig, TcR and MHC sequence analysis: http://imgt.cines.fr:8104/

7 The Kabat Database of Sequences of Proteins of Immunological Interest—superb site for finding the sequence you require: http://immuno.bme.nwu.edu/

8 The British Society for Immunology's home page: http://immunology.org/

9 Cells—the American Type Culture Collection: http://www.atcc.org/

10 Cells—the European Collection of Animal Cell Cultures: http://www.biotech.ist.unige.it/cldb/descat5.html

11 The cytokines web: http://cmbi.bjmu.edu.cmbidata/cgf/CGF_Database/cytweb
http://www.copewithcytokines.de/

12 Flow cytometry sites including free software: http://www.bio.umass.edu/mcbfacs/flowcat.html
http://facs.scripps.edu/

13 The Antibody Resource Page. Far too many useful sources too list; well worth a visit: http://www.antibodyresource.com/

14 Replacement methods for animals in monoclonal antibody production: http://altweb.jhsph.edu/science/mab/ardf/intro.htm

15 Epitope mapping: http://www.mimotopes.com/index.html
http://www.mgen.uni-heidelberg.de/MB/tech.html

16 Pedro's BioMolecular Research Tools—yet another source of much information, not so much immunology but great for the biomolecular: http://www.biophys.uni_duesseldorf.de/Bionet/Pedro/research_tools.html

17 Inbred strains of mice: Michael F.W. Festing, MRC Toxicology Unit, Hodgkin Building, University of Leicester, UK. Hundreds of strains with detailed information on each: http://www.informatics.jax.org

18 Molecular probes—masses of information on linking fluorescent tags to antibodies: http://www.probes.com/handbook/toc.html

19 Pierce on line—the handbooks and useful guides: http://www.piercenet.com/

20 SIGMA—that wonderful catalogue and more on your computer: http://www.sigma-aldrich.com

21 Vector Laboratories—helpful tutorials as well as good product information: http://www.vectorlabs.com/home/home1.htm

22 R and D systems for cytokine products: http://www.rndsystems.com/

23 HMS Beagle—an everyday changing science magazine with lots of practical information: http://biomednet.com/hmsbeagle/

APPENDIX C

Equipment and manufacturers index

| Equipment index

(Numbers indicate listing in address index.)

A

ABTS 45
Actinomycin D 45
Adhesive tape, double-sided 6 mm 31
Adjuvants
 Bordetella pertussis 40
 Freund's, complete and incomplete 14
 saponin 45
Aerosil 380 45
Agar, Difco-Bacto, for haemolytic plates 14
Agar, McConkey, for bacterial culture 14
Agar, Noble Special, for electrophoresis 14
Agarose 45
 compounds linked to agarose 45
 Jacalin 47
Albumin
 bovine 45
 chicken 45
 dog 45
 donkey 45
 goat 45
 guinea-pig 45
 hamster 45
 horse 45
 human 45
 mouse 45
 pig 45
 pigeon 45
 rabbit 45
 rat 45
 rhesus monkey 45
 sheep 45
 standard albumin solution 45
 turkey 45
Albumin, ^{125}I 22
Alkaline phosphatase 45
Alsever's solution, sheep blood in 14, 22
American-type culture collection 2
Amino acid mixture, tritium labelled 3
p-Aminobenzoic acid 31
Aminopterin 22

Ampholines 43
Ampholytes 9, 43
Animals (laboratory) 20
Antisera
 antibodies
  biotinylated 3, 35, 45
  monoclonal (various) 12, 22, 45
 anti-C3 serum 45
 anti-human blood groups 45
 anti-human D 45
 anti-human IgG, IgM and IgA, class-specific sera 45
 anti-human IgG subclasses 37
 anti-human serum albumin 45
 anti-mouse IgG subclasses 43, 45
 anti-sheep erythrocyte 19
 customer request, in goats or sheep 19
 general 45
 goat anti-rabbit gammaglobulin 45
 normal rabbit serum 19
 rabbit anti mouse IgG–FITC conjugate 7, 43, 45
 sheep anti-rabbit γ-globulin 22
 standard antigen solution, i.e. IgG Cohn fraction 2–45
Anti-thyroid antibody detection kit 19
Aquacide 11
Assay systems 39
Aurodye 25
Automatic cell-harvesting machine 46
Automatic pipettes 4, 22
2,2′-azino-di-(3-ethyl benz-thiazoline sulphonic acid) 45
Avidin 19, 45
Avidin substituted with fluorochrome, enzyme, radioisotope labels 3, 35, 45

B

BCA for protein estimations 38
Beads, polyacrylamide for immobilizing immunoglobulins 15
Biogel A 9

II Manufacturers index

USA suppliers are given in italics below the UK supplier where appropriate. It is worth noting that biotechnology companies are well known for regularly changing their name and location. Information in this list is correct at the time of publication.

1 Abbott Diagnostics Ltd
Abbotts House, Norden Road,
Maidenhead,
Berks SL6 4XF
01628 784041

Abbott Laboratories Limited
Diagnostics Division,
7115 Mill Creek Drive (2nd Floor),
Mississauga, Ontario L5N 3R3
(905) 858 2450

2 *American Type Culture Collection*
10801 University Boulevard,
Manassas, Virginia 20110-2209
(703) 365 2700

3 Amersham Pharmacia Biotech (APBiotech)
Amersham Place,
Little Chalfont,
Bucks HP7 9NA
0870 606 1921

4 Anachem Ltd
Anachem House,
20 Charles Sreet,
Luton,
Beds LU2 OEB
01582 745040

Gilson Inc.
3000W Beltline Highway,
Box 620027,
Middleton WI 53562
(608) 836 1551

5 Anderman and Co. Ltd
145 London Road,
Kingston upon Thames,
Surrey KT2 6NH
020 8541 0035

Zeton-Altamira
149 Delta Drive, Suite 200,
Pittsburgh, PA 15238
(412) 963 6385

6 Baxter Health Care
Wallingford Road,
Compton,
Newbury,
Berks RG20 7QW
01635 206000

Baxter Health Care
Scientific Products Division,
1620 Waukegan Road,
McGaw Park, IL 60085
(847) 473 6134

7 Becton-Dickinson
Between Towns Road,
Cowley,
Oxford OX4 3LY
01865 777722

BD Bioscience
1 Becton Drive,
Franklin Lakes, NJ 07417-1880
(201) 847 6800

8 Bibby-Sterilin Ltd
Tilling Drive,
Stone,
Staffs ST15 OSA
01785 812121

9 Bio-Rad Laboratories
Bio-Rad House,
Maylands Avenue,
Hemel Hempstead,
Herts HP2 7TD
0800 181134

Bio-Rad Chemical Division
Group Headquarters,
Bio-Rad Laboratories,
2000 Alfred Nobel Drive,
Hercules, CA 94547
(800) 424 6723

10 British Biotechnology
Watlington Road,
Cowley, Oxford OX4 5LY
01865 748747

11 Calbiochem-Novabiochem UK Ltd
Boulevard Industrial Park,
Padge Road,
Beeston,
Nottingham NG9 2JR
01159 430840

Calbiochem-Novabiochem Corp.
10394 Pacific Centre Court,
San Diego, CA 92121
(858) 450 9600

12 Cambridge Bioscience
25 Signet Court,
Stourbridge Common Business Park,
Swann's Road,
Cambridge CB1 2BL
01223 316855

13 DAKO Ltd
Denmark House,
Angel Drove,

Ely,
Cambs CB7 4ET
01353 669911

DAKO Corp.
6392 Via Real,
Carpinteria, CA 93013
(805) 566 6655

14 Difco Laboratories Ltd
PO Box 14b,
Central Avenue,
West Molesey KT8 2SE
020 8979 9951

BD Bioscience
1 Becton Drive,
Franklin Lakes, NJ 07417-1880
(201) 847 6800

15 Dynal Biotech UK
11 Bassendale Road,
Croft Business Park,
Bromborough,
Wirral CH62 3QL
0151 346 1234

Dynal Inc.
5 Delaware Drive,
Lake Success, NY 11042
1-(800) 638 9416

16 Elkay Lab Products UK Ltd
Unit 4, Marlborough Mews,
Crockford Lane,
Basingstoke,
Hants RG24 8HL
01256 811118

Elkay Products Inc. (Kendall)
15 Hampshire Street,
Mansfield, MA 02048
1-(800) 962 9888

17 European Collection of Cell Cultures
CAMR Centre for Applied Microbiology and Research,
Porton Down,
Salisbury,
Wilts SP4 0JG
01980 612512

18 Pall Gelman Laboratories
Europa House,
Havant Street,
Portsmouth PO1 3PD
02392 302600

Pall Gelman Laboratories
600 South Wagner Road,
Ann Arbor, MI 48103-9019
(734)665-0651

19 Glaxo-Smith Kline
Wellcome Research Laboratories,
South Eden Park Road,
Beckenham,
Kent BR3 3BS
020 8658 2211

Glaxo-Wellcome Inc.
PO Box 13398,
Research Triangle Park,
North Carolina 27709
(919) 483 2100

20 Harlan Sera Laboratories
Hillcrest,
Dodgeford Lane,
Belton,
Loughborough LE12 9TE
01530 222123

Harlan Bioproducts for Science
PO Box 29176,
Indianapolis, IN 46229
(800) 9-SCIENCE

21 Phillip Harris Scientific
Novara House,
Excelsior Road,
Ashby Park,
Ashby-de-la Zouch LE65 1NG
0845 6040497

22 ICN Pharmaceuticals
Cedarwood, Chineham Business Park,
Crockford Lane,
Basingstoke,
Hants RG24 8WD
01256 707744

ICN Pharmaceuticals Inc.
ICN Plaza,
3300 Hyland Avenue,
Costa Mesa, CA 92626
(714) 545 0100

23 Ilford Imaging UK Ltd
Town Lane,
Mobberley,
Knutsford,
Cheshire WA16 7JL
01565 684000

Ilford Imaging USA Inc.
West 70 Century Road
Paramus, NJ 07653
(201) 265 6000

24 Invitrogen Ltd
3 Fountain Drive,
Inchinnan Business Park,

Paisley PA4 9RF
0141 814 6100

Invitrogen Corporation
1600 Faraday Avenue,
PO Box 6482,
Carlsbad, California 92008
(800) 955 6288

25 **Janssen CILAG**
PO Box 79,
Saunderton,
High Wycombe,
Bucks HP14 4HJ
01494 567567

Janssen Pharmaceutica
PO Box 200,
Titusville, NJ 08560-0200
(609) 730 2000

26 **Jencons (Scientific) Ltd.**
Cherrycourt Way Industrial Estate,
Stanbridge Road,
Leighton Buzzard,
Beds LU7 8UA
01525 372010

Jencons Inc.
800 Bursca Drive,
Suite 801,
Bridgeville, PA 15017
(412) 257 8861

27 **Leica Microsystems (UK) Ltd**
Davy Avenue,
Knowlhill,
Milton Keynes MK5 8LB
01908 246246

Leica Microsystems Inc.
2345 Wankegan Road,
600015 Bannockburn, USA
(800) 248 0123

28 **Life Sciences International UK Ltd.**
Unit 5, Ringway Centre,
Edison Road,
Basingstoke,
Hants RG21 6YH
01256 817282

Forma Scientific Inc
Mill Creek Road,
Box 649,
Marietta, Ohio 45750
(740) 373 4763

29 **Lorne Laboratories**
7 Tavistock Industrial Estate,
Ruscombe Business Park,

Ruscombe Lane,
Reading,
Berks RG10 9NJ
0118 934 2400

Worthington Biochemical Corp.
730 Vassar Avenue,
Lakewood, NJ 08701
(732) 942 1660

30 **Marathon Laboratories Supplies**
Unit 6, 55–57 Park Royal Road,
London NW10 7TJ
020 8965 6865

31 **Merck Laboratory Supplies**
Hunter Boulevard,
Magna Park,
Lutterworth,
Leicester LE17 4XN
01455 558600

Gallard Schlesinger
777 Zeckendorf Blvd,
Garden City,
New York 11530
(516) 229 4000

32 **Millipore UK Ltd.**
The Boulevard,
Blackmoor Lane,
Watford,
Herts WD1 8YW
01923 816375

Millipore Corporation
Corporate Headquarters,
80 Ashby Road,
Bedford, MA 01730
1–800 MILLIPORE

33 **National Diagnostics**
Unit 4, Fleet Business Park,
Itlings Lane,
Hessle,
Kingston-upon-Hull HU13 9LX
01482 646022

National Diagnostics Inc.
305 Patton Drive,
Atlanta, Georgia 30336
(404) 699 2121

34 **National Institute for Biological Standards and Controls**
Blanche Lane,
South Mimms,
Potters Bar,
Herts EN6 3QG
01707 654753

National Cancer Institute
Bethesda, USA

35 Nycomed-Amersham plc
Amersham Place,
Little Chalfont,
Bucks HP7 9NA
01494 544000

Nycomed Amersham Inc
2636 South Clearbrook Drive,
Arlington Heights, IL 60005
(847) 593 6300

36 Organon Laboratories Ltd.
Cambridge Science Park,
Milton Road,
Cambridge CB4 4FL
01223 432700

37 Oxoid
Wade Road,
Basingstoke,
Hants RG24 8PW
01256 841144

Oxoid Inc.
Suite 100
1926 Merivale Road
Nepean, Ontario K2G 1E8

38 Perbio Science UK Ltd
Century House,
High Street,
Tattenhall,
Cheshire CH3 9RJ
01829 771744

Pierce Chemical Co.
PO Box 117,
Rockford, IL 61105-0117
1-(800) 874 3723
815-968-8148

39 Perkin Elmer Life Sciences Ltd
204 Cambridge Science Park,
Milton Road,
Cambridge CB4 0GZ
01223 437400

Perkin Elmer Life Sciences Inc.
549 Albany Street
Boston MA 02118
(800) 446 0035

40 PHLS Centre for Applied Microbiology and Research
Porton Down,
Salisbury,
Wilts SP4 0JG
01980 612100

American Type Culture Collection
10801 University Boulevard,
Manassas, VA 20110-2209

41 Porvair International Ltd.
Estuary Road,
King's Lynn,
Norfolk PE30 2HS
01553 622000

42 Sanyo-Gallenkamp plc
Monarch Way,
Belton Park,
Loughborough LE11 5XG
01509 265 265
0116 263 0530

Sanyo Scientific
900 North Arlington Heights Road,
Suite 320,
Itasca, IL 60143
1-(800) 858 8442

43 Serotec
22 Bankside Station Approach,
Kidlington,
Oxford OX5 1JE
01865 852700

Serotec Inc.
NCSU Centennial Campus, Partners
1017 Main Campus Drive,
Suite 2450
Raleigh, NC 27606
1-(800) 265 7376

44 Shandon Southern Products
Chadwick Road,
Astmoor,
Runcorn,
Cheshire WA7 1PR
01928 566611

45 Sigma-Aldrich
Fancy Road,
Poole,
Dorset BH17 7NH
01202 733114

Sigma Chemical Co.
3050 Spruce Street,
PO Box 14508,
St Louis, MO 63103
(314) 771 5765

46 Thermo LabSystems
Acton Court,
Ashford Road,
Ashford TW15 1XB
01784 251225

Thermo LabSystems
8 East Forge Parkway,
Franklin, MA 02038

47 **Vector Laboratories**
Unit 3 Accent Park,
Bakewell Road,
Orton Southgate,
Peterborough PE2 6XZ
01733 237999

Vector Laboratories
30 Ingold Road,
Burlingame, CA 94010
1-(800) 227 6666

48 **Whatman Lab Sales Ltd**
Whatman House,
St. Leonards Road,
Maidstone,
Kent ME16 OLS
01622 676670

Whatman Inc. (Whatman)
9 Bridewell Place,
Clifton, NJ 07014
(201) 773 5800

49 **X O-GRAPH Imaging Systems**
X O-GRAPH House,
Hampton Street,
Tetbury GL8 8LD
01666 501501

50 **Carl Zeiss Ltd**
PO Box 78,
Woodfield Road,
Welwyn Garden City,
Herts AL7 1LU
01707 871200

Carl Zeiss, Inc.
Microscopy and Imaging Systems,
One Zeiss Drive,
Thornwood, NY 10594
1-(800) 233 2343

Further reading

Coombs, J. & Alston, Y.R. (1998) *International Biotechnology Directory 1999*. Macmillan Press, London.

Haugland, R.P. (2001) *Handbook of Fluorescent Probes and Research Chemicals*, 8th edn. Molecular Probes Inc., Eugene, Oregon. (This handbook is available as a free CD-ROM or on the web at: www.probes.com/handbook.)

Linscott's Directory of Immunological and Biological Reagents, 11th edn. Linscott's Directory Int., Box 188, S-79124 Falun, Sweden. (Also available on the web at: www.linscottsdirectory.com.)

INDEX

interleukin-5 (IL-5; T-cell replacing factor; TRF; eosinophil differentiation factor; EDF) 310–12
  proliferation assay 311–12
  reverse plaque-forming cell assay 310–11
interleukin-6 (IL-6; B-cell differentiation factor-2; BCDF-2; interferon-beta-2; IFN-beta-2) 312–13
  hybridoma proliferation assay 313, 317
  immunoglobulin secretion 312–13
  production 301, 312
  reverse plaque-forming cell techniques 313
interleukin-7 (IL-7) 314
interleukin-8 (IL-8) 314–16
interleukin-9 (IL-9) 316–17
interleukin-10 (IL-10) 317
interleukin-11 (IL-11) 317
interleukin-12 (IL-12) 317–18
interleukin-13 (IL-13) 318
interleukin-14 (IL-14) 318
interleukin-15 (IL-15) 319
interleukins 305–9
  see also cytokines
iodination
  antibody labelling 140, 143–4, 174
  cell-surface iodination:lactoperoxidase technique 229–30
^{131}I-iododeoxyuridine 273, 280
Iodogen labelling 140, 143–4, 174
ion-exchange chromatography 8–16, 62
  antibody isolation 63
  DEAE 119, 120
  DEAE-cellulose 8, 21
ionic strength gradient 10–13
iron powder phagocytosis 188 9

jacalin–agarose 19, 23–4
jacalin storage buffer 349
Jerne plaque assay 263–5

K cells 211, 212, 214
keyhole limpet haemocyanin (KLH) 135–6

lactate dehydrogenase (LDH) assay 225
lactoperoxidase iodination technique 229–30
Langmuir plot 73–4
large granular lymphocytes 214
laser scanning confocal microscopy 257–9
latex agglutination 107–8
lectins 277
leucocytes 335
limiting dilution analysis (LDA) assay 291–4
liquid scintillation 166

liver
  pig-liver powder, preparation 124–5
  serum absorption 122–3
Lowry technique 367
lymph nodes 185–6
lymphocyte antigens *see* cell-surface antigens
lymphocyte membranes 231 9
lymphocytes
  see also B lymphocytes; T lymphocytes
  antibody production *see* plasma cell 241–5
  antigen-binding 233–5
  antigen response 134–5
  antigen-responsive normal T-lymphocyte lines, propagation 193–6
  antigen-specific precursors, frequency estimation 289–94
  apoptosis 294–9
  autoradiographic labelling 235–9
  B-cell depletion for T-cell enrichment 189–92
  bursa of Fabricus 185–6, 338
  cell counting 338
  cell harvesting 279
  cell proliferation 261–99
  cell-mediated cytolysis (CMC) 286–8, 293–4
  cell-mediated cytotoxicity *see* cell-mediated cytotoxicity
  chicken
    labelling 236–9
    preparation 184–5
  circulation 273–7
  colorimetric microassay 280–81
  complement receptors 240
  confocal microscopy 257–9
  detergent solubilization 362–4
  dye exclusion test 340–41
  dye-monitored proliferation 283
  Fc receptors 239–41
  fluorescent labelling 275–6
  function 261–99
  granzyme B, cytotoxicity marker 288
  homing 273–4
  human, preparation 182–4
  human T-lymphocyte lines *see* T lymphocytes
  intraorgan distribution 274–5
  karyotype analysis 200–1
  large granular 214
  limiting dilution analysis (LDA) assay 291–4
  lymph nodes 185–6
  lymphocyte antigens *see* cell-surface antigens
  microculture 281–5
  mitogenic response 277–81
  mixed-lymphocyte reaction (MLR) 283–4, 285–6, 291